WEIGHTS FOR
WEIGHT LOSS

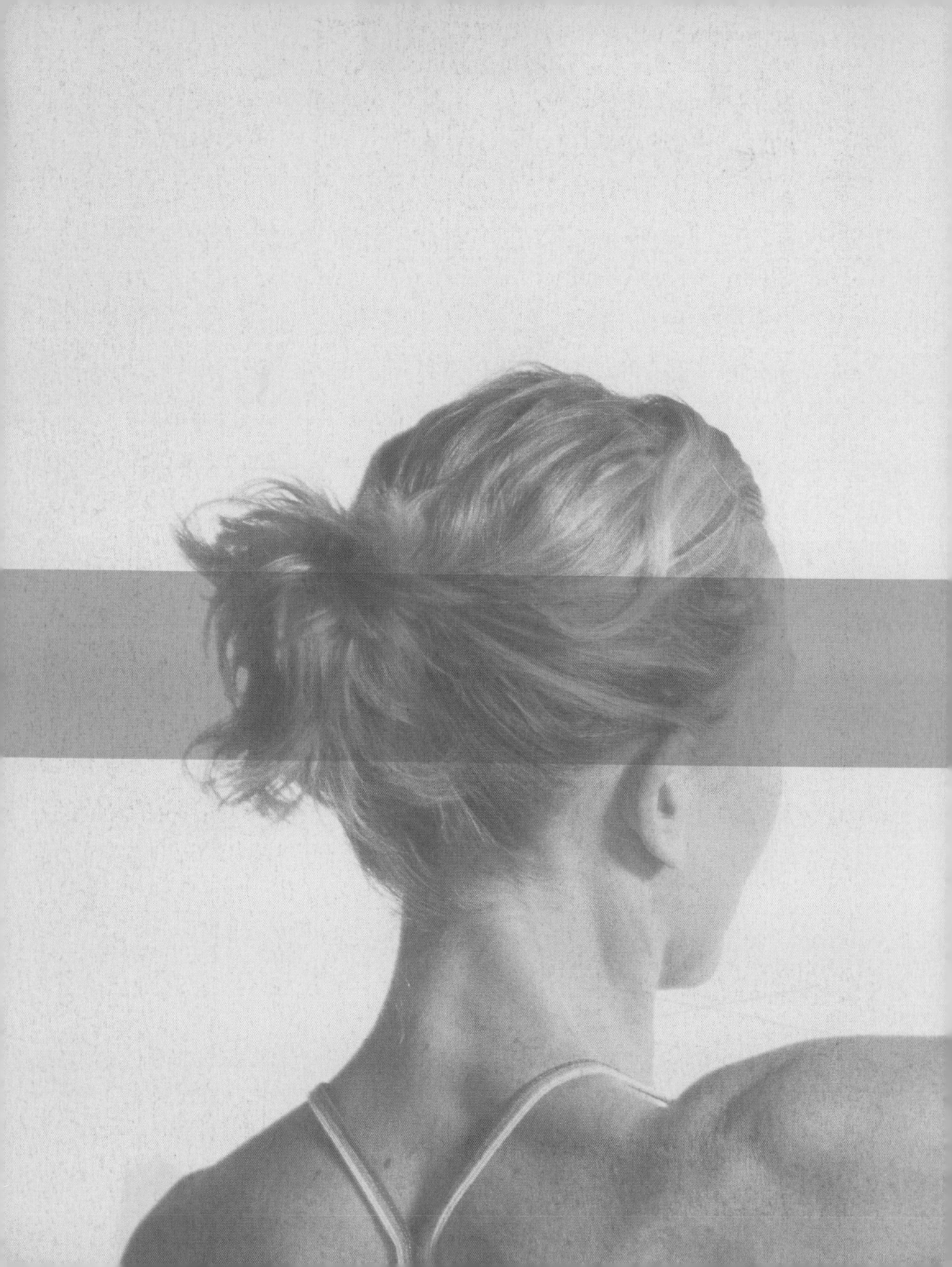

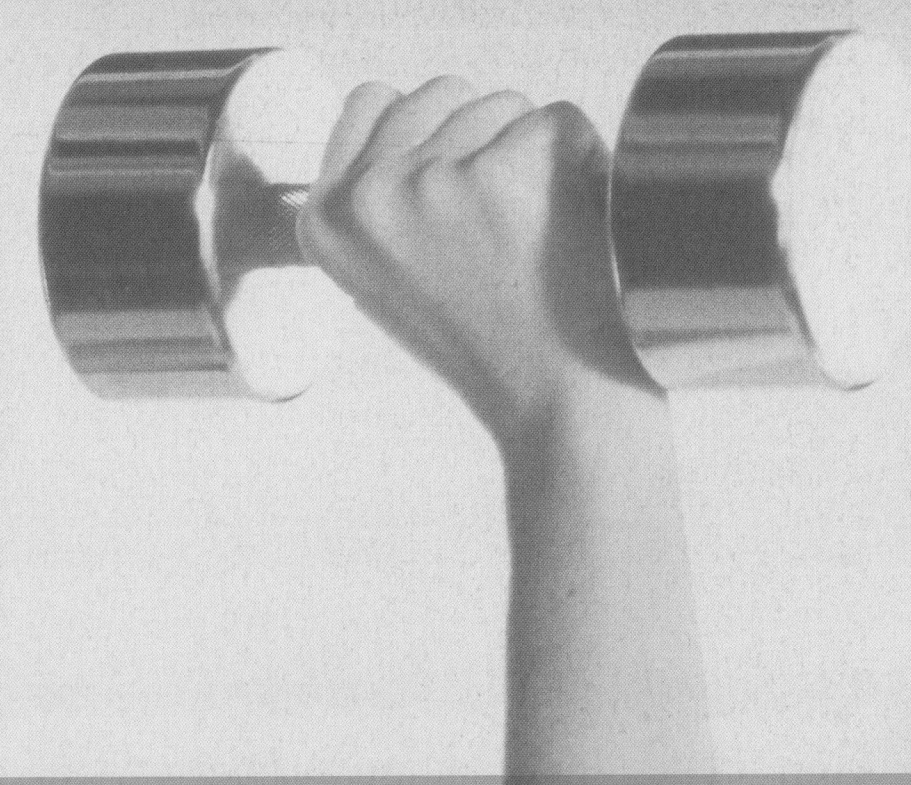

WEIGHTS FOR
WEIGHT LOSS

The fast track to a slimmer, stronger, firmer body

SAM MURPHY

Kyle Cathie Limited

First published in Great Britain in 2006 by
Kyle Cathie Limited,122 Arlington Road,
London NW1 7HP
general.enquiries@kyle-cathie.com
www.kyle-cathie.com

10 9 8 7 6 5 4 3 2 1
ISBN 1 85626 660 5
ISBN (13-digit) 978 1 85626 660 4

Additional photography: page 18 Stockbyte / Royalty Free / Getty
Images, 144 Samboli / Alamy, 149 Dynamic Graphics Group / IT
Stock Free / Alamy, 150 Dynamic Graphics Group / IT Stock Free /
Alamy, 153 Jon Feingersh / Getty Images

Project editor Caroline Taggart
Editorial assistant Vicki Murrell
Copy editor Sarah Epton
Designer Rebecca Herriott
Illustrator Peter Cox
Production Sha Huxtable and Alice Holloway

A CIP record for this title is available from the British Library.

Colour separations by Colourscan
Printed and bound in Singapore by Tien-Wah Press

CONTENTS

INTRODUCTION

So you want to lose weight, shape up and shed body fat? Then you need to be strong. I'm not talking about being strong enough to resist chocolate cake or a second helping of Sunday roast (although that inevitably helps!) – but about physical strength.

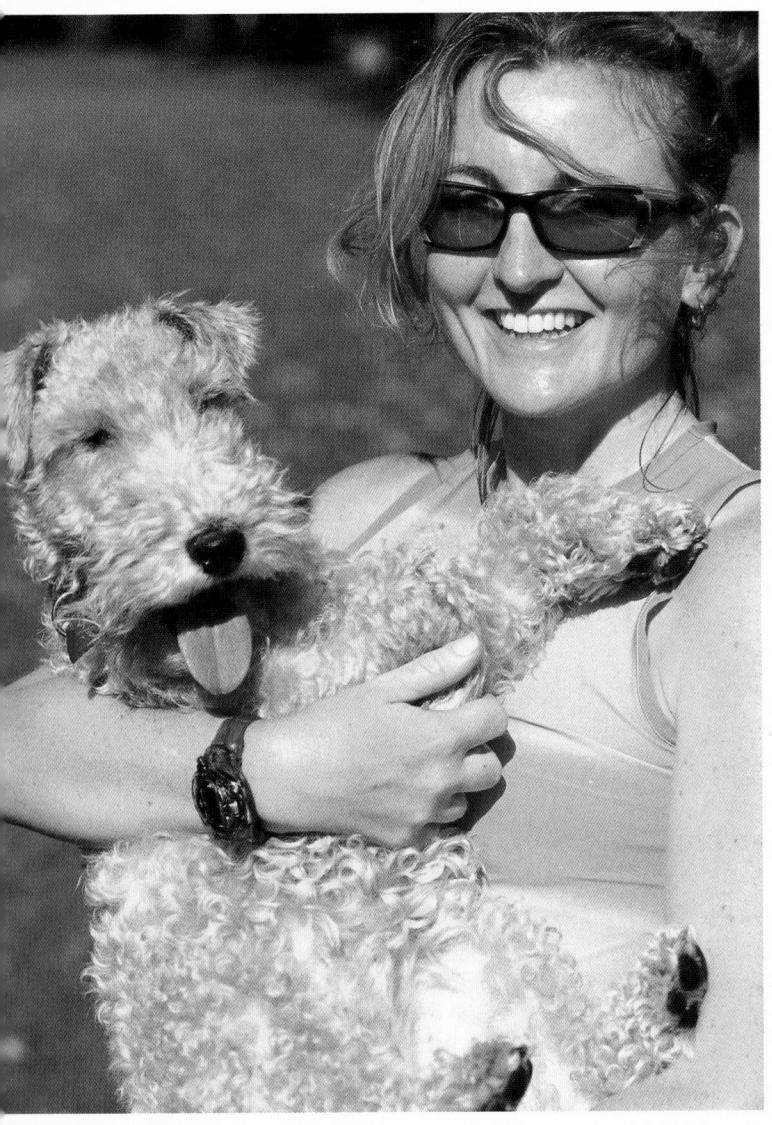

When we set our sights on weight loss, most of us turn to the kind of activities that get the heart pumping – like running, swimming, cycling or aerobics classes. And while there is no doubt about the value of cardiovascular activity (for weight loss and general health), strength – or resistance – training is the unsung hero when it comes to maximising daily energy expenditure and fat loss – and *really* streamlining your body shape.

But if you are serious about using weights for weight loss, that means dispensing with the ubiquitous can of baked beans as a makeshift dumbbell – many women squander their time in the gym by using weights that simply aren't challenging enough to trigger changes in the body. Others fail to benefit because they use poor technique or don't have any structure to their weights workout.

This book will show you how to incorporate strength training into your fitness regime (even if you don't yet have one!) in a safe, enjoyable and above all *effective* way. You won't believe what a difference it will make to your weight loss efforts, your body shape and size. But what's just as gratifying is the sense of empowerment you'll feel when you can lift a couple of heavy shopping bags (or kids) without a second thought…

Because there is no definitive 'strength training prescription' that gets the best results for every individual, *Weights for Weight Loss* will also help you to understand how your body type and shape is likely to respond to strength training, what other factors might influence the results you get and, most importantly, how to manipulate your workouts to maximise your own personal benefits.

There are a lot of myths and misconceptions about weight training out there but rest assured that you won't end up with big, bulging muscles, nor will you lose your aerobic fitness or flexibility. What you *will* lose is fat – revealing your new, firmer, more defined shape. You'll also reduce your risk of osteoporosis and back problems, stave off age-related declines in metabolism, muscle mass and general function, maintain full range of motion in your joints and, perhaps most surprisingly of all, lower your risk of heart disease, high blood pressure, diabetes and some cancers.

And all this can be achieved with just three strength-training workouts a week. You don't even need to go to a gym or pick up a dumbbell, as it's perfectly possible to train with alternative – or even no – equipment. The workouts in this book will show you how. You will also find the information you need to make smart eating choices so that you can lose body fat without starving yourself or feeling deprived and *keep* it off. After all, anyone who tells you that you can

successfully shed fat without addressing what you eat is stringing you along.

Weights for Weight Loss works because it is based on the sound scientific principles underpinning strength training, metabolism and energy balance. No false promises. No complicated diet plans or baffling exercise regimes. Just a definitive weights workout that will reward you with a leaner, firmer, stronger body. Worth the weight…?

GIVE ME STRENGTH

What strength training is all about and why everyone should be doing it…

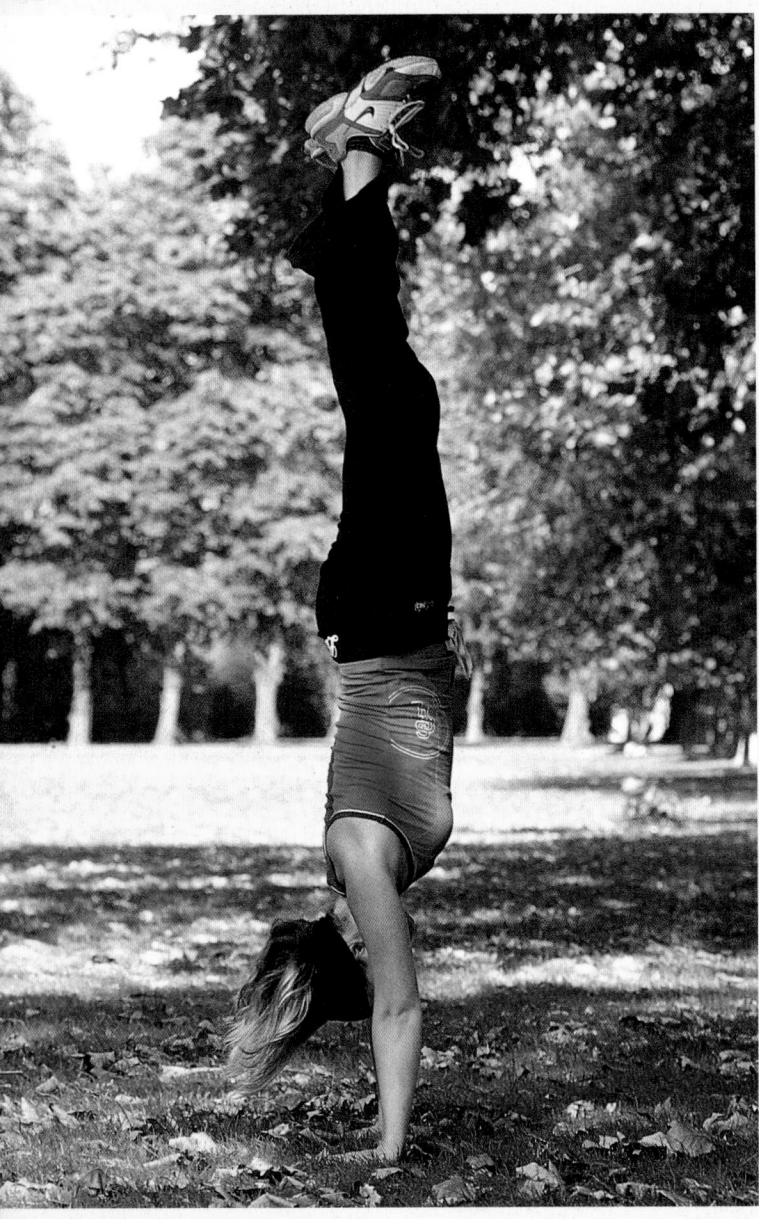

What exactly is strength? Put simply, it's the ability of a muscle to exert force and overcome resistance. That might not sound like something you are eager to devote your time to improving but there are a multitude of benefits to be gained from becoming stronger which go far beyond being able to shift heavy objects. How about looking leaner, improving muscle definition, getting a firmer, shapelier body, enhancing body composition and boosting your calorie expenditure for starters? And there's more…

A few years back strength training didn't get much of a look in when people extolled the virtues of exercise. It was all about aerobic workouts. But there is now irrefutable evidence that strength training is not just desirable but *essential* for optimal health.

Getting the picture that it is well worth making strength training part of your life? Just in case you're not convinced, here are 12 compelling reasons – weight loss aside – to persuade you…

It helps your heart

If you think that the aerobic system isn't involved in resistance training, you are mistaken. For starters, it fuels recovery, not just between repetitions and sets of exercises but also following the session itself. It instigates heart-healthy changes in the cardiovascular system – such as allowing more blood to get to the muscle and enabling waste products to be cleared more efficiently. Of course, the heart itself is a muscle and strength training has been shown to increase the size of the heart chamber responsible for pumping blood around the body. This allows more blood to be delivered to the exercising muscles with every beat.

It lowers the risk of diabetes

Diabetes is one of the fastest increasing diseases in the Western world. Traditionally, aerobic exercise has been recommended to improve glucose metabolism but in a recent study four months of strength training increased glucose uptake by an average of 23% – indicating that it could be equally as effective. It also seems that strength training improves glucose metabolism both in subjects with normal glucose metabolism and those who already have an abnormal response. Researchers aren't exactly sure how it helps but recent studies suggest that resistance training increases the number and efficiency of glucose receptors in muscles so that the body doesn't need to produce as much insulin.

It reduces blood pressure

Strength training used to be thought to increase blood pressure but, increasingly, evidence shows that it can reduce blood pressure both acutely (as the result of a single session) and chronically (in the long term). This is especially good news because hypertension is associated with heart disease, stroke and kidney problems. Improved strength also reduces stress on the heart. In a twelve-week study

subjects worked out with weights to strengthen the lower body muscles. By the end of the study period their blood pressure rose significantly less during lifting activities.

It bulks up your bones

Building bone density is the first line of defence against the debilitating disease osteoporosis that affects one in three women over the age of 50. Research shows that bone mineral density (BMD) is highly related to the strength of the muscles attached to those bones. In a research study, twice-weekly resistance training over the course of a year resulted in a 6.3% increase in bone mineral density of the lumbar spine. The surprising thing about this is that the women were post-menopausal – when bone density is usually plummeting. The control group in the study (who did no strength training) lost 3.7% of their bone density during that same year.

While weight bearing activities like running and high impact aerobics are great for bone density, they only influence the particular parts of the skeleton that are loaded by the activity. As well as preserving bone density strength training reduces the risk of osteoporotic fractures, by improving balance and muscle strength, thereby reducing the risk of falls.

It preserves your joint health

Strength training isn't just good for muscles – it strengthens the connective tissues too – such as ligaments, tendons and cartilage – while movement keeps the joint structures bathed in sticky synovial fluid. All these factors keep joints healthy and can even alleviate the symptoms of osteoarthritis.

It may improve your cholesterol profile

First, a quick cholesterol recap: HDL good, LDL bad! High levels of low density lipoprotein (LDL) and total cholesterol are associated with a higher risk of coronary heart disease, while high density lipoprotein (HDL) cholesterol is positively beneficial to heart health, helping to prevent the development of athersclerosis. There's been conflicting evidence regarding whether strength training can help to improve cholesterol profile but it certainly seems that post-menopause (when heart-protective oestrogen is out of the picture) resistance training can be very beneficial. In research from the University of Oklahoma post-menopausal women who took part in twelve weeks of resistance training using resistance bands, experienced a significant rise (13%) in HDL cholesterol levels despite the fact that they did not lose weight or body fat. The poorer the initial cholesterol profile the greater the subject's improvement.

It keeps you regular

Yup, strength training can improve your digestion! A study that involved thirteen weeks of strength training, including exercises for the abdominals, found a staggering 56% acceleration in gastrointestinal tract time (GITT). The reason this is desirable is because a long GITT is associated with colon cancer, not to mention digestive problems.

It's the way to an easier life

If you think strength training is all about aesthetics, think again. Put it this way: if you can lift a 10kg weight, that 5kg bag of shopping isn't going to pose a challenge. Being stronger helps you get through daily tasks with less effort and more energy. In fact, anyone reading this who has had children has already experienced the effects of 'progressive overload' strength training: first off when the baby was growing inside you and then after his or her birth, when you continued to nurse, pick up and carry your little bundle of joy despite his or her rapidly advancing weight.

It can make you a better athlete

Even if your main fitness focus is an endurance activity such as running or cycling there is solid evidence that strength training can aid your performance. As well as making connective tissues more robust it also increases muscle power and makes movement patterns more efficient, so that you waste less energy. Being stronger will make you less injury-prone – an important consideration for most sportspeople.

It makes you happier

Strength training can put a smile on your face! And the harder you work the happier you'll get, according to research from the Royal Prince Alfred Hospital in Sydney. Depressed adults were put on a high or low intensity-training strength programme for eight weeks. At the end of the study period a reduction in depressive symptoms was directly associated with the amount of strength gained. Over half the high intensity group reported a 50% improvement. Sleep quality improved significantly in all the subjects too. But you need to keep it up: recent research found that as little as a week of no exercise resulted in an 85% drop in mood scores among regular gym rats!

It improves your body image

Strength training doesn't just improve your body, it also improves how you *feel* about your body. I can definitely attest to the feeling of empowerment you get when you can lift an Olympic bar in the gym when all the other girls are wielding 2kg dumbbells – or when you can place that six-pack of Evian on the checkout without so much as a grunt!

It keeps you youthful

The average adult loses between 2.25 and 3.2 kilograms of muscle mass every decade from around twenty years of age and experiences a 2–5% reduction in metabolic rate. As you'll find out in the next chapter, these two factors combine to form a potent fat-gaining force. But resistance training can prevent this. When you consider that muscle accounts for 16–22% of resting metabolic rate, it's easy to see how important it is not to let that muscle waste away.

So there you have it. But what about dropping excess kilos, shaping up and losing body fat? The next section looks more closely at exactly how weight training works for weight loss.

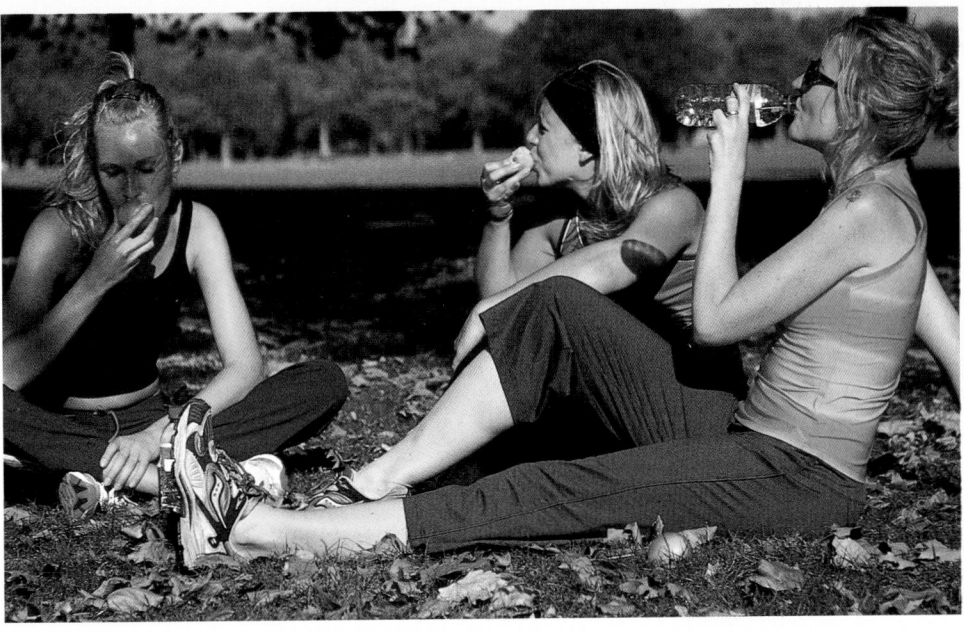

HOW WEIGHTS WORK FOR WEIGHT LOSS

The lowdown on strength training and its effect on fat loss, energy expenditure and body shape

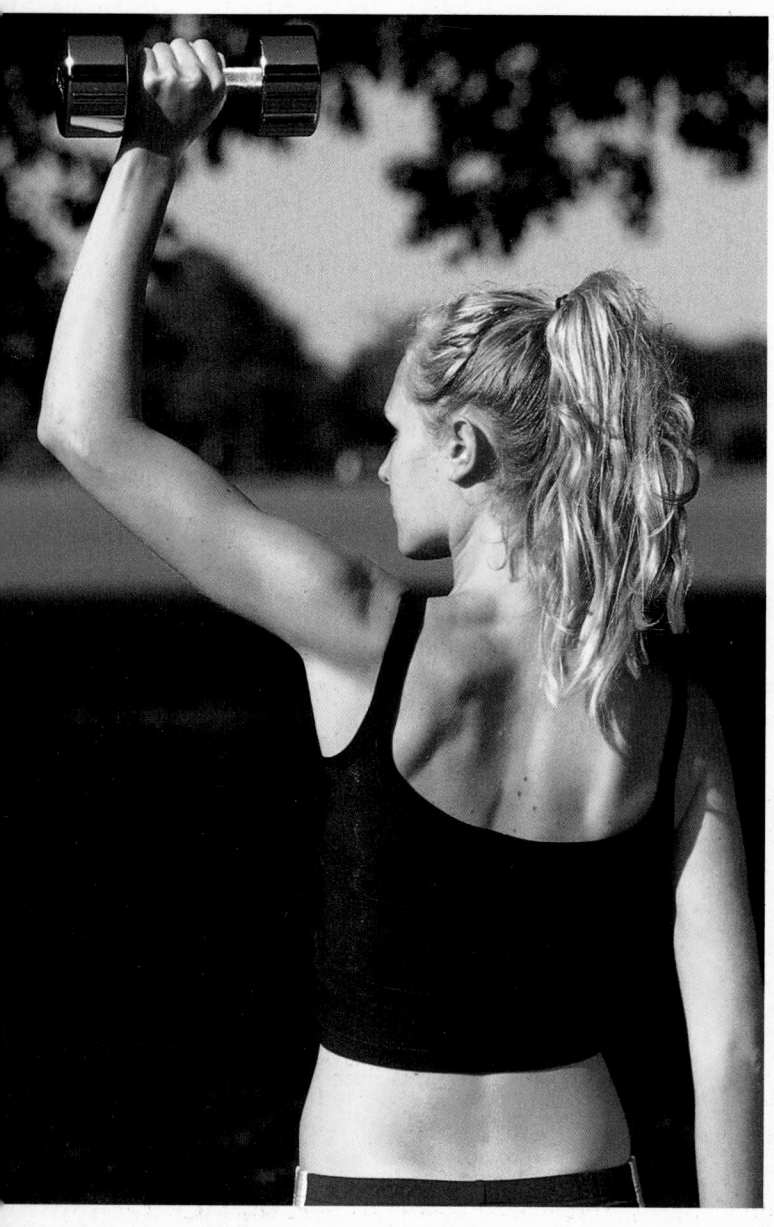

So you want to lose weight. Surely you need to eat less and burn calories through exercise then? Absolutely. But if you are steering clear of weight training, believing that because it doesn't get you hot and sweaty it can't be much good for burning calories, then you are selling yourself short.

Strength training will help in three ways. It will burn calories, it will give you stronger muscles, which are more able to cope with the demands of weight-bearing aerobic exercise, and it will help you maintain your lean muscle mass as you decrease calorie intake so you don't lose precious metabolically active muscle tissue. The single biggest contributor in determining your total daily energy (calorie) expenditure is your resting metabolic rate (or RMR – the amount of energy your body expends just 'ticking over' on a typical day). A low RMR is an independent predictor of future weight gain but the single most important factor in *determining* your RMR is the amount of lean muscle tissue you have in your body – which is why weight loss experts now recommend combining aerobic exercise and strength training with diet to produce successful results.

Another important benefit of strength training is that it will allow you to *enjoy* becoming more active. Being overweight is not an impediment to successful strength training and in fact, brand new research on young people found that it was actually the most overweight kids who fared best in the gym. Strength training is a great first step to becoming more active and healthy as there's no bouncing about, no excessive stress on joints and no need to feel self-conscious. Whether you do it at home alone, or in a busy gym, strength training is a very individual pursuit that you can tackle with dignity and focus. Let's look at how it works for weight loss…

The high cost of strength training

Exercise at any intensity – whether it's walking, running, weight lifting or circuit training – burns calories and utilises fat. The number of calories and the proportion of fat is what varies – but while lower-intensity exercise burns a higher proportion of fat, higher-intensity exercise burns more calories overall – and weight training can certainly be considered to be a high-intensity activity (when done properly, of course).

But it isn't just the calorie 'cost' of the sessions themselves that make weight training such a crucial part of the weight loss equation. Studies suggest that resistance training has an effect on average daily metabolic rate and energy expenditure through other means too. In an eighteen-week intervention study from the University of Limburg in Holland, average daily metabolic rate increased by 9.5% and energy expenditure by 10% as a result of twice-weekly training. Less than half of this increase could be attributed to the calorie cost of the workouts themselves, so positive effects on metabolism must explain the rest.

What are you made of?

There are two important factors at work. Firstly, research shows that by increasing your 'fat-free mass' (the proportion of your body weight made up of anything other than fat), your body burns more calories on a daily basis. Therefore, altering your body composition to include less fat and more muscle is a good thing for weight loss (not to mention heart health). At the very least, resistance training causes a short term hike in resting metabolic rate.

Secondly, all exercise has an 'afterburn' effect, known as 'excess post-exercise oxygen consumption' (EPOC) – a period during which additional energy is needed to help the body replenish depleted fuel stores following a workout. This recovery period following exercise is almost entirely fuelled by fat oxidation (oxidation just means burning or 'use'). The intensity of the exercise and length of the session dictates the amount of energy used – the greater the intensity the better. Research has shown that fat oxidation can last up to three hours post resistance exercise and burns a significant number of extra calories.

Lose the fat, keep the muscle

The case for weight training becomes even stronger when you bring reduced calorie intake into the equation. When you cut calories, more than a quarter of the kilos you lose aren't fat – they consist of water, muscle tissue and even bone. Now, the relevance of this is that muscle is a demanding type of tissue – it needs to be fed calories constantly to keep it functioning.

The more muscle you have, the more calories you burn whether you are walking along the street or doing barbell squats. Fat, in contrast, is quite happy to just sit there without making any demands for energy.

A study, from the University of Texas, Austin, looked at the effects of twelve weeks of either high-intensity endurance or resistance training on resting metabolic rate in men aged 18–35. After training both exercise groups showed significant declines in body fat. Resting metabolic rate did not significantly change after either training regime but there *was* a definite increase in energy expenditure. These results suggest that both endurance and resistance training may help prevent the attenuation of RMR normally seen during dieting.

STRONG WORDS

WHY NOT JUST DIET?

Calorie restriction has been shown to have a very positive effect on weight loss in the short term. But, in a study review looking at research on calorie cutting and weight loss over 25 years, it was found that the average person regained 35% of the weight they'd lost within a year. Diets that restrict calories to 1200 or below can reduce metabolic rate by as much as 20%. It's also been shown that exercise causes 'protein sparing' (literally, your body tries to hold on to its protein stores), which helps to maintain muscle mass.

And finally...

There's yet another reason why strength training is such a string to your weight loss bow. It has a remarkable effect on the shape and outline of your body. Fat is like a big sponge while muscle is dense, like stone. A kilo of fat takes up as much as five times more space than a kilo of muscle which is why you'll look so much trimmer after strength training.

And here's the scientific evidence on six ways weights work for weight loss...

A flatter tummy

In a study in the journal *Medicine & Science in Sports & Exercise* strength training three times a week, using two sets of each exercise, reduced levels of fat both under the skin on the abdomen and in between the organs in the abdominal region. In all, the female subjects lost 1.7kg of pure fat in 25 weeks.

Reduced body fat

In research published in the *Journal of Strength and Conditioning Research* women over 30 were assigned to a twelve-week weight-training programme, working out three days a week. Both body fat and skinfold girths (measurements of the amount of skin that can be 'pinched' at specific body sites) were lower, while fat-free mass increased.

Better body composition

In a study published in the *Journal of the American Dietetic Association*, the effect of weight training on resting metabolic rate, fat-free mass, strength and dietary intake was

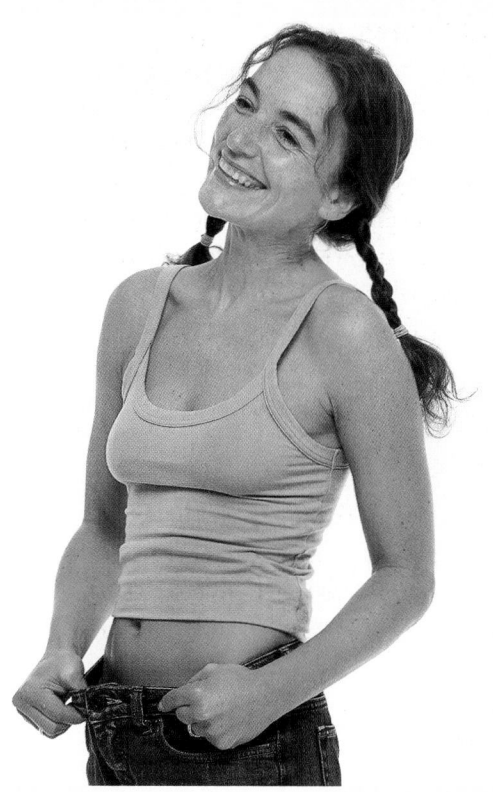

expenditure increasing by over 220 calories per day. RMR also increased by 6.8%. Even after adjusting the figures for the calorie cost of the training sessions themselves total daily energy expenditure was *still* significantly higher, meaning that both RMR and increased physical activity contributed to the higher figure.

Higher fat-free mass

A Japanese study found that fat-free mass and the amount of high-intensity physical activity performed were the strongest determinants of total daily energy expenditure, accounting for 51% of it.

Greater afterburn

A study in *Medicine & Science in Sport & Exercise* found that 45 minutes of resistance training elevated metabolism for two hours afterwards, resulting in an additional expenditure of 155 calories.

assessed for twelve weeks in young women. The women showed a significant increase in fat-free mass of 2kg, a highly respectable decrease in body fat percentage of 2.6% and significant increases in strength. RMR did not change significantly and neither did body weight. So, in this case, it seems that weight training had a beneficial effect on body composition.

Higher total energy expenditure

In a study from the University of Alabama that looked at older adults, 26 weeks of resistance training resulted in total daily energy

Hopefully, you are now convinced that weight training is something you simply can't leave out of your weight loss strategy. But stop right there! Before you skim over this section in your keenness to get on with the *Weights for Weight Loss* programme, I think it is important to understand a little about what muscles are and how they work. I'm not asking you to sign up for a physiology course but the whistle-stop tour in the next section will help you learn how to get the most out of resistance training and make you understand why doing biceps curls with a can of baked beans in each hand is, frankly, a waste of time.

BONING UP ON MUSCLES

Are you sitting comfortably? Then I'll begin…

What is muscle?

At the most basic level, muscle is simply the tissue in the body that initiates movement. That's not to say it does such a remarkable thing all on its own (the cardiovascular, nervous and hormonal systems are all involved) – but muscle is what actually enables us to move, by contracting and pulling on bones. There are more than 430 skeletal muscles in the body and virtually every move we make involves the action of more than one of them.

A closer look

Let's take a muscle, say, the biceps muscle in the arm (the one Popeye is always flexing), and have a closer look. A muscle is made up of thousands of long thin fibres (the term muscle fibre and muscle cell are used interchangeably) – about the diameter of a human hair. Each individual fibre is surrounded by connective tissue and groups of fibres are arranged into bundles (consisting of up to 150 fibres each), also encased in connective tissue. Then the whole muscle is sheathed in yet another layer

The make-up of a muscle

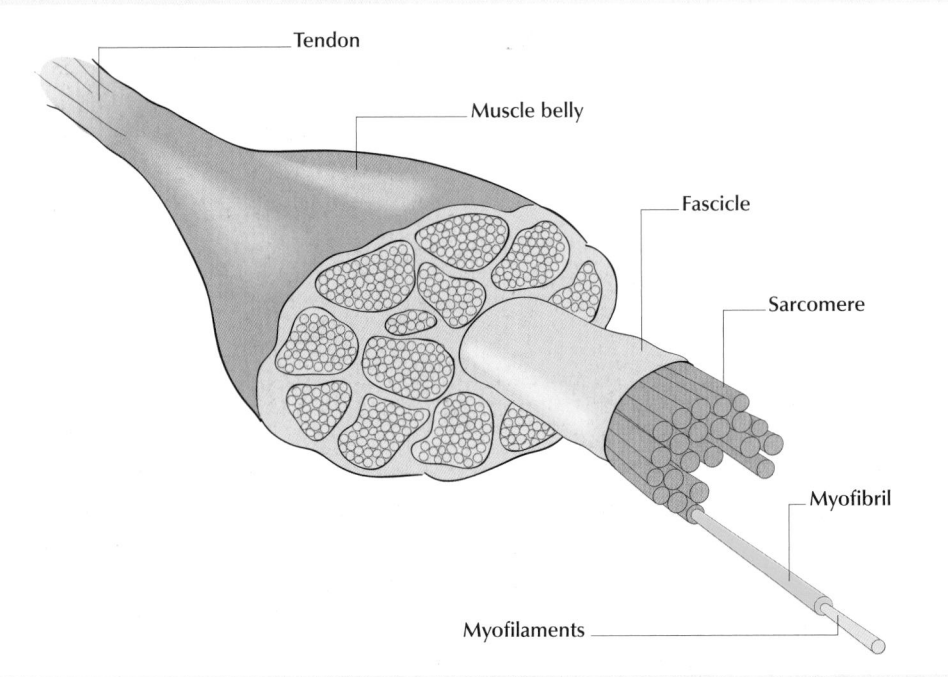

Tendon

Muscle belly

Fascicle

Sarcomere

Myofibril

Myofilaments

of connective tissue – the epimysium. All these layers of connective tissue join up to the tendon – which is what makes the structure so robust – and it is via these tendons that muscles pull on bone. To cause movement, each end of the muscle is attached to a different bone – one end is called the insertion, the other end the origin. So, for example, the biceps muscle is attached at one end to the radius (a bone in the forearm) and at the other end to the scapula or shoulder blade. When the biceps contracts the forearm moves towards the shoulder, as in a biceps curl.

The muscle fibre is divided into a series of blocks called sarcomeres. As far as muscle contraction is concerned the most important components of each sarcomere are the myofibrils (basically, these are strands of two proteins, called actin and myosin, which are arranged in bundles lengthways along the muscle fibre). These myofibrils are the key structures responsible for facilitating muscle contraction – since it is the action of one locking on to the other that draws the sarcomeres closer together, shortening the muscle and pulling on the tendon… and the bone… and causing movement.

How does muscle get stronger?

Muscle will only be as strong as it needs to be. If you rarely lift a finger, let alone a dumbbell, then your muscles will have adapted to cope with this low level of demand and, consequently, will find more taxing activities a challenge. To make a muscle stronger you need to 'overload' it. That is, you need to put it under more stress than it is accustomed to. Now, correct me if I'm wrong, but I wouldn't have thought getting a can of baked beans out the cupboard causes you to buckle under the weight… So neither is it (nor a 1kg hand weight or a bottle of mineral water) sufficient to create overload or instigate the adaptations needed to make your muscles stronger.

A muscle's 'pulling power' is dependent on the number of actin-myosin bonds (those protein strands) per myofibril. If you want to pull harder, you need more of 'em. So how do you get them? Tiny amounts of damage, caused by training, initiate the creation of further strands being added to the myofibril, and, indeed, more myofibrils being added to the fibre. More myofibrils mean the fibre gets physically bigger, as it has more 'bundles' packed along its length. And the increased thickness of the muscle fibre gives it a greater ability to develop force.

It is worth knowing that while you can make the fibres *bigger*, it is not believed that you can change the *number* of fibres within a muscle – that is determined by your genetics.

Hitting a nerve

The second thing that changes in order to increase strength relates to the communication between the central nervous system and the muscles (the neuromuscular system). A special type of nerve cell, called a motor neuron, acts as the 'governor' to a specific group of fibres (which could be anything from several hundred to just a handful) and it is this that gives the signal to contract. Muscles that have to do very precise actions may have just one fibre per motor neuron but bigger muscles with less particular jobs will have several hundred fibres being served by one motor neuron. A motor neuron and the muscle fibres it activates are collectively called a motor unit. When the motor neuron receives a message from the central nervous system (ground control) saying 'Move!', it, in turn, tells all its muscle fibres to contract.

The motor neuron makes all the fibres within the motor unit contract and develop force at the same time… But don't think that each *muscle* consists of just one motor unit – in fact, a muscle consists of *scores* of motor units and they don't all contribute to every movement. The number that is recruited is proportional to the force needed to initiate the movement – the greater the force, the more motor units recruited.

If you were to try to lift an iron bar, for example, most of the motor units in the biceps would be recruited, whereas if it were just a cup of tea only a small number would

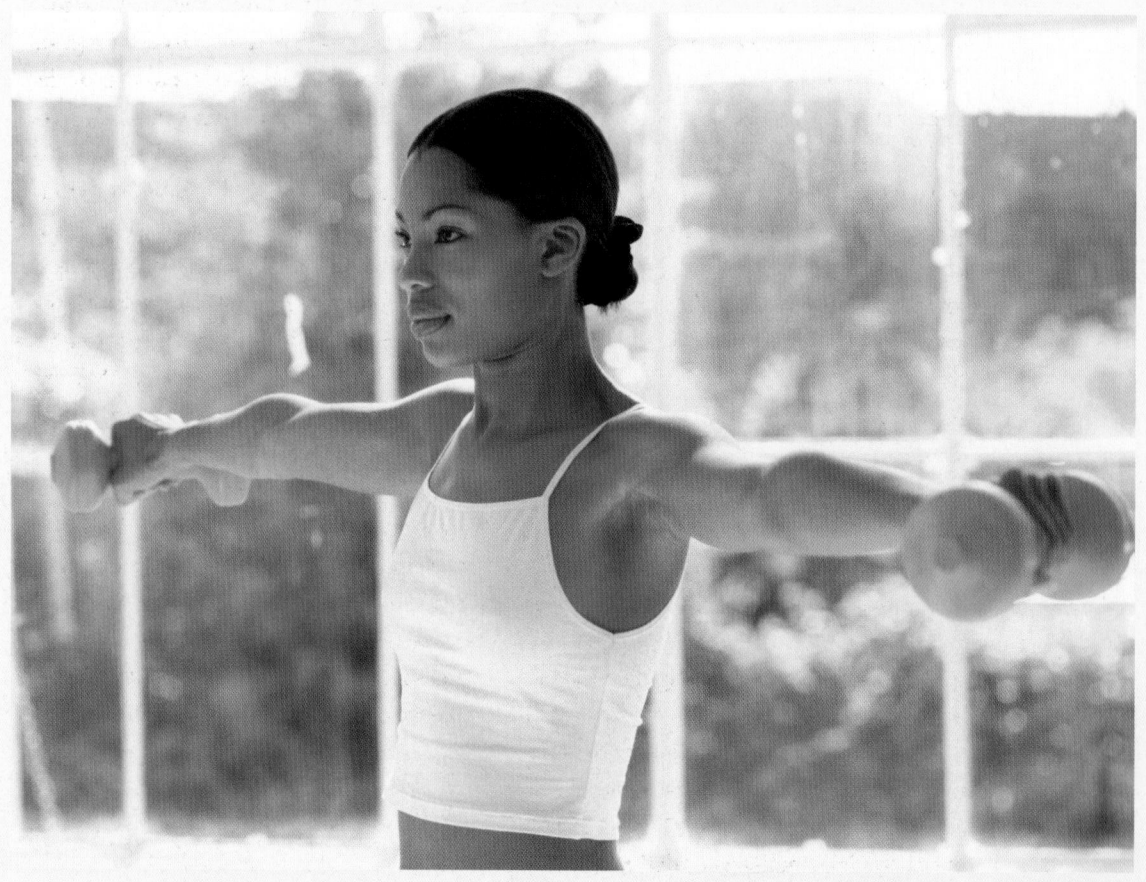

get involved. Whatever the movement the motor units involved are not continually active. Instead, they switch on and off at different times but they do this so fast that you get a smooth contraction (think of a Mexican wave).

All systems go

The question of how many motor units will be fired at any one time is determined by your training experience and efficiency, not to mention your genes. At first, the mechanism is very crude – and the nervous system tends to underestimate how many 'workers' it needs for the job. But, as you train regularly, you become more effective and fire up more motor units every time, so you get more 'hands on deck' and, consequently, greater strength. In strength training newbies, strength gains over the first few weeks of training are mostly to do with improved neuromuscular pathways rather than physiological changes in the muscle – which set in later. That's why you can't expect to see an increase in muscle size (known as hypertrophy) in the first couple of months. But, however much you train, you cannot change the number of fibres per motor unit. This varies between individuals and is one of the reasons why some people can achieve greater muscle size and strength far more easily than others.

But whether it is just a couple of motor units or a few hundred that take part, the order in which they are recruited is always the same. This 'sequential order' is related to the type of muscle fibre that the motor unit contains. Yup! There ain't just one type of fibre to get your head around...

Fibre types

Fibres are broadly divided into type 1 and type 2 – and the distinction relates to whether the fibre develops force slowly or rapidly. We all have some of both but the type that predominates varies from person to person and muscle to muscle and this will influence – to some extent – the kind of activity you are best suited to. Postural muscles, such as the soleus in the calf, have a high percentage of slow-twitch fibres, to allow them to provide stability; while dynamic muscles, such as the quads in the front of the thigh, have a mixture of fast- and slow-twitch fibres, to allow them to execute both low-intensity (such as walking) and high-intensity (like jumping) activities. Endurance athletes tend to have a lot of type 1, or slow-twitch fibres. (Muscle biopsies have revealed as much as 99% slow-twitch fibres in the calf muscles of marathon runners.) These fibres are highly resistant to fatigue due to their ability to process lots of oxygen but they tend to be recruited mainly at low intensities of effort (such as picking up that cup of tea). Type 2 or fast-twitch fibres, on the other hand, are associated with muscle power, strength and speed – and only kick in when the intensity of the effort required increases.

The major muscles

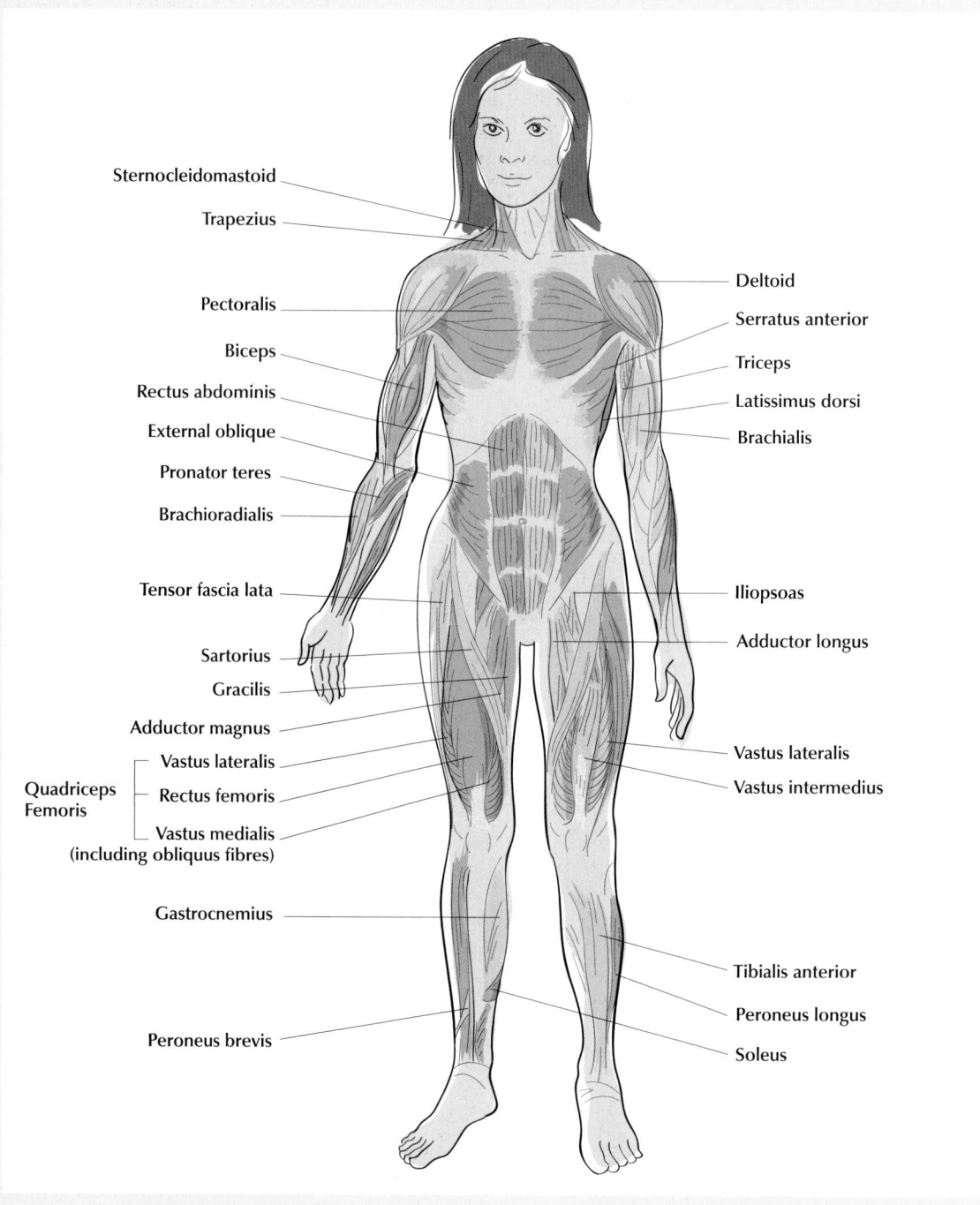

Sternocleidomastoid

Trapezius

Pectoralis

Biceps

Rectus abdominis

External oblique

Pronator teres

Brachioradialis

Tensor fascia lata

Sartorius

Gracilis

Adductor magnus

Quadriceps Femoris
- Vastus lateralis
- Rectus femoris
- Vastus medialis
(including obliquus fibres)

Gastrocnemius

Peroneus brevis

Deltoid

Serratus anterior

Triceps

Latissimus dorsi

Brachialis

Iliopsoas

Adductor longus

Vastus lateralis

Vastus intermedius

Tibialis anterior

Peroneus longus

Soleus

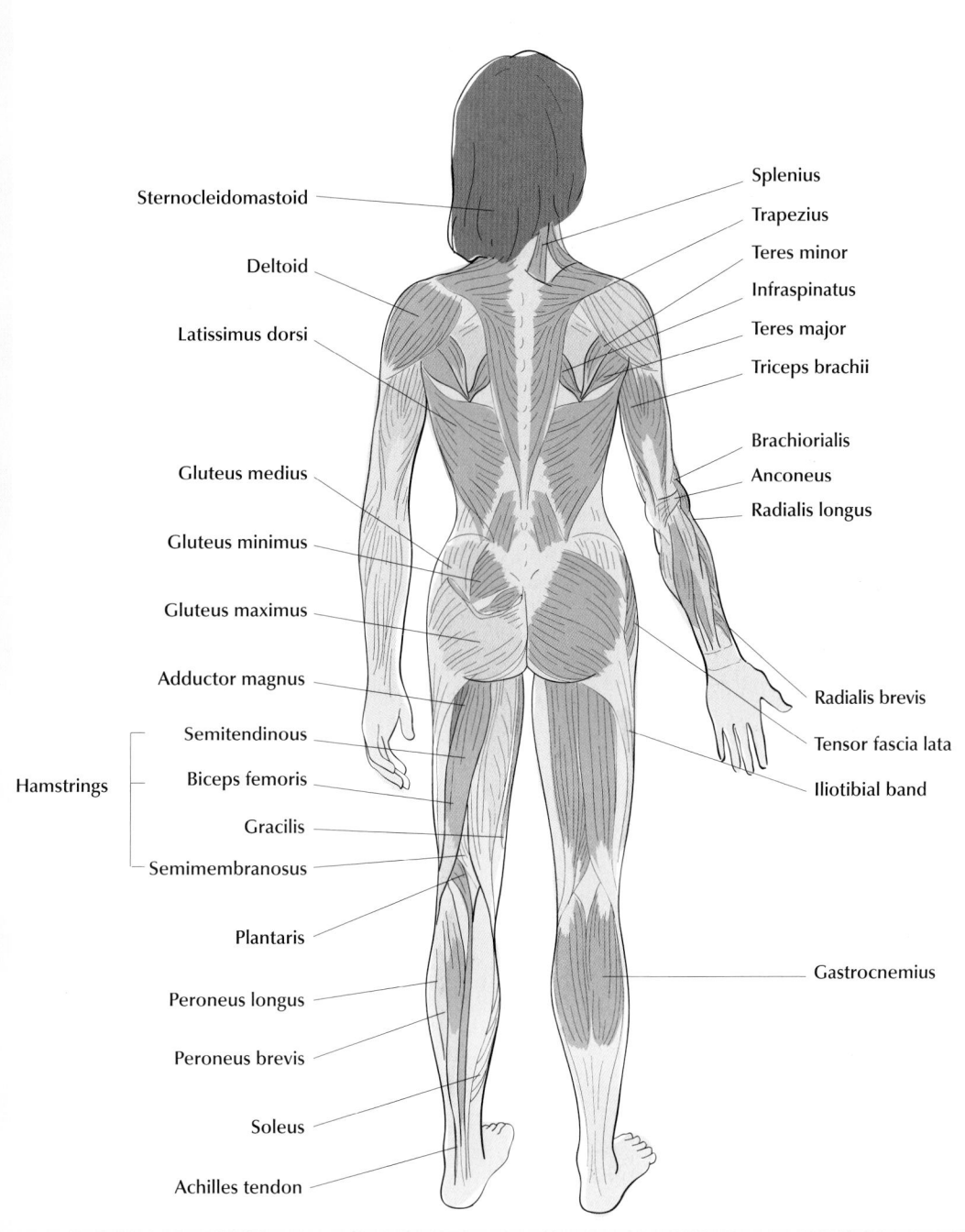

Sternocleidomastoid

Deltoid

Latissimus dorsi

Gluteus medius

Gluteus minimus

Gluteus maximus

Adductor magnus

Semitendinous

Biceps femoris

Gracilis

Semimembranosus

Hamstrings

Plantaris

Peroneus longus

Peroneus brevis

Soleus

Achilles tendon

Splenius

Trapezius

Teres minor

Infraspinatus

Teres major

Triceps brachii

Brachiorialis

Anconeus

Radialis longus

Radialis brevis

Tensor fascia lata

Iliotibial band

Gastrocnemius

What it all means

And here's the important bit, as far as strength training is concerned. (At last!) Since the motor units are recruited in sequential order, from slow twitch to fast twitch, it follows that the only way to train a muscle in its entirety (getting the maximum number of motor units involved) is to expose it to high – and increasingly challenging – loads to ensure they all get 'a piece of the action'. That is why doing lots of reps with a light weight won't build strength or size. No muscle fibre – fast or slow twitch – is overloaded. In a nutshell, light weights don't present enough load to change the physiology of any fibre.

Makes sense? Well, just to confuse things, there are two types of type 2 fibres – known as type 2a and type 2b. While 2b are the true power rangers, the type 2a fibres sit on the fence and, depending on the type of training you do, can be made to act either more like endurance-based type 1 or power-based type 2b fibres. In other words, they can be trained for stamina or strength. This is very important when it comes to programme planning, as you can't have your cake and eat it – at least, not within one particular muscle. That's why knowing the basics of muscle physiology is so useful, when you want to train for real results.

Why stronger doesn't mean bigger

There is probably one question that you are still asking by this point. Is it possible to get firmer and stronger, without getting bigger muscles? The answer is yes. If you were to look at a muscle in cross-section, you'd see that there is space between those bundles of long thin fibres. In an untrained muscle, there is lots of space. When you train, the fibres get bigger. But that doesn't mean the muscle *itself* gets bigger, as the muscle fibres simply take up more of the free space in the muscle by becoming more tightly packed. This – along with a host of other physiological adaptations – is why muscles 'firm up' when you train them. And no amount of reps with those baked bean tins is going to get you there. This will not actually instigate the adaptations that allow the fibres to get thicker, so will achieve neither definition nor firmness.

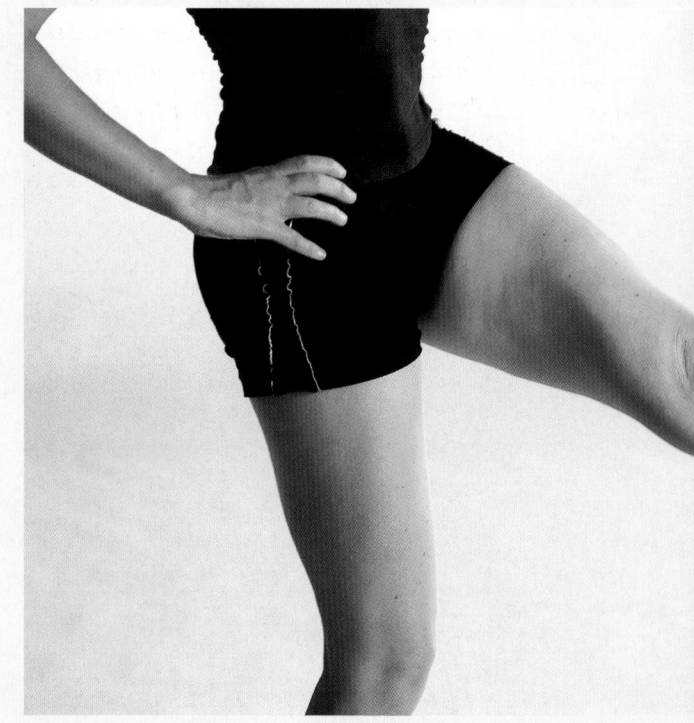

If you don't want to increase the overall size of the muscle you can stop increasing the overload, once the muscle has gained sufficient strength and firmness, to maintain this new level of 'tone' (see right) without adding volume. Continue to 'overload' the muscle, though, and it will increase slightly in diameter, as the fibres and myofibrils thicken.

The results

So now we know a little about how muscles function, let's look at how to train them to get the results we want. How strength training affects you as an individual depends on a number of factors – most importantly, arguably, the way you train (in terms of frequency, weight, number of reps and sets) but also your genes, gender, age, what other physical activity you do, your diet and even your technique. The next chapter will help you gain an idea of how your body is likely to respond.

STRONG WORDS

CAN YOU JUST 'TONE UP'?

We all use the word 'tone' as though it is a specific training goal but, really, all tone means is 'a state of slight tension' – in other words, the muscle is slightly active, rather than totally passive. If muscles are accustomed to being active they tend to have a higher level of tone than in people who are inactive and don't use their muscles much. Tone is related to shape, or definition, in a muscle because when a muscle contracts it shortens and bulges as the fibres overlap one another, giving more shape. So, yes, strength training will improve your muscle tone.

However, definition – or lack of it – is very often more to do with too much body fat covering the muscle rather than a lack of muscle shape. It may also be due to poor flexibility. Pat Fox, strength and conditioning specialist at South Bank University, points out that working through a full range of motion, and practising flexibility work, are essential to achieve a streamlined non-bulky look.

HOW WILL WEIGHTS WORK FOR ME?

The factors that affect the results you are likely to get from strength training and how to get the best results for you

This may come as some surprise to you but even if you and your best friend do exactly the same workout, with the same amount of weight, the same number of times a week, there is no guarantee that you will get the same results.

Lots of factors affect how your body responds to weights. Gender is probably the biggest factor because of the huge differences in levels of testosterone and other anabolic (muscle building) hormones in men and women; but women's natural testosterone levels can also vary from person to person. Your age, training status, body shape and size, predominant type of muscle fibres, diet and good old DNA will all also have an influence on the results you can achieve.

Two scientists, Paul Thompson and Eric Hoffman, demonstrated the wild variation in response to working with weights by recruiting 700 male and 700 female newbies to lift weights for twelve weeks. The biceps

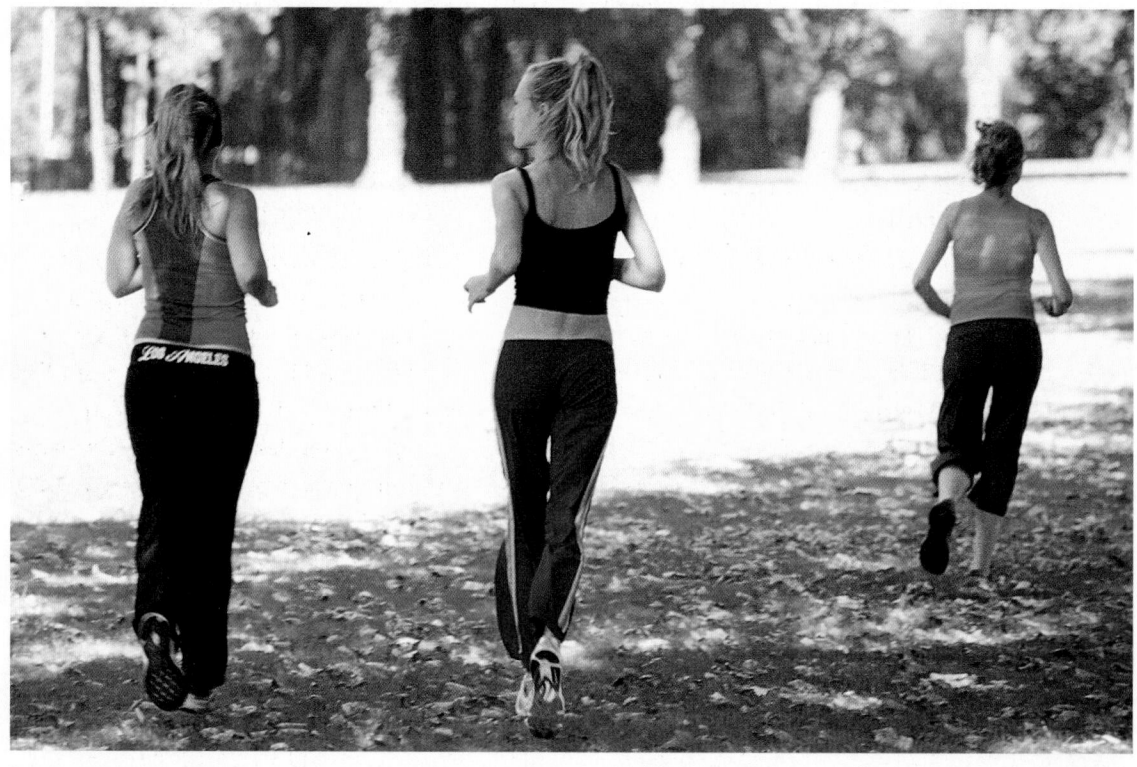

and triceps muscles of the subjects were scanned using magnetic resonance imaging (MRI) to precisely measure muscle size, while special machines were used to assess strength in each of these muscles at the start of the study. At the end of the study, during which time these muscles were trained intensively, some subjects had built size but not strength. Others had built considerable strength but not size. Still others had gained both and a handful didn't seem to have got either stronger or bigger, proving that there is undoubtedly a genetic component involved in how your body will respond to weights. (That's not to say you can't influence the way your body responds by manipulating some of the training variables – but we'll come on to that later.) First let's look at factors specific to the fairer sex…

How being a dame affects the results

On average, a woman has around 50–60% of the absolute strength of a man in the upper body and about 70% of the lower body strength. Women tend to be smaller, shorter and lighter – and carry more body fat – than men. Even when you factor in the smaller body size, the higher level of body fat remains, because women have a supply of 'essential' fat to cope with the demands of pregnancy and lactation. So overall, a woman's body composition is geared towards more fat and less muscle than a man's. On average, skeletal muscle accounts for about 38% of total body weight in men and 31% in women.

STRONG WORDS

GIRTH CONTROL

In studies looking at the effect of weight training on women the greatest increase in various body girths, as a result of between twelve and twenty weeks of training, was 0.4–0.6cm, proving that strength workouts are hardly going to give you strapping shoulders and bulging calves. A quite considerable *decrease* in body girths where fat tends to be stored, such as the hips, thighs and abdomen, is commonly found. In one twelve-week study, tummy girth decreased by 0.2–1.1cm, while a ten-week programme resulted in hip, thigh and abdominal circumferences decreasing by 0.2–0.7cm.

We girls also tend to have a smaller hip to shoulder ratio, a wider pelvis and a greater 'Q' angle; the angle at which the thighbone travels from the hip to the knee. With smaller muscle fibres – and a tenth of the muscle-building hormone testosterone that a man has – women aren't primed for building big, bulky muscles. But they absolutely *can* get stronger, firmer and shapelier – and tip the body composition balance towards less fat and more muscle through working with weights.

The average woman can expect to see a strength improvement of 25–30% within six months of starting a resistance training programme.

Confession time

Despite the title of this book, I have to admit that resistance training may not help you shed body weight. Disappointed? Well, consider this – would you rather fit your 58kg frame into size 14 jeans, or your 64kg frame into a size 10? The truth is, muscle weighs a lot more than fat (a third again as much, in fact) but I promise you will look and feel trimmer and slimmer by altering your body composition to consist of more muscle and less fat, regardless of whether you lose weight. You *will* see a change in your body silhouette and you *will* see shape and tone. That goes for whether you are a classic pear-shaped woman, an apple, a stick insect or an hourglass. Happily, there is no physiological reason that any body type cannot increase muscle mass and decrease fat mass and gain better body definition. But, of course, you can't actually change the basic structure of your body – think of it as the 'blank canvas' you have to work with…

What's your type?

Scientists refer to your body shape as your somatotype. William Sheldon's somatotyping system, developed in the 1950s, is still widely used though it has been rather oversimplified.

Sheldon talked in terms of the relative dominance of certain body characteristics when he defined his three somatotypes. Endomorphy referred to roundness, mesomorphy referred to muscularity and ectomorphy referred to linearity. He used a scale of 1–7 for each type to give an overall score. So, for example, a score of 1-7-1 would indicate an extremely mesomorphic person. Nowadays, people use the system to brand one person as an 'ectomorph', another as an 'endomorph'. But, if it were really that simple, wouldn't an endomorph who lost lots of weight become an ectomorph? Body typing is only useful if it reflects body qualities that cannot be changed, such as the ratio of your shoulder-to-hip width or the length of your bones.

Sheldon's somatotyping is not the only method used to classify body types: another system refers to glandular dominances, in which the 'thyroid' type replaces the ectomorph, the 'adrenal' type replaces the mesomorph and the 'pituitary' type replaces the endomorph. This body typing system introduces a fourth category for women only, termed 'gonadal', which is associated with the stereotypical 'pear-shaped' female – narrow shoulders and wide hips. Regardless of the system used few of us represent textbook versions of one particular somatotype – but we do tend to have more features from one type than another.

Here are some of the classic characteristics associated with each type of dominance…

Endomorphs – Pear shaped – shoulders that are narrower relative to hips – rounded, soft. Short limbs, long torso. Short musculature. If you circle your wrist with your opposite thumb and middle finger and the digits don't meet you may be endomorphic. Picture a trapezius.

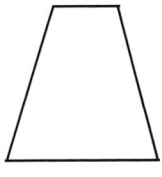

Mesomorphs – broad shouldered, thick chested, narrow waisted and muscular with a long torso. Usually well proportioned. Triangular shaped body (wider shoulders than hips). Finds it easy to build muscle mass. If you circle your wrist with your opposite thumb and middle finger and the digits just touch it indicates a dominance of mesomorphy. Visualise an upside down trapezius.

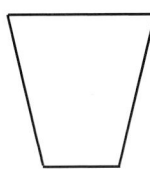

Ectomorphs – short upper body, long arms and legs, long narrow feet and hands and very little fat storage. This body type has a narrow chest and narrow shoulders and long, thin muscles; quite 'straight up and down' (not much of a waist). Narrow bones – if you circle your wrist with your opposite thumb and

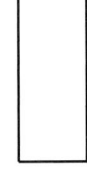

middle finger and the digits overlap you are most likely an ectomorph. Visualise a rectangle.

How does your body type affect your training?

It's all very well knowing that you are, say, mainly mesomorphic but what does it mean when it comes to training? After all, it's only worth knowing if it has some influence on what you should actually do. A lot of nonsense is written about this – such as if you are endomorphic you should concentrate on aerobic exercise while if you are ectomorphic you should do less aerobic exercise and more weights. This kind of advice totally disregards the issue of heart health and the importance of a balanced programme and implies that you can't be a slim endomorph or an overweight ectomorph, which simply isn't the case.

A classic illustration of this is the notion that it is 'difficult' for a pear-shaped endomorph to gain muscle, especially in the lower body. In fact a larger frame – whether it be at the hips or shoulders – indicates a *greater* potential for muscular development, as the surface area of the muscle needs to be larger to span the greater distance from origin to insertion.

Since body fat storage predominates around the pelvic frame, however – whether that be around the abdominal region or the hips, buttocks and thighs – a wider pelvic girdle gives greater potential for fat storage too, which explains the tendency for an endomorphic body shape to have a high propensity for body fat storage.

Working from the inside out

The factors we've discussed so far are beyond your control – such as your sex, body type and limb length. Another major reason that people don't get the results they expect from strength training is that they inevitably take their own postural idiosyncrasies, muscle imbalances, weaknesses and tightnesses with them into the gym. In other words, few – if any – of us are starting off with a truly blank canvas.

Say, for example, you start doing lots of chest exercises to strengthen and tone your pectorals but already have a rounded shoulder posture. Without the inclusion of flexibility work for the pecs, and strengthening of the opposing muscle groups in the back, you will simply exacerbate the existing postural problem. Or you begin doing squats with tight hip flexors and poor knee mechanics and end up with a sore back and knee pain.

While I am not claiming that you can reverse the maladaptions of a couple of decades in a matter of weeks, it is still a wise idea to spend a little time on improving posture and redressing imbalances before you even pick up a weight – which is why the *Weights for Weight Loss* programme begins with the Foundation Workout on page 58. It does exactly what it says on the tin – it lays the foundation for you to become stronger without reinforcing poor postural and movement habits, enabling you to develop long, lean and balanced muscles that work efficiently and are injury-resistant. Even if you feel you are in good shape I still recommend that you follow the Foundation Workout for two to three weeks before moving on to the more demanding programmes. See 'Three easy steps to better body awareness', right, to get you off on the right foot. You can start practising these moves RIGHT NOW!

STRONG WORDS

LONG LIMBS, LONG MUSCLES

When it comes to relative strength, shorter-limbed people have an advantage over the lankier-limbed, because the latter have to exert a force over a longer distance. (For example, in a bench press the bar has to travel further until the arms are straight.) It's also harder for the longer-limbed to gain definition and shape, as the muscle itself (which, you'll remember, attaches at both ends to bone) is physically longer and therefore more spread out. But in most cases, this is the exact long, lean look many women want to achieve.

Three easy steps to better body awareness

Mastering these three techniques will put you on track to better posture and body awareness ensuring you get the most out of every move in the *Weights for Weight Loss* Workout. It will also minimise your risk of injury, both during exercise and in normal daily activities.

The trunk muscles

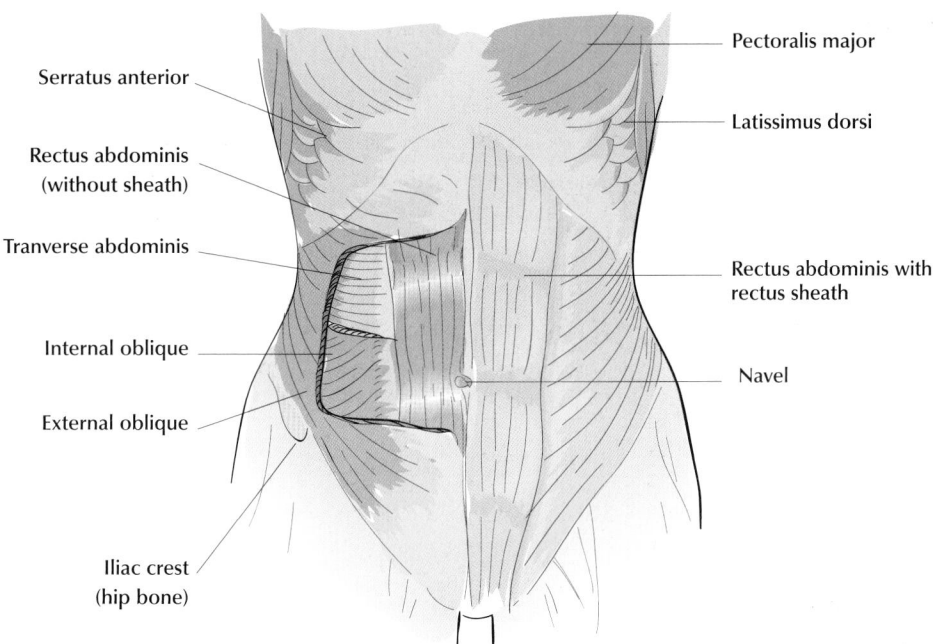

Serratus anterior

Rectus abdominis (without sheath)

Tranverse abdominis

Internal oblique

External oblique

Iliac crest (hip bone)

Pectoralis major

Latissimus dorsi

Rectus abdominis with rectus sheath

Navel

Engaging the core

Engaging the core is really just a posh way of saying 'pull your tummy in'. But you have to learn how to identify and 'engage' or 'switch on' the right muscles. These are the deep muscles of the back, waist and abdominals – known collectively as the 'core' muscles (see illustration on previous page) – whose role it is to protect and support the spine and provide a solid base for movement. Engaging the core muscles is fundamental to good posture, stability, a flatter abdomen and more efficient movement.

1 To get a feel of the muscles you are trying to get to (as they lie deep below the surface of the tummy) kneel, sit or stand and place your fingertips 5cm in and 2.5cm down from your hipbones and feign a cough – you should feel the muscles contract involuntarily under your fingertips. Got it?

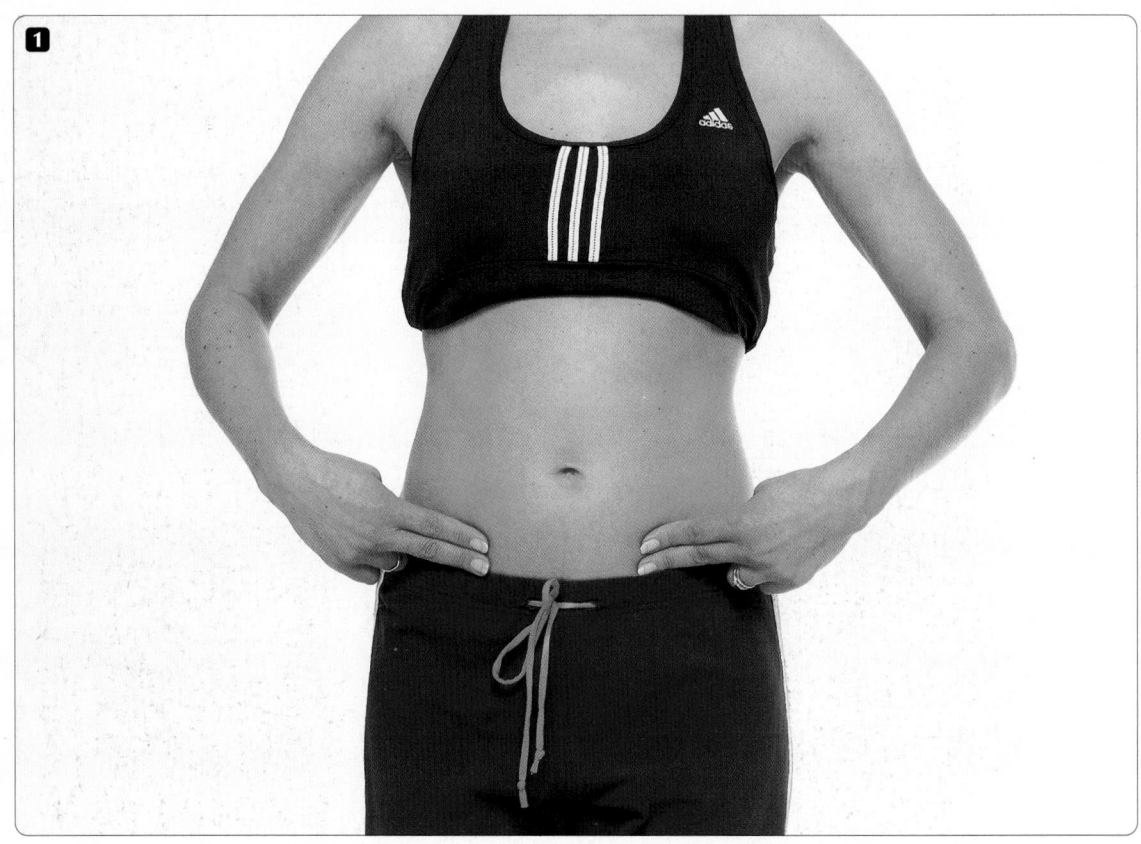

2 Now inhale and, as you exhale, start pulling up the pelvic floor (as if you were trying to stop yourself from peeing). This works because the lower fibres of the deep-set transversus abdominis muscle actually intermingle with the pelvic floor muscles. Continue to pull in and up, using those muscles you located in the cough, imagining you are doing up a zip from your pubic bone to your navel.

3 It may help to take one hand to your lower back (palm away) and the other to your tummy (palm touching). You should feel the tummy pull away from the front hand but you don't want to feel the back pushing into the hand behind you. The spine remains still as the core engages but don't hold your breath. Build up to progressively longer holds and practise regularly throughout the day.

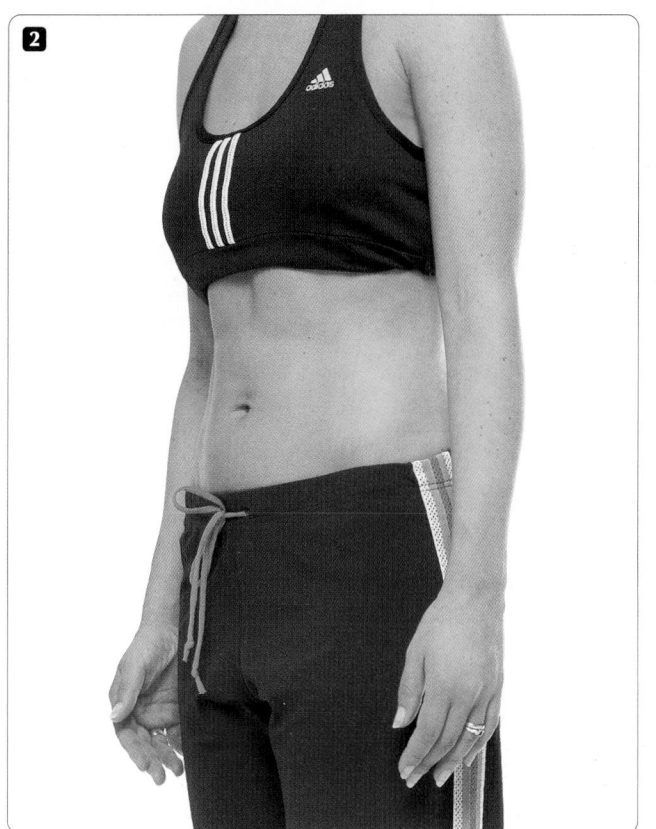

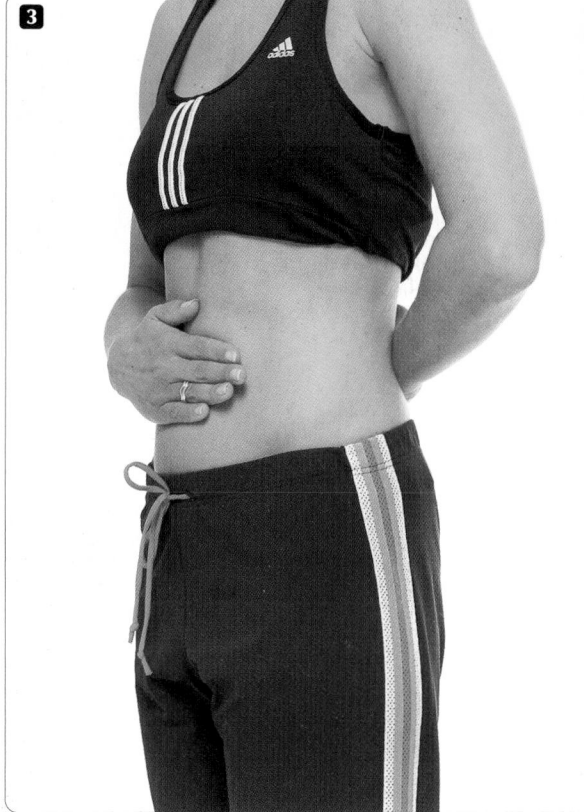

Setting the shoulder blades (scapulae)

Setting the shoulder blades makes your upper body more stable, injury resistant and ensures that bigger, stronger muscles don't take over the job of the smaller ones and cause imbalances. Draw the shoulder blades back and slightly down, anchoring them at the top of the back of the ribcage. You should feel the chest lift and open slightly. A good way of getting the feeling is to hold a resistance tube in each hand behind your back and gently draw the hands away from each other until you feel a tension in the middle of the upper back. That is how the shoulder blades should feel when they are 'set'.

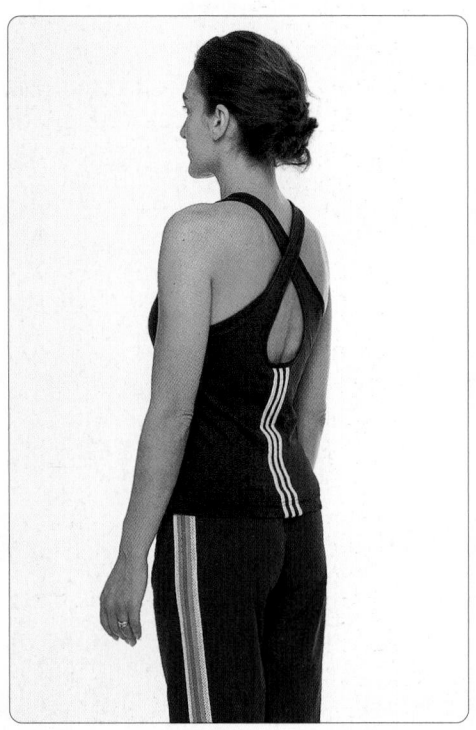

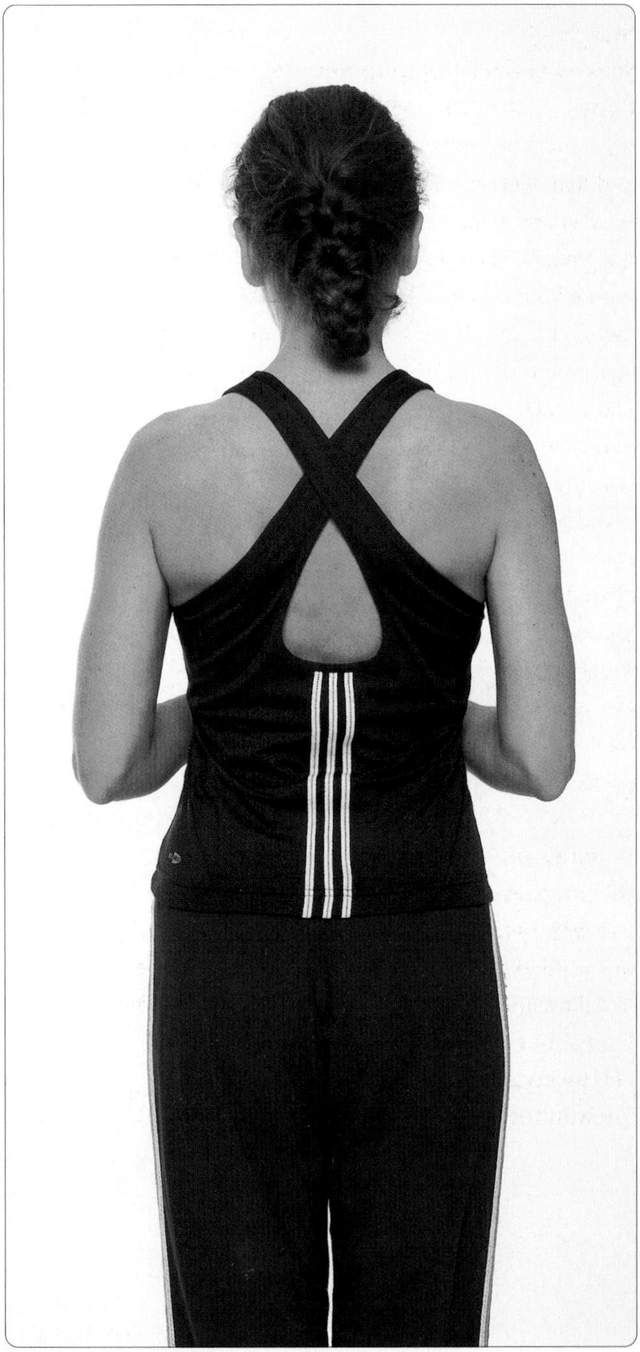

Standing tall

Stand with feet below your hipbones. Ensure the weight is evenly distributed between the front and back of the feet and between the left and right feet. Pull up through the arches of the feet and ensure all toes have contact with the ground. Pull up through the legs and ensure your buttocks have some tension in them but aren't clenched. Keep the hips square and level. Lengthen through the spine and engage the core, imaging the torso 'growing' out of the pelvis. Drop the rib cage, drawing the lower ribs down towards the pubic bone. Relax the shoulders, draw the spine deep into the back and gently open the chest and front of the shoulders by turning your thumbs to face the front (your little finger should be parallel to your trouser seam). Keep the neck long, the chin slightly retracted, and allow the head to sit squarely on top of the spine. Breathe freely.

Whether you are going to follow any of the programmes in this book, or intend to create your own workout with the knowledge you've gained – it is important to follow the 'rules' of training and know a little about strength training terminology and protocols. You'll find all you need to know in the next chapter.

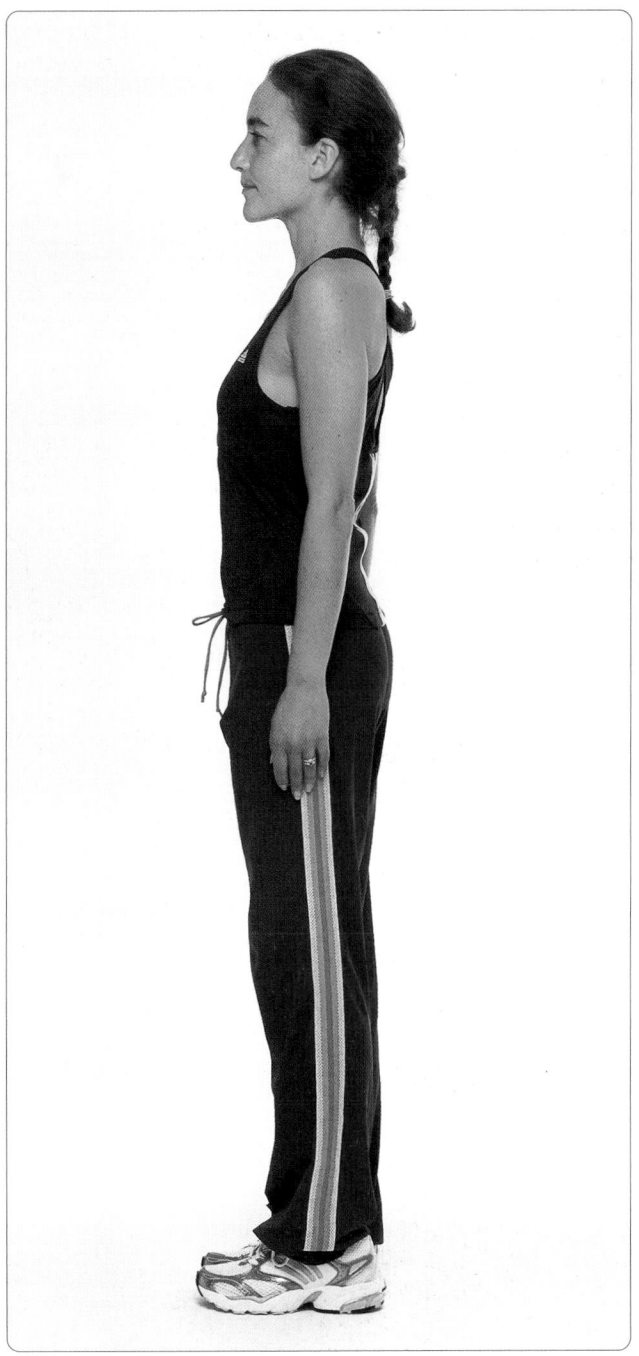

THE RULES

Follow the rules to ensure you train safely and effectively
– and get the results you want.

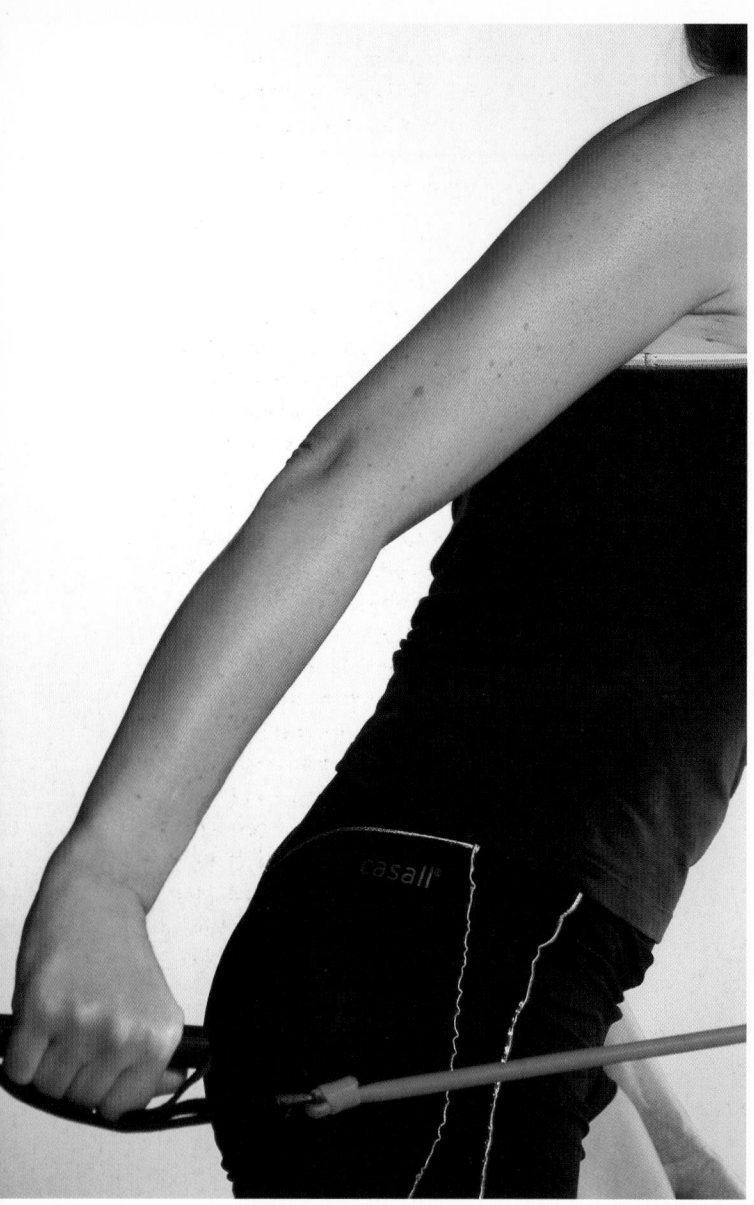

Can there *really* be a whole section on how to lift weights? Surely lifting and lowering a dumbbell can't be that complex! Well no, not once you know the ground rules. But even once you have got to grips with these, it doesn't mean they are set in stone. As you have probably guessed by now, there is no set, definitive formula for strength training that works for all goals and all people.

Crack an egg and you can make an omelette or a meringue, you can scramble it, poach, fry or boil it. It's how you cook it, what you add and what kind of utensils you use to cook it that makes it turn out one way or another. And it's exactly the same with strength training!

There's an acronym that strength and conditioning specialists use, known as the 'SAID' principle. It stands for 'specific adaptation to imposed demands' and what it means is that the type of demand you place on your body dictates the type of changes that will occur. As a simple example, if you took up running, putting in four sessions of 45 minutes a week, your body would respond very differently from if you took up yoga – or weight training. The SAID principle also holds true *within* strength training. For example, lots of reps with a light weight and brief rests will have a very different outcome from short, heavy sets with long rests, as we will find out in just a moment.

Getting with the programme

The American College of Sports Medicine's resistance training guidelines include the following advice (don't worry if you don't understand some of the terminology used – it is all explained over the following pages):

• Use both concentric and eccentric muscle actions.

• Use both single- and multiple-joint exercises (isolated and compound moves).

• Order exercises to optimise the quality of the workout (by training large before small muscle groups, doing multiple-joint exercises before single-joint exercises and higher-intensity before lower-intensity exercises).

• Beginners training for strength should use a weight corresponding to their 8–12 repetition maximum (RM).

• For intermediate to advanced strength training, use a wider loading range i.e. instead of just doing between 8–12 reps you can do between 1–12, experimenting with heavier weights with fewer reps.

• When you can comfortably perform 1 or 2 more repetitions than the number you set yourself, increase the weight by 2–10%.

• The recommendation for training frequency is 2–3 days a week for novice and intermediate training and 4–5 days a week for advanced training.

STRONG WORDS

A MOVING TALE

Muscle contractions are divided into three main types. An *isometric* contraction is when the muscle is producing a force but not changing in length. A perfect example of this is core stability work, such as the navel to spine hold on page 64 – you are holding the core stabilisers firm, while other parts of the body move. Isometric contractions will strengthen muscles but only in and around the position in which the contraction is held. For example, if you did that exercise where you 'sit' with your back against a wall with your knees bent at a right angle, you'd only see increased strength in the thigh muscles at 90 degrees and perhaps 20 degrees either side of that.

In strength training you commonly have muscle contractions where the muscle first shortens and then lengthens as it exerts force, known as isotonic actions. For example, when your biceps contract to bend your arm the muscle shortens. This is called a *concentric action*. And then, when you lower the arm back down, the biceps have to control the descent of the arm – the contraction is happening while the muscle lengthens. This is called an *eccentric* action.

- Higher-volume, multiple-set programmes are recommended for maximising hypertrophy, with loads corresponding to 1–12 RM, with emphasis on the 6–12 RM zone using 1- to 2-minute rest periods between sets performed at a moderate speed.

- For local muscular endurance training, it is recommended that light to moderate loads (40–60% of 1 RM) be performed for high repetitions using short rest periods.

- All strength training should use the principle of periodization, in which a planned training programme is divided into phases, each of which has a specific purpose or focus.

The ACSM points out that their guidelines need to be considered within the context of individual needs. It's also worth bearing in mind that even if you did find the 'perfect' formula – it wouldn't last long because, if there is one crucial ingredient to a successful strength training programme, it is variety that stops both you and your muscles from getting bored!

That's progress

Another crucial element is remembering that, as you get stronger, you need to increase what's known as the 'training load'. It sounds obvious but I am always amazed by the number of people who get stuck in a rut with those 5kg biceps curls or twenty crunches. Once your body becomes comfortable with the workout you are presenting it you need to increase the challenge. Otherwise, you will fail to continue making improvements. This is known as 'progressive overload'. Now, increasing the training load can be achieved in a number of ways. The most obvious one is to increase the weight but you can also increase the number of reps or sets, or the frequency with which you exercise that muscle group. Note that word 'progressive' however – it means that you should increase the training load by a small amount – not pile it on all at once!

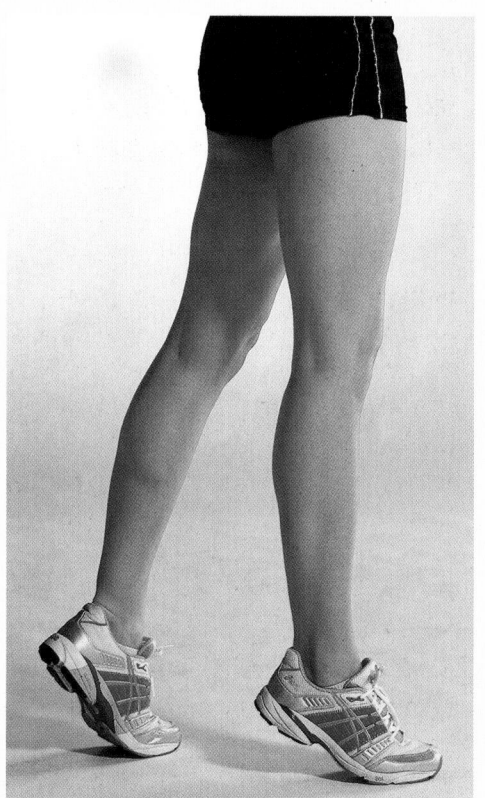

What are my strength training options?

As I promised in the introduction, you don't need to be a gym member to get into strength training. You can work with any type of resistance – including your own body weight (when working against gravity), elastic tubing, dumbbells, barbells, medicine balls – or, of course, the weight-training machines designed to train each muscle group. All have their place in a balanced programme and practicalities – such as space, availability, convenience or cost – may dictate what you choose to work with but the gold standard is generally considered to be free weights.

Free vs fixed weights

A free weight is one that isn't attached to anything, such as a dumbbell or barbell, while a 'fixed' weight moves in the plane and range dictated by the machine it is attached to. Because you aren't supported by anything as you exercise with free weights they demand greater effort and recruit more muscles in order to stabilise other joints while the movement is taking place. They also mimic real life more than fixed machines. After all, when you get a heavy box off a high shelf there isn't a machine providing stability and support for you... Also, training with free weights burns more calories – as you engage more muscles in order to stabilise the body and assist the movement – not to mention having to lift and carry the weights around.

So what's the benefit of machines? Well, there are some movements that it is difficult to perform without the help of a machine (the lat pulldown is a good example) – and, of course, variety is the spice of life.

Traditionally, resistance training machines are recommended to beginners for ease of use and safety. Granted, you are less likely to clunk yourself on the head if you use the triceps pushdown machine rather than do a supine French press, for example. And you are also far less able to do the exercise 'wrong,' as the direction and range of motion is controlled and limited by the machine. But many experts now argue that this isn't necessarily a good thing and believe that using a combination of free weights, body weight and stability balls better teaches people to stabilise themselves and control their range of motion. Also, since machines are designed to fit 'Mr Average', they won't always fit you – although the array of adjustments that can be made to help you 'fit' better into a machine is impressive on today's hi-tech machinery.

At the end of the day, it's your choice. Research in the journal *Medicine & Science in Sport & Exercise* found no significant difference in strength gains in a free-weight bench press compared to a chest press machine so, if you like the familiarity of the machines, you aren't selling yourself short in strength terms. Weights machines can also help build confidence and are less intimidating for newcomers than the free weights area in a gym.

Exercise balls, medicine balls and resistance tubing

Exercise balls or Swiss balls (basically, overgrown Spacehoppers with no ears) have become ubiquitous in gyms these days, and for good reason. Any exercise you do on the ball will be more challenging than it is on a stable surface. As well as coping with the exercise itself, your body has to work to keep you stable so you don't end up on the floor. It's also a great leveller – you will soon find out if your right side is stronger than your left, or if, despite your strength, you are sorely lacking in balance and coordination. In general, a 55cm ball is perfect if you are under 1.65cm – otherwise, you need a 65cm ball. The thing to look for is a ball that, when you sit on it, supports your hips slightly higher than your knees. Pump it up nice and firm.

Medicine balls are also making a comeback in modern gyms, probably due to the surge of popularity of one-to-one training. You can't get quite so much out of medicine ball workouts on your own (as many of the best moves involve catching, passing and throwing) but they can add challenge to abdominal moves and are good for more explosive speed work.

Resistance tubing – with or without handles – has many advantages. It takes up hardly any space, you can easily manipulate the resistance by creating more or less tension in the band, it is inexpensive and offers a great alternative to dumbbells and machines but there are some limitations. One idiosyncracy of resistance tubing is that the hardest bit of

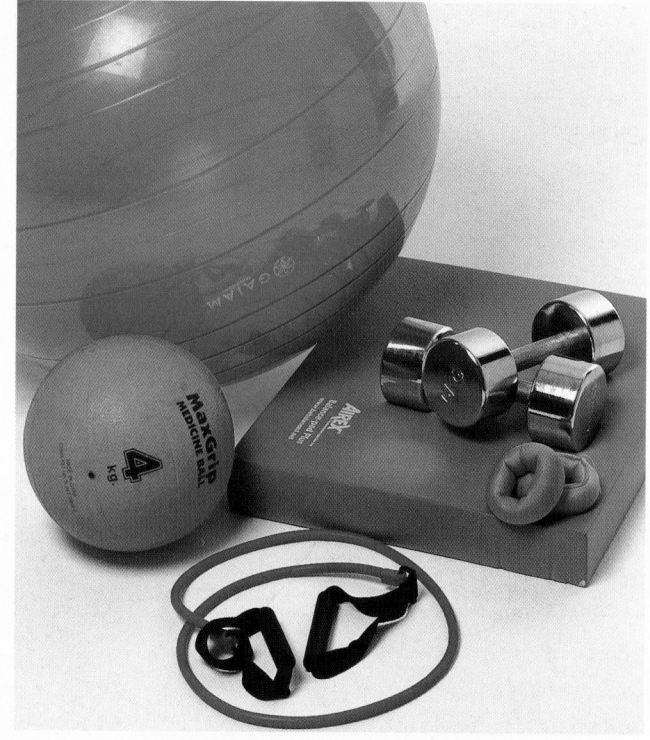

the move is at the end of the range while, if the same move is performed with a dumbbell, the toughest bit is in the middle of the range (often described as the 'sticking point'). It also isn't possible to perform every type of exercise with tubing providing the resistance, simply because you can't get the direction of the movement to work against gravity. A simple, cheap addition – a door attachment, which allows you to hook the tube over a closed door frame – expands your repertoire considerably. Exercises using a range of equipment (and no equipment at all!) are offered in the *Weights for Weight Loss* workouts.

Working order

As the ACSM guidelines stress, strength exercises need to be cleverly sequenced. In other words, don't work your muscles in a random order. Individual exercises are often described as either 'compound' or 'isolated'. A compound exercise is one that uses lots of muscle groups to execute the action (such as a squat) while an isolation exercise hones one specific muscle or muscle group (like a hamstring curl). In order to get the most out of every exercise, it's important to structure your workout so that you start with the multi-muscle exercises and then narrow in on the more isolated moves. For example, you'd do push-ups before you did triceps pushdowns.

Even if you are doing mainly isolated muscle group exercises, think big to start with and work down to the smaller muscles. Another good principle to factor in is to alternate a pushing move with a pulling one. For example, if you've just been pulling in a seated row, follow it with pushing in a chest press. Bearing in mind the importance of rest, you can also alternate upper and lower body exercise to allow the muscles to recover without squandering your time – but remember to still employ the other principles outlined above. A recent study from Brazil found that, whatever order muscles are worked in, the final exercises in a workout tend to be the poorest – so don't let those big, calorie-hungry muscles off the hook by saving them till last!

Many fitness practitioners recommend that the abdominal muscles are trained last, since

BODY TYPES AND WAYS TO WORK OUT

The advice relates to the somatypes described in Chapter 3. It is just a guideline and should be read within the context of the rest of the information in this chapter.

Mostly ectomorph

Use weights that you can lift only six to ten times and rest for at least two minutes between sets. Train at least three times a week, focusing on compound movements to recruit multiple muscle groups with each exercise. Train consistently, too, as any strength you gain will be harder to hold on to than for other body types. It's also wise to change your programme regularly.

Mostly mesomorph

Mesomorph guys are the kind who just walk into the gym and gain muscle. As a woman that is less likely to happen but you will probably find that your body responds very quickly and visibly to weight training. If you have the classic broad-shouldered, narrow-hipped mesomorph shape, focus on the lower body to prevent looking too muscular up top. Or, to get the physiological benefits of strength training and aid weight loss without gaining size, you could focus on muscular endurance as opposed to strength. By doing lots of repetitions, you get all the fibres involved through a process called 'motor unit rotation' (basically, the knackered ones move aside to let the fresher ones do the work). Aim for twenty to thirty repetitions, moving swiftly from exercise to exercise and set to set with little rest. Please note, though, that this does not constitute pure strength training.

Mostly endomorph

Endomorphs don't find it as easy as mesomorphs or as hard as ectomorphs to build muscle. Use moderate weights that you can lift nine to fifteen times at a swift training pace (allowing 1 minute rest between sets and exercises). Train two or three times a week, and focus on shaping the upper body to create balance to a pear-shaped lower half.

they are needed to provide stability and support throughout all the other exercises, although some argue that working them beforehand will 'switch' them on so that they function more efficiently during subsequent exercises. You don't have to do all your abdominal and core stability work at once, anyway. You could start with some simple exercises to warm up and switch on the core stabilisers and then complete your abs workout at the end of your strength training regime. The best advice is to experiment and find what works best for you. If you have a lower back problem, however, you should definitely do them at the end so that you have sufficient core strength to support the spine during your workout.

Talking technique

To get the longest leanest look your body will allow, you need to work through the full range of motion of each particular joint in your strength training. Continually working in a shortened range can actually cause the muscles to drop sarcomeres (the little 'blocks' that each muscle fibre is made up of) and become physically shorter and therefore bulkier. Working through a full range enhances strength development too. A study published in 2005 in the *Journal of Strength and Conditioning Research* compared the progress of women training through a partial range and a full range and found that the latter was far superior.

One of the best ways to ensure good technique is to watch yourself perform the exercise in the mirror. I know some people hate to do this but it really can be helpful in allowing you to see and feel correct posture simultaneously and store that information. Another important consideration is to know what muscle groups you are working, where they are and what the movement is that they are meant to be executing. I don't think I have ever been to the gym without spotting someone performing an exercise so badly that it is a complete waste of time.

Regardless of what muscle group you are working, I think it's a good idea to focus on your core muscles. Using your core will make executing the movement easier, it will protect your back from injury and make the core muscles themselves stronger and more efficient.

As for speed of movement, the usual advice is to ensure each repetition takes about two seconds on the lift and four on the lower and the whole exercise is performed with control. But this isn't always the ideal. If, for example, you were aiming to improve your explosiveness in a muscle group (say, to aid your leaping height in netball or your dive in squash) then the SAID principle comes into its own: the notion that you get what you train for. In that scenario, a more rapid motion would be better. There is no harm in experimenting with speed of movement, provided you maintain control and don't use momentum to swing the weights.

Breathing

Breathing is a Very Good Idea when you are strength training! Yet many people automatically hold their breath when they move a weight around. Try not to acquire this habit, even if you can't quite master the commonly recommended breathing rhythm of exhaling on the effort and inhaling on the release. The important thing is to get oxygen into your lungs and get carbon dioxide out. And bear in mind, you may well find lifting weights easier if you can learn to exhale on the toughest bit of the movement.

Some experienced weight lifters and bodybuilders use a technique called the Valsalva Manoeuvre when lifting exceptionally heavy weights. This technique enables the weightlifter to increase the pressure within the abdominal and chest cavity by forcibly breathing out while keeping the throat closed to trap and pressurise air in the lungs (sorry to be graphic but like when you're trying to have a poo when you are a kid). This manoeuvre should most definitely be avoided in weight training as it sends blood pressure soaring, can cause dizziness or fainting and is positively dangerous for those with existing high blood pressure or cardiovascular disease.

Putting a routine together

So let's start to put the framework for your weight-training regime in place. There are six main considerations:

- How much am I going to lift?

- How many reps and sets will I perform?

- How much rest will I take?

STRONG WORDS

WHEN IS ONE-SET TRAINING WORTHWHILE?

If you are a total beginner, it seems that one set will suffice to make significant strength gains. A study from Appalachian State University found that almost any overload at all could instigate change in subjects who were totally inexperienced at strength training. In addition, one-set training has been shown to be sufficient to offset the loss in muscle tissue associated with losing weight. Research published in the journal *Medicine & Science in Sports & Exercise* found that adding one-set strength training to aerobic exercise and diet attenuated muscle loss while still allowing fat loss to take place. And finally, if your main goal is to develop your aerobic fitness (say, for example, you are training for a half marathon or a charity bike ride), one set may be enough to create a base of muscular strength and more robust connective tissues. It is worth mentioning that one-set groups in research studies do get stronger just not as strong as the multiple-set groups. For example, in one study they gained 6% in thigh strength compared to 15% for the multiple-set group.

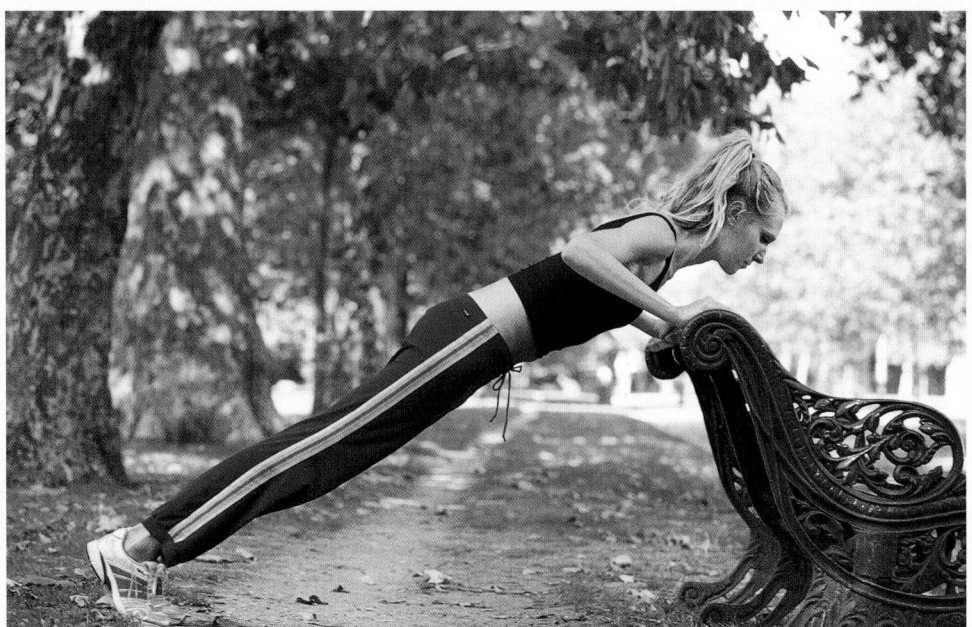

- How often will I train?

- What exercises will I do?

- How will I progress?

Before giving the advice that follows, I think it's worth pointing out that there does have to be a certain amount of experimentation in this. Not everyone will get the same physiological response to a set protocol. If you aren't seeing results, look at changing what you are doing to see if that works better. But only change one thing at a time and stick with it for three to four weeks – change everything at once and you won't know what worked… or didn't.

Load, reps, sets and rest explained

The issue of how much weight to lift, how many times to lift it and how much rest to take are all interrelated. Lifting the heaviest load you can manage, for example, will probably mean lifting it just three to four times and taking lots of rest, while a weight that is only half of what you could ultimately shift could be lifted more times and wouldn't necessitate so much rest. Strength specialists use percentages of what's called the 'One Repetition Maximum' (1RM) to define how heavy the load should be to gain a particular result. The 1RM is the heaviest weight you could lift once (theoretically, at least, as it's not always easy to measure). So 80% of 1RM is a weight that equals 80% of the weight you could lift only once.

Throughout this book I shall talk about 'sets' and 'reps' to refer to the number of times you do an exercise. A rep or repetition simply means lifting and lowering a weight once. A set is a pre-determined number of reps which you might do just once or repeat a number of times with a rest between each set.

Doing the numbers

Studies have found that working at 80+% of the maximum load is best for strength and power, while general muscular hypertrophy (growth) involves working at 60–80% of IRM, but with a greater overall volume of reps and sets. Working below 60% of 1RM has been shown not to increase strength at all, although it will build muscular endurance.

But how does that relate to actual numbers of repetitions – and numbers of sets? (This is useful to know as it removes the necessity of having to test out your IRM in every exercise.) Research suggests that six or fewer reps provide the most strength and power gains, while six to twelve reps produce strength and size gain. In a study from Goethe University, subjects did three sets of just six to nine repetitions but at an effort level at which they couldn't actually perform another repetition, and gained significant strength. Beyond 20 repetitions, you are looking at predominantly endurance gains. Remember, though, that muscles can't count. So don't do a specific number just because you said you would. If your technique has gone AWOL before you've finished the planned set, then stop.

Is one set enough?

Not so long ago the virtues of 'single set' training were widely extolled but recently the tide has turned and generally – as concluded by a largescale study at the University of Queensland – multiple sets are a better bet. A study in the *Journal of Strength and Conditioning Research* from Appalachian State University found that, in untrained women, multiple sets yielded greater strength gains and other positive adaptations than single-set training. In the Goethe University study women with basic weight training experience gained more strength after a three-set programme compared to a one-set programme. What's more all the subjects in the study performed the same number of repetitions and the same exercises, making comparisons between one and three sets clear and simple.

STRONG WORDS

HOW LONG WILL IT TAKE TO SEE RESULTS?

In previously untrained people, eight to twelve weeks is needed to see changes in actual fibre size. Initial improvement in strength is largely attributed to better nerve-muscle communication but it's also due to more efficient help from 'synergist' muscles (those that assist the movement) and increased inhibition of opposing or 'antagonist' muscles – so that they don't impede the working muscle's contraction.

As far as fat loss – and increased muscle gain – is concerned, the volume of training you do plays a part in maximising calorie expenditure, so the more 'work' you do the better. One of the key factors in improving strength is that the muscle needs to be fatigued in order to trigger the physiological mechanisms that cause size and strength gains. Fatigue is much greater in multiple set protocols. Secondly, research shows that we reach maximum power in the second or third set of an exercise, not the first. Traditionally, multiple sets means three but there's no reason to stop there – four or five sets may be beneficial, depending on your personal goals and needs.

And the rest

In general, the higher the percentage of your 1RM you are working at, the longer the rest period between sets should be. Insufficient rest means optimal effort cannot be put into the next set, while too much rest deactivates the muscle. In the Goethe University study, the rest interval between sets was two minutes. The researchers suggest that the protocol they used may have improved strength because the two-minute rest meant that the second and third sets took place under a certain amount of pre-fatigue, triggering motor unit rotation, whereby the tired muscle calls in more motor units to help with the workload, as those already used in the first set are whacked.

The inclusion of more motor units increases the overall stress on the muscle and also, due to the activation of a larger number of nerves,

improves neuromuscular efficiency, which has a bearing on strength. If you don't want to waste time hanging around between exercises, you can, of course, use your rest time to work on a completely different muscle group, to allow the worked one to recover.

The general principle to follow is that the higher the number of reps you are doing, the more you are focusing on endurance and, therefore, the shorter the rest period should be – perhaps 45–60 seconds. The fewer reps you are doing the heavier the weight and the more important it is to make a full recovery for the next set. You may therefore be looking at as much as three to four minutes' rest between sets. If you are working in the middle range – say, six to ten reps – to gain both strength and some firmness and growth – I recommend that you allow two minutes' rest between sets.

What's the frequency?

So you've decided on reps and sets – you know what weight you are going to lift. How many times a week are you going to get with the programme? As we've seen, the ACSM recommends two to three times per week for beginners and intermediates – and up to five days per week for advanced exercisers. A study from the University of Alabama looked at the relative strength gains of a group of subjects who worked either one day a week, performing three sets to failure, or three days a week, with one set to failure. On upper and lower body strength the three-day a week group achieved greater gains in strength and lean body mass implying that, although the total exercise volume stayed the same, the more frequent training was more successful. But the differences were not that great (the one-day a weekers gained 62% of the strength that the three-day a weekers did) and the researchers also found that the more experienced a subject is in strength training, the more the emphasis needs to be placed on volume.

A baseline frequency of two sessions a week seems to allow existing gains to be maintained. What is perhaps most surprising about the results of this study, though, is the fact that even *one* day a week of training made such a significant difference to strength gains. Even if you can't commit to three or more sessions, the evidence shows that strength training is far from a waste of time.

More isn't necessarily better

Incidentally, if you *do* choose to train more frequently, it is possible to have too much of a good thing. The body needs 48 hours to recover and adapt to the stress of the training you have placed upon it. So do not strength train the same muscle group on consecutive days. If you do, then you take away the 'window of opportunity' that your body has to make the necessary repairs and changes in order to cope with that same workload next time round. There is no need to train any muscle group more than three times a week. You can still train daily, but ensure that you alternate between different muscle groups to allow each one to come to the next training session refreshed.

This is what is known as a 'split routine' – where you turn up to train, say, the shoulders, chest and triceps on Mondays and the legs, back and biceps on Tuesdays. Whether you adopt a split routine or not is largely determined by how much time you want to spend in the gym. It's fine to train the whole body in one session, each time you work out, if you prefer to do so.

Anything goes!

Before we leave the *how much, how often, how hard?* question behind, what is perhaps most crucial to remember is that almost *anything* works, at least initially. And, interestingly, it is as you become a more experienced strength trainer that variety – in intensity, volume of training, speed of movement and exercise choice – becomes even more important in continuing to reap benefits.

Exercise choice and making progress

So let's now think about choosing the right exercises to perform. Since the goal is to increase lean muscle mass, calorie expenditure and, hopefully, maximise metabolic rate and afterburn – we want to emphasise those compound or multi-muscle group exercises. After all, the more muscles that need to get involved, the harder we are working and the more energy we are expending. We also, presumably, don't want to spend seven hours a week working out with weights, so using compound exercises is more time-efficient. But there are always specific muscle groups that we want to tone up so, in addition to the twelve main moves in the *Weights for Weight Loss* workouts, there are targeted toning segments that focus on tightening and shaping some of the classic problem areas. These also offer you some variety as you progress – as you can swap exercises from the main workout for targeted toning moves – or add in a few of the latter for a more challenging and longer session.

In order to make continued successful progress, it's a good idea to use the periodization strategy described in the ACSM guidelines (see page 36). In other words, you apply progressive overload logically, rather than randomly.

The first step in a periodized programme is to lay the foundations on which you intend to build. That is why I recommend you embark on your strength training journey with the 'Foundation Workout'. Follow it for two to six weeks, depending on your existing fitness level, before moving on to the *Weights for Weight Loss* workouts. You'll find out more about how to progress beyond the twelve-week programmes later on.

Warming up

Regardless of the number of reps and sets you plan to do, you should always start your weights workout with a warm-up. It doesn't need to take long – and the benefits you'll reap make it well worth it – your muscles will work more efficiently when they are warmer, be less prone to injury, according to a study published in the *American Journal of Sports Medicine*, and quicker to recover.

The first part of the warm-up aims simply to increase heart rate and body temperature – it's the 'get things moving' phase… If you are in the gym, a few minutes walking on the treadmill, rowing, stepping or cycling will do the trick. Otherwise, brisk marching on the spot, with some side steps and knee bends, is fine.

Then, in the second phase, mobilise (circle, bend, extend) your major joints by taking them gently through their full range. Start with the neck, then the shoulders, trunk, hips, knees and ankles. Finish by gently mobilising the back.

Don't stretch your muscles before your weights workout. There is evidence that stretching prior to exercise actually reduces force output for up to an hour. But prior to each exercise you perform, it's a good idea to 'rehearse' the exercise with no weight at all or a very light weight, just to gear up the neuromuscular pattern involved.

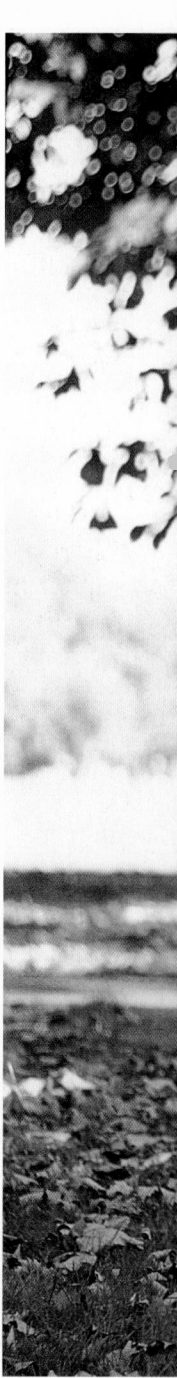

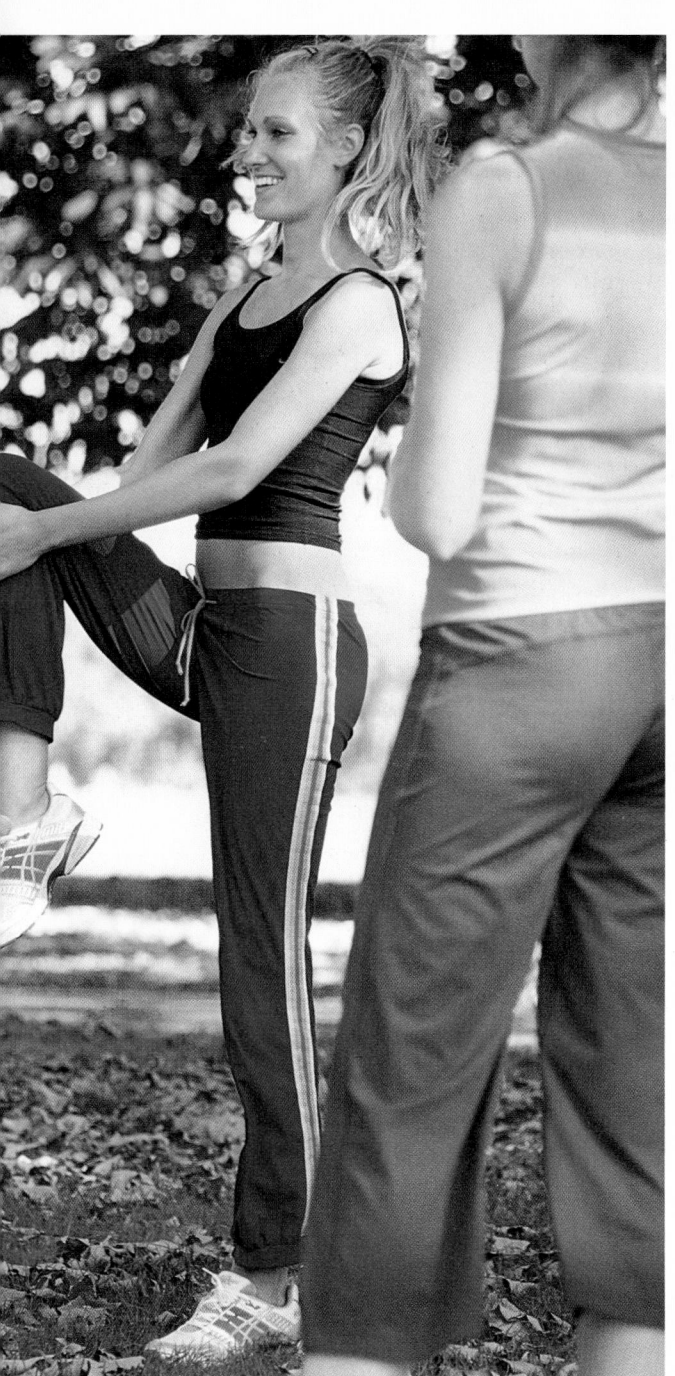

Cooling down

Strength training differs from aerobic exercise in that heart rate doesn't remain elevated for a prolonged period – it rises and falls because you intersperse work with rest. So a cool down to gradually take the body back to a 'resting state' isn't really necessary. However, it *is* important to stretch. At the very least, this helps restore muscles to their natural resting length following a period of intense activity. And if you do it correctly, and often enough, it will also help you improve your range of motion and increase suppleness.

Stretching know-how

Do you find that despite doing your stretching, your flexibility never seems to get any better? If so, it may be that you aren't following the golden rules, in terms of how far to stretch, how long to hold it and what technique to employ. Recently revised American College of Sports Medicine guidelines suggest 15–30 second holds are needed and that each stretch should be repeated two to four times. (In other words, those slap-dash four-second stretches that we are all occasionally guilty of won't contribute to flexibility!) Flexibility also varies from joint to joint – you may have fantastic range of motion in your neck and shoulders, for example, while your hamstrings are as tight as guitar strings. Or you may be more flexible on your right side than your left. Whatever the case, work harder on the less flexible muscles and stiffer joints otherwise you'll simply maintain your imbalances.

Your muscles should always be warm when they are to be stretched, so if you are not slightly warm, breathless and sweating, then spend a few moments raising your heart rate and body temperature again with some gentle aerobic exercise. Stretch until you feel tension and a slight 'irritation' in the muscle but not pain. As the muscle relaxes, you can move slightly deeper into the stretch and hold again. Use your breath to help you develop the stretch: inhale as you ease off, and exhale as you move deeper into the stretch. Do not bounce in and out of your 'end' position, however.

Finally, do it after *every* session. Not just once in a blue moon... The ACSM guidelines recommend stretching a minimum of two to three days a week, with five to seven days being the ideal.

The post-strength training stretch

The following routine addresses all the muscles you'll be working on in the Foundation and *Weights for Weight Loss* workouts. Hold each position for 15–30 seconds (per side, if appropriate) and perform each stretch twice. Add 1–2 repetitions on the tight side if there is a noticeable discrepancy between left and right.

① HAMSTRINGS

Stand face on to a support between knee and hip height. Extend one leg and place it on the support, with the foot relaxed. Your supporting leg should be perpendicular to the floor. Now hinge forward from the hips (keep the arch in your lower back), with the pelvis level and the knee of the extended leg straight. Feel the stretch along the back of the supported thigh. To emphasise the outer hamstring, bring the leg slightly across the midline of your body and rotate the hip joint slightly inwards. To emphasise the hamstrings closest to the middle of the body, turn out at the hip joint and take the leg slightly away from the midline of the body. Finally, bend the knee slightly to emphasise the belly of the muscle. You don't need to pull your toes back towards you – the only reason this intensifies the stretch is because it stretches the sciatic nerve, too.

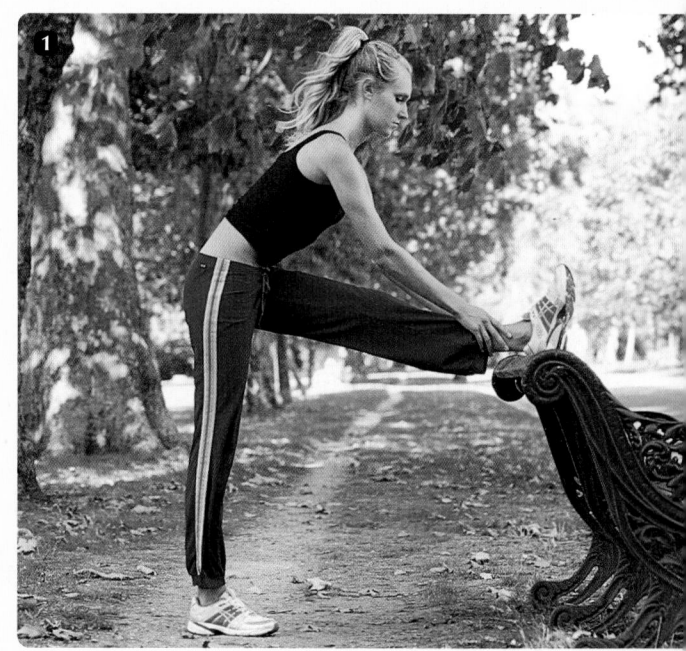

[2] UPPER AND LOWER CALVES, FEET AND ANKLES

Stand facing a support, with feet a stride length apart, back leg straight and front leg bent. Press the back heel into the floor so that you experience a stretch in the middle of the calf muscle. Turn your toes slightly inwards to focus on the outer side of the calf. Hold. Now bring the back leg forwards a little, bend the knee and flex the hips, so that the stretch moves down to the lower part of the calf and Achilles tendon. Finally, with both legs still bent, place the toes of the front foot up against the support to stretch the muscles along the sole of the foot.

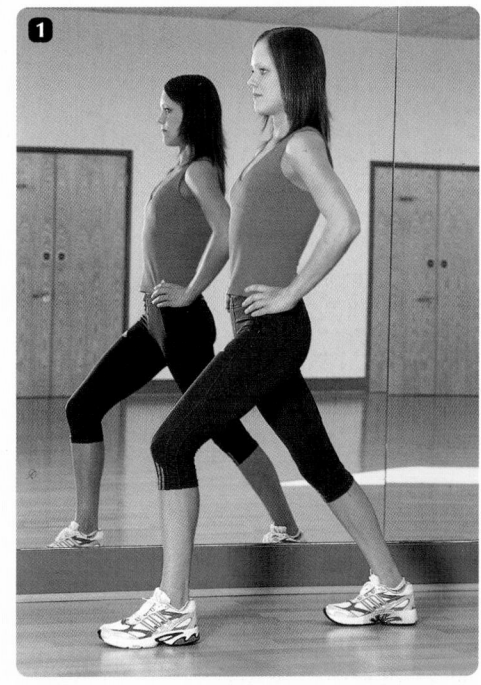

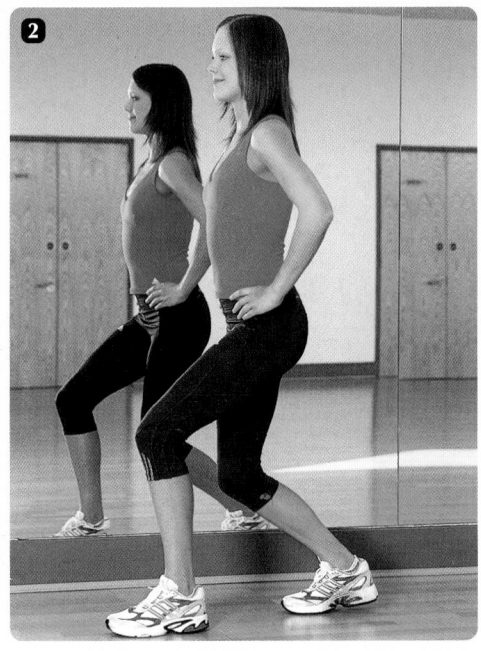

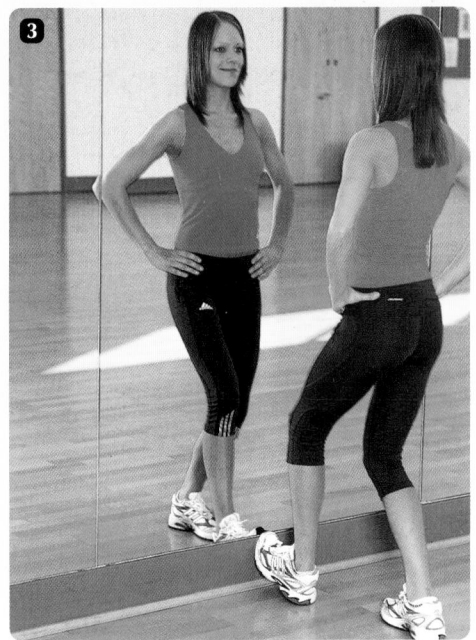

③ QUADS

Stand tall with feet parallel. Lift your right foot, taking your right hand behind you to grab it and bring it towards the bottom. Bring the pelvis into a neutral position and gently press the foot into your hand, keeping the knees close together. It doesn't matter if your stretching thigh is in front of the supporting one, as long as you feel a stretch.

④ INNER THIGHS

Sit on the floor with your knees drawn into your chest and feet flat on the floor. Drop the knees out to the sides and use your elbows to gently press the legs open. Don't round the back, sit up tall. If necessary, sit on the edge of a rolled-up towel to prevent your back rounding. Hold, then extend the legs out to the sides and hinge forward from the hips.

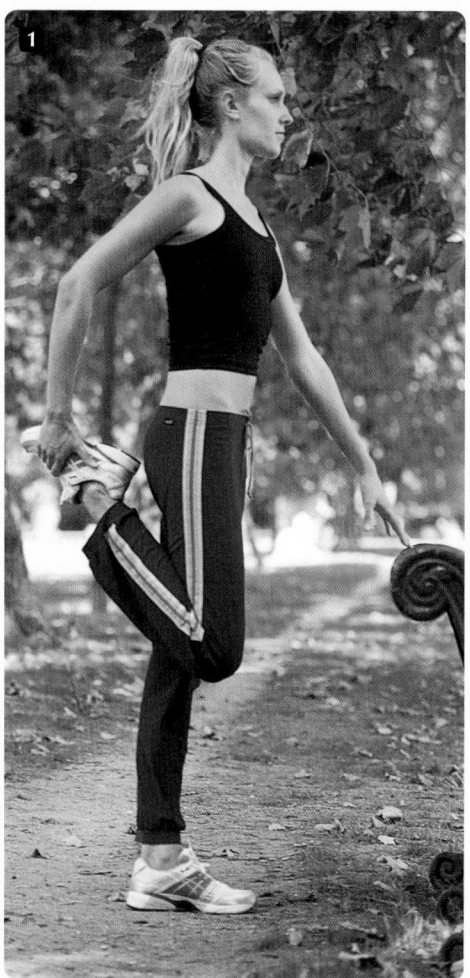

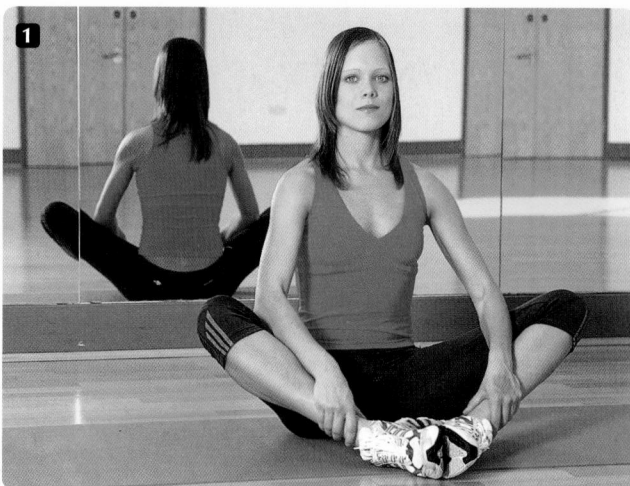

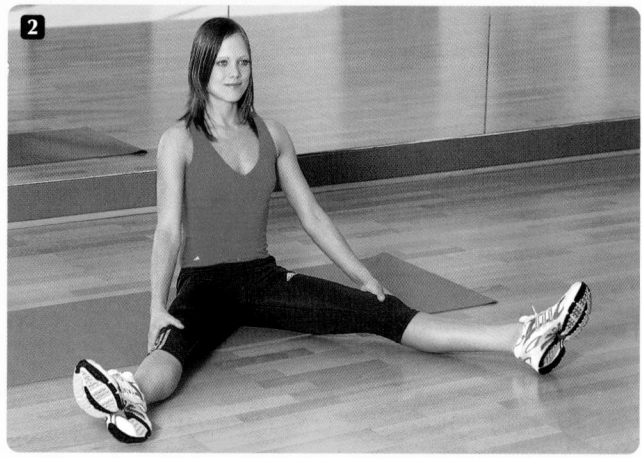

5 HIPS/GLUTES

Sit against a wall with your legs outstretched. Cross your left foot over your right thigh and put the foot flat on the floor. Now place your right arm around the left knee and gently pull it around towards the right shoulder (rather than hugging directly to chest), sitting up tall.

6 HIP ROTATORS

Lie face up on the floor and bring one knee into your chest, leaving the other leg flat on the floor. Now grasp the ankle of the bent leg and holding the knee in place with your other hand (like a hinge), gently pull the ankle towards you until you feel a deep stretch in the hip area of the lifted leg.

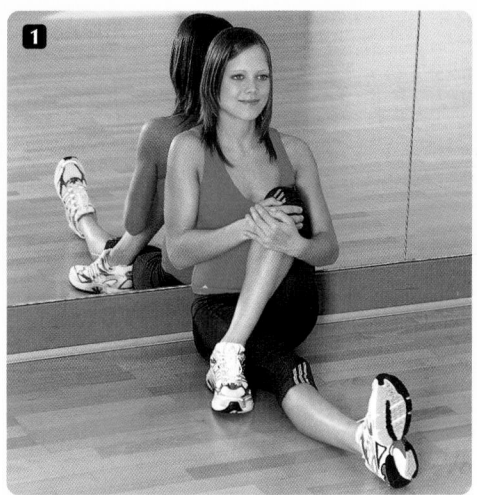

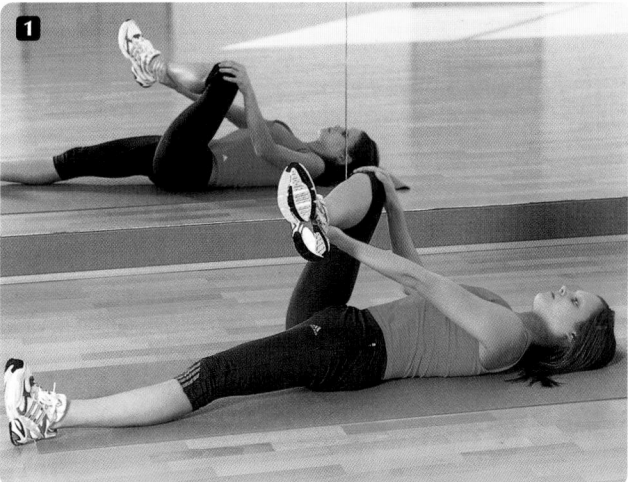

7 SIDE STRETCH (OBLIQUES, QUADRATUS LUMBORUM)

Stand with your feet below the hipbones and arms above your head, hands interlinked. Drop the torso directly to the right side (as if you were sandwiched between two plates of glass), keeping the core engaged and the arms stretching upwards. Feel a stretch along the left side. Pause, then return to the start position and sink down to the left side.

8 CHEST (PECTORALIS MAJOR)

Stand with your feet below the hipbones, with your hands interlinked behind you, palms facing each other. Keeping the shoulders back and down, draw the arms away from you, until you feel a stretch along the front of the chest. If you don't feel a stretch through this action, do the chest stretch on page 61…

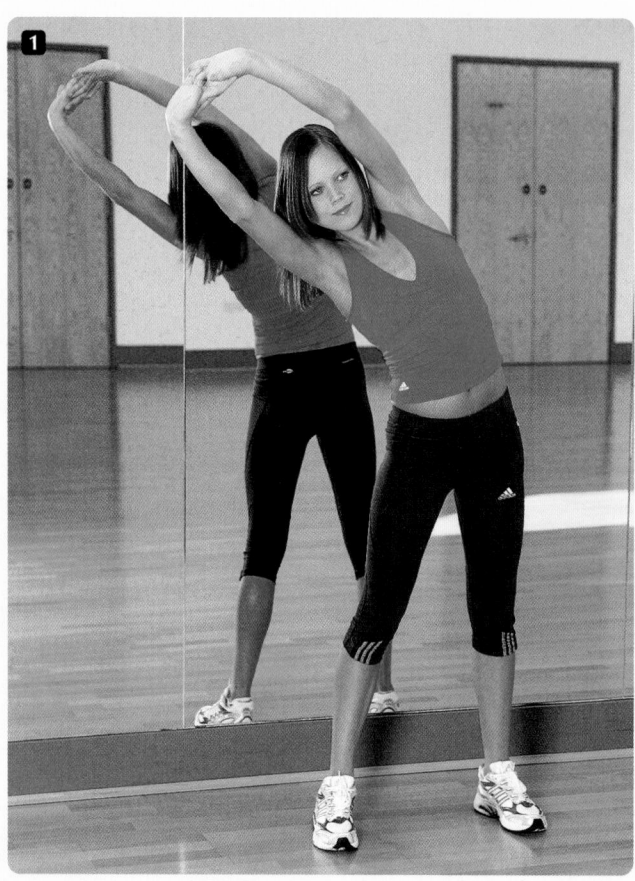

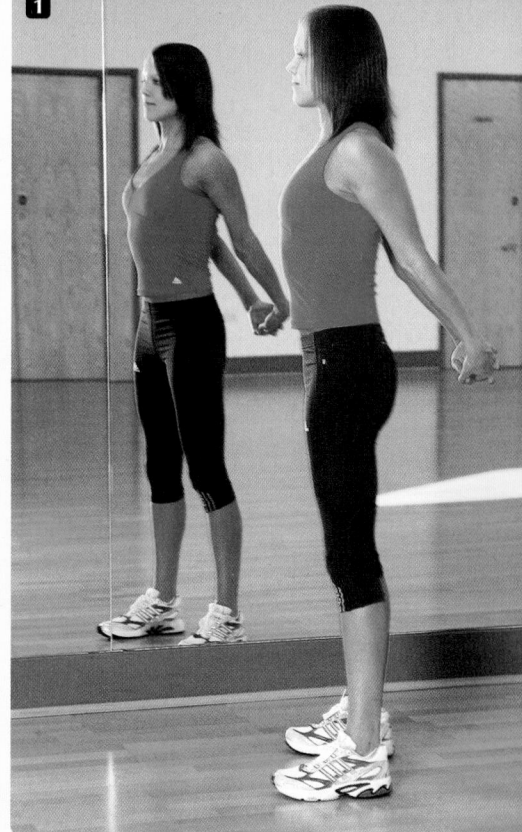

9 UPPER BACK (LATISSIMUS DORSI, RHOMBOIDS, TRAPEZIUS)

Stand with your feet below the hipbones and knees bent – clasp your hands together in front of the body, palms facing you, and push the arms away from you, feeling a stretch along the back of the shoulders and upper back. Try to make your upper back into a 'C' shape as if you were resisting being pulled forward by your hands and your knees.

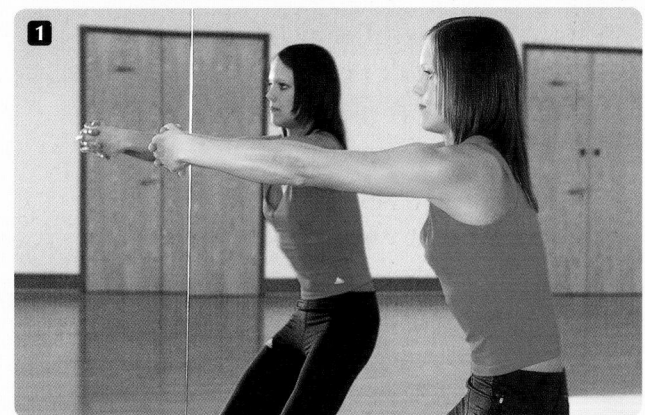

10 BACK OF UPPER ARM (TRICEPS)

Raise your right arm overhead and allow it to drop down behind your back. Now take the left hand up to the right elbow and gently push the arm back until you feel a stretch along the back of the right arm. Swap sides.

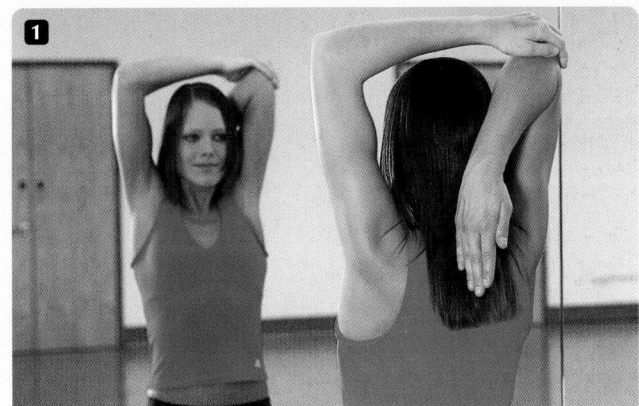

11 FRONT OF UPPER ARM (BICEPS)

Stand side on to a wall in a split stance with the leg closest to the wall in front of the other. Place your right hand against the wall at shoulder height, with the fingers pointing backwards. Now, keeping the hand pressed firmly against the wall, lean forwards until you feel a stretch along the front of the arm from shoulder to wrist. Swap sides.

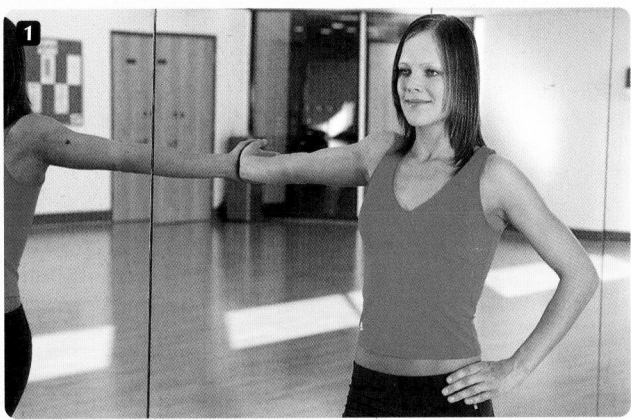

12 SHOULDERS (DELTOIDS)

Bring your left arm across the body, just below shoulder height, and use your right hand (holding above the left elbow) to gently press the arm across the chest. Don't hunch the shoulder up. Swap sides.

13 NECK (STERNOCLEIDOMASTOID, SCALENES, SPLENIUS)

Stand tall and take your head directly to the right side, not allowing it to tilt upwards or downwards. Then rotate the head to the left and drop it forwards. Change sides.

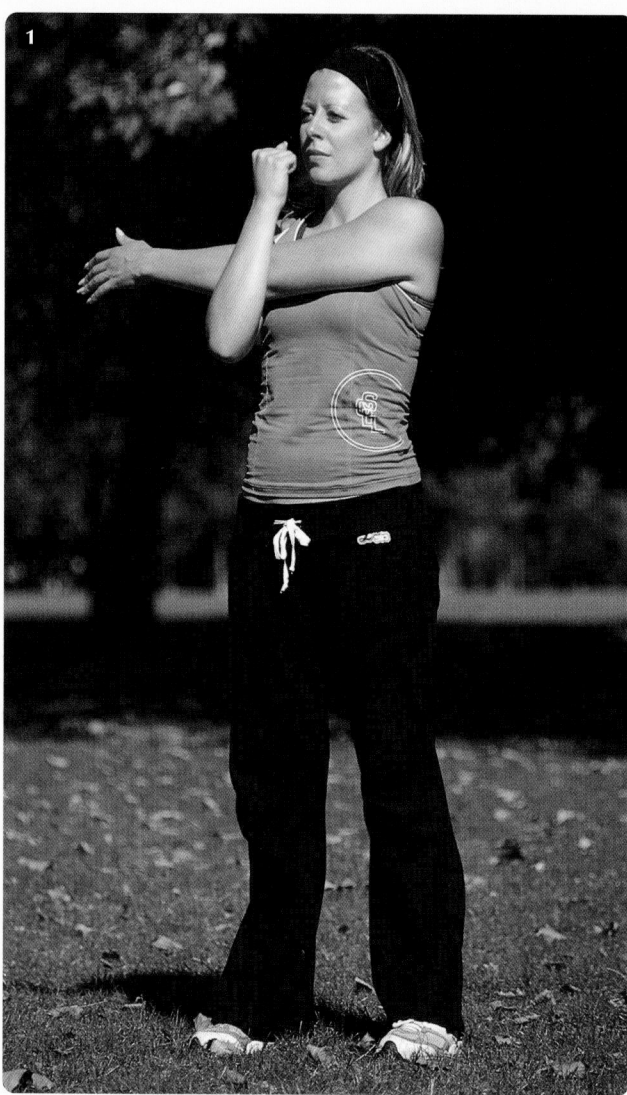

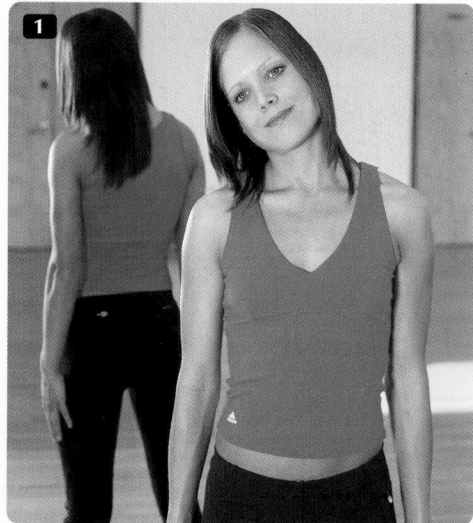

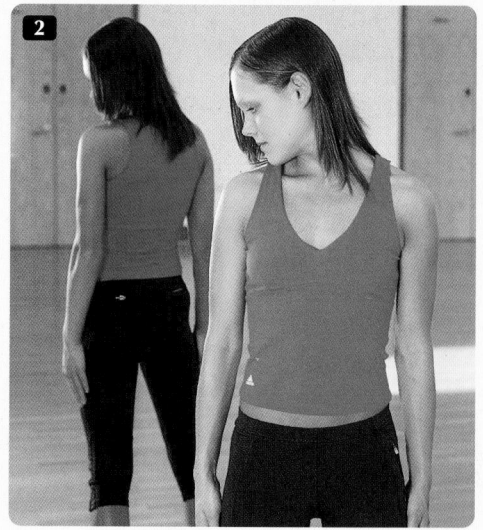

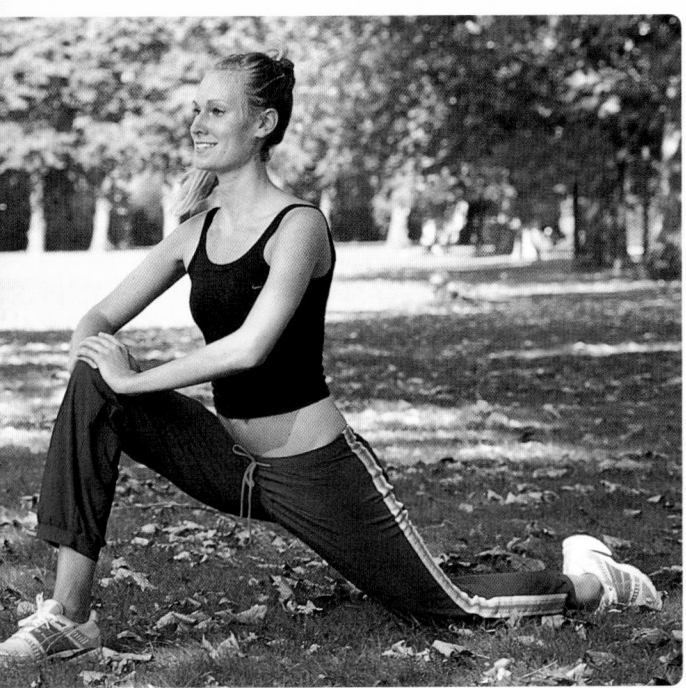

14 HIP FLEXORS (ILIOPSOAS)

From a lunge position, with the right foot forward, take your left knee to the floor with the lower leg extended behind it (the knee well behind the hip) and the toes facing down. Tighten the tummy muscles and extend forwards from the hips, until your left knee is at 90 degrees. You should feel a stretch along the front of the hip joint and thigh.

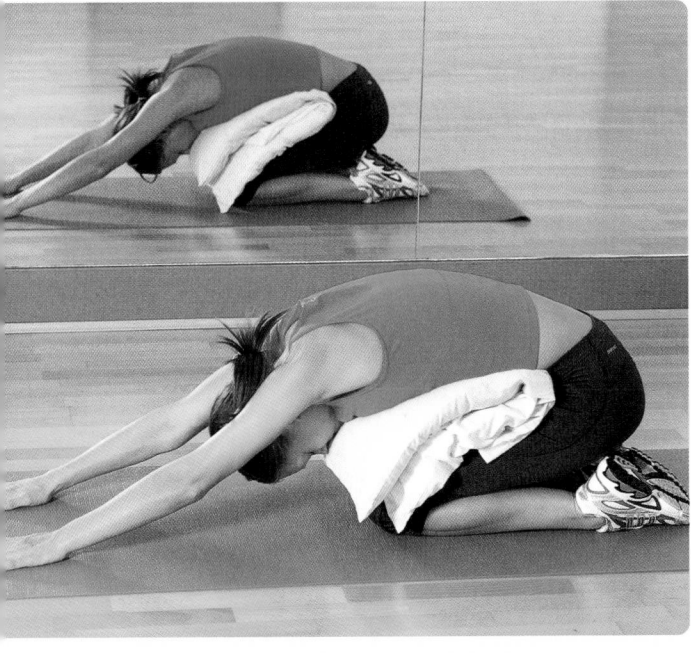

15 LOWER BACK AND ERECTOR SPINAE MUSCLES

Kneel on the floor with a couple of cushions or a pillow on your lap. Bend the torso forwards, walking your hands out in front of you and taking your buttocks back to rest on your heels. Let the cushions support the front of the body so that the spine can really flex and stretch out.

WEIGHTS FOR WEIGHT LOSS WORKOUT

Time to put words into action and start getting stronger, firmer and slimmer.

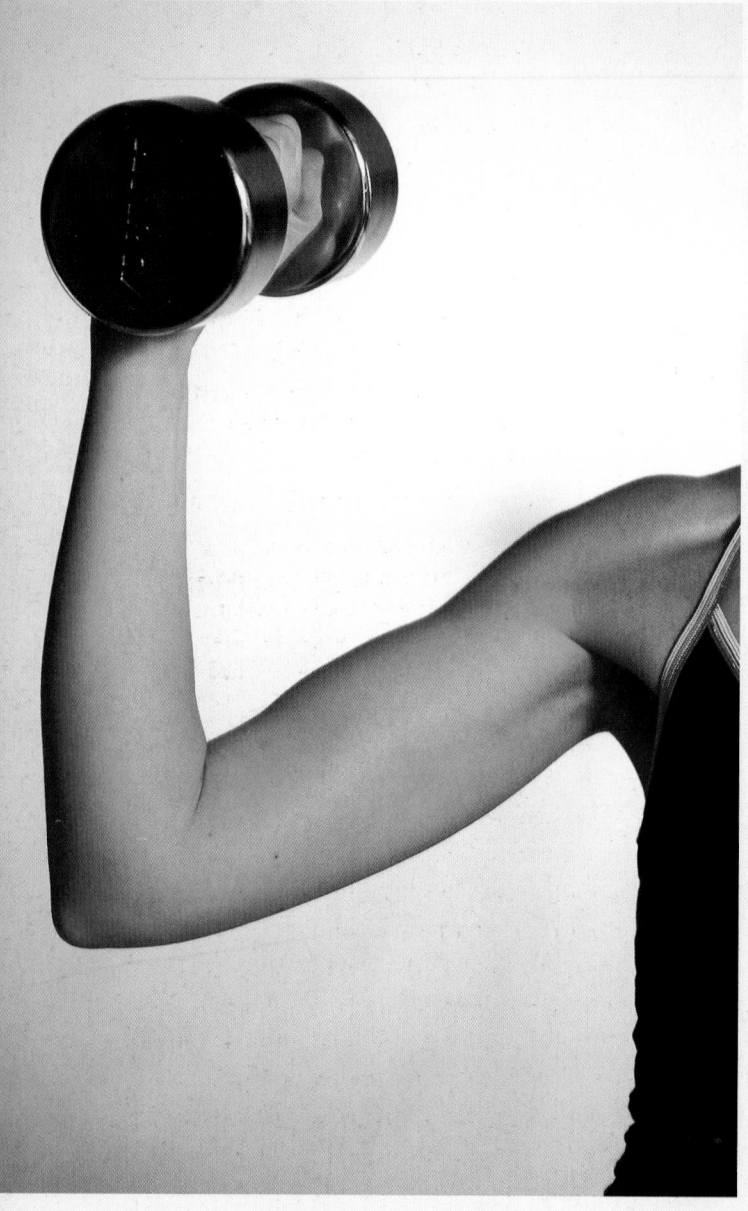

This section of the book is where we put the principles of strength training into practice – you'll find a choice of workouts to suit your needs and preferences and to offer variety but they all have one thing in common: results! In order to track your progress, you are going to need some idea of your starting point. Taking a few simple measurements will help you gauge your progress over the next few weeks and months. But *please* bear in mind, not all the benefits you reap from weight training will be immediately noticeable or measurable.

Measurements to take

Make a note of your results, as well as the date you took the measurements…

Weight

It's fine to weigh yourself, but remember that muscle weighs more than fat so even as you lose body fat, you may not end up lighter on the scales.

Body fat percentage

This is optional as you will need to get it measured professionally at a gym, health centre or perhaps at your doctor's. Bear in mind that the two most commonly used measurements, skinfold girths and bioelectrical impedance assessment (BIA – where a mild elecrical current is sent through the body) both have wide margins of error. To minimise this, get the same person to take skinfolds each time you get measured and get your BIA reading done when you are well hydrated and at the same stage of your menstrual cycle each month.

Girths

WAIST – Measure around the narrowest part of your midriff at the end of a natural exhalation.

NAVEL – Measure around the midriff directly over the bellybutton.

HIPS – Measure across the top of the buttock cheeks.

THIGHS – Measure 20cm up from the top of your kneecap and take a circumference measurement of your thigh.

UPPER ARM – Measure 10cm up from your elbow crease and take a circumference measurement.

Building a firm foundation

The Foundation Workout is the starting point for all newcomers to strength training – and those who haven't exercised for a while. It's all about working from the inside out, serving as a stepping stone to the more challenging workouts that follow. Don't be disheartened that little or no weight is used in the exercises – it is because they are working the 'tonic' muscles of the body, whose role it is to support, stabilise and protect the joints when the larger, more dynamic (phasic) muscles are

DOING THE FOUNDATION WORKOUT

- Warm up first.
- Wear something loose and comfortable.
- Breathe freely throughout.
- Use an exercise mat ideally or at least a thick towel or rug to support the spine.
- You will need a resistance tube or band, a step or stair, a wall and a cushion or rolled-up towel.
- Build up gradually to the number of reps and sets suggested if you can't do it straight away.
- Do the exercises in the order shown.
- Rest for 30 seconds between sets EXCEPT for on the stretches, in which there is no need to take a rest. On some moves you can use the rest time to work the other side of the body so that you don't waste time.

called into play. The goal is to improve their responsiveness and muscular endurance rather than their brute strength.

At the very least, this workout will improve your posture, enable you to move more gracefully, help ease muscular tension or joint pain and help redress imbalances. And best of all, it will ensure you get the best possible results from your strength training programme. Before you start, recap on the three steps to better body awareness on page 29.

The foundation workout

The rotator cuff muscles

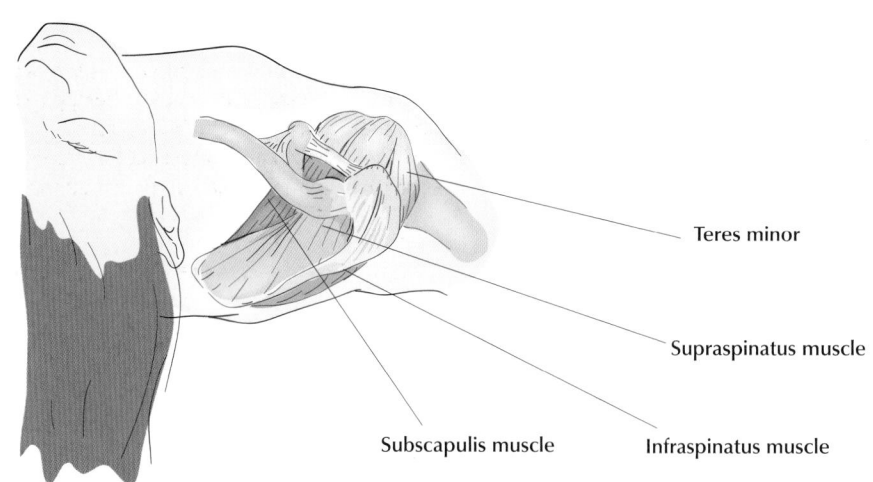

Teres minor

Supraspinatus muscle

Subscapulis muscle

Infraspinatus muscle

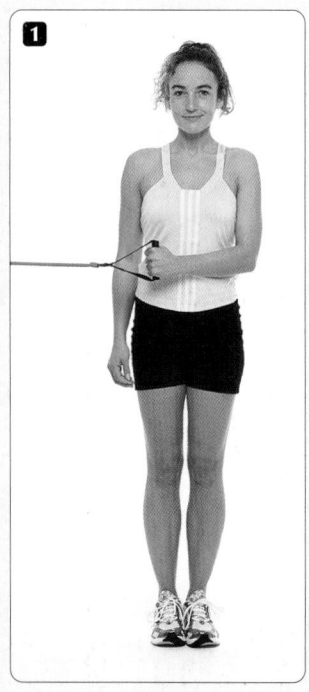

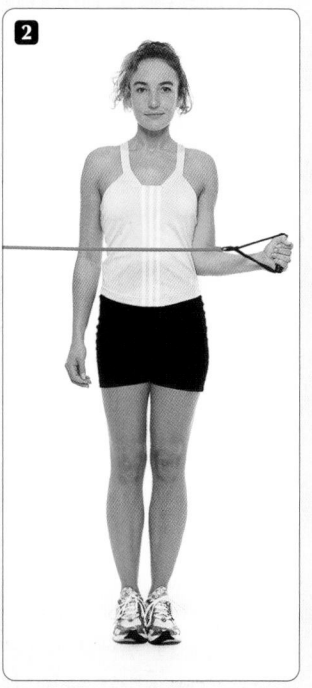

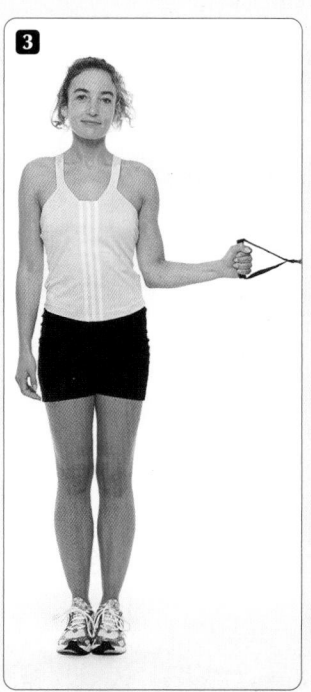

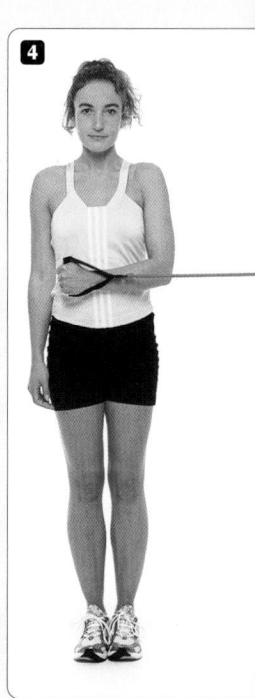

1 ARM HINGE

What's the point?

The rotator cuff is a group of small postural muscles that serve to stabilise the shoulder joint, like guy ropes around a tent. Strengthening them will reduce the overpowering of the larger muscles, help protect your shoulder joints when you lift weights and improve your shoulder position, preventing impingement and contributing to better posture.

How to do it:

1 Take a resistance band and hook it around a closed door handle, or something else sturdy of a similar height. Take a few steps away so that the band has some tension and position your arm so that the upper arm is close to your side and the forearm at a right angle across your body.

2 Now, 'set' your shoulder blades and open the chest. Pulling against the resistance, 'hinge' the arm open to the side, keeping the upper arm close to the torso. Pause then return to the start position and repeat until you complete the set.

3 Now turn around so that the resistance is coming from the other way (i.e. your arm is in the 'open' position at the start…

4 …and the resistance comes when you bring it across the body). Again, ensure that you 'set' your shoulder blades – and align your upper back and shoulders before you start. Use a maximum pain-free range of motion.

How many?

Do 2–4 sets of each position – 8–10 reps per set on each side.

2 HEAD AGAINST A BRICK WALL

What's the point?

To strengthen the 'thoracic extensors', the muscles that maintain the natural curve of the upper spine, and counteract 'protracted head syndrome', an unhappy combination of neck flexion, head extension, a concave chest and rounded shoulders!

How to do it:

1 Stand a few centimetres from a solid wall and rest your back, shoulders and head against it.

2 Now push off, so that only the back of your head is in touch with the wall but still in line with your spine. You may feel as if you have created a double chin, but that's OK! Keep your shoulders relaxed and the core engaged.

How many?

Hold for 8 seconds and repeat 5 times.

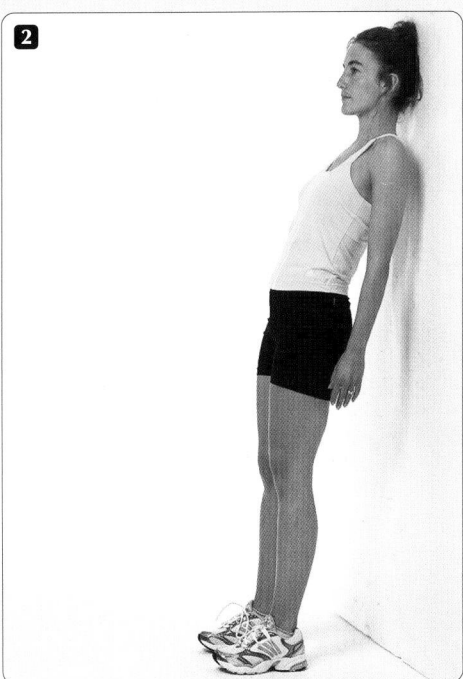

3 CALF DROP AND RAISE

What's the point?
To improve lower leg muscle balance and strengthen calf muscles during the lowering phase of movement, where they tend to be weak.

How to do it:
1 Stand on the edge of a step or stair with your feet half on and half off – and holding on to something for balance.

2 Rise swiftly and fully up on to the toes…

3 …then lower yourself down moderately slowly, allowing the heels to drop as far below the level of the stair as they can. This part of the exercise is really important, so go to the end of your natural range of movement. Then rise explosively upwards again and repeat the slower descent.

How many?
Do 3 sets of 15 reps.

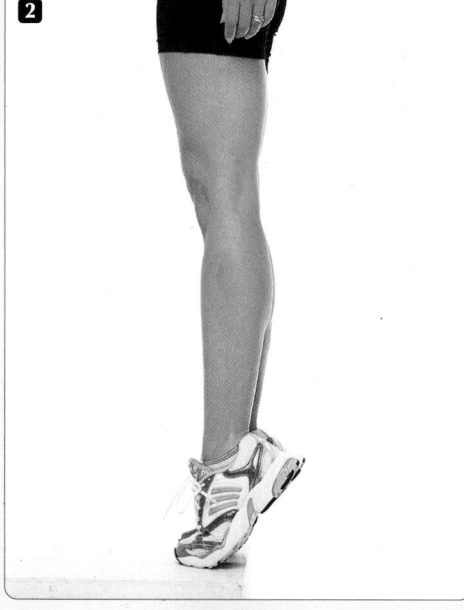

TIP: Why not do your chest stretches between sets of the calf drop and raise to save waiting around?

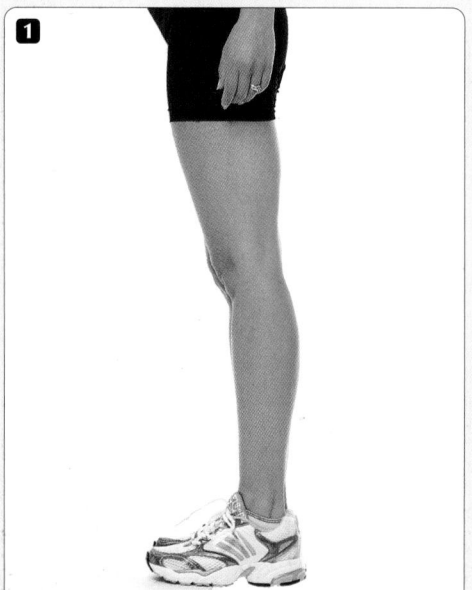

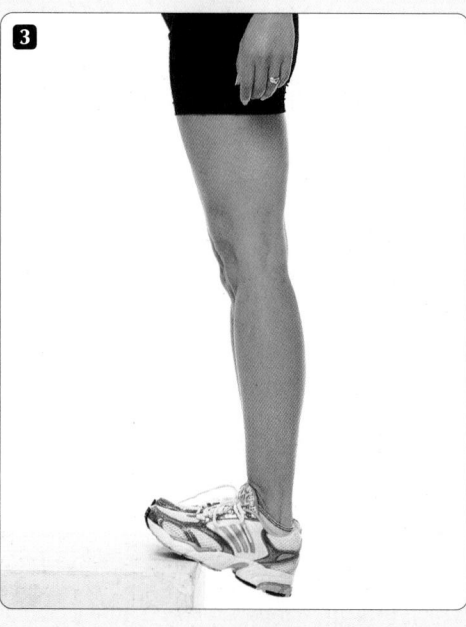

4 CHEST STRETCH

What's the point?
To stretch the shoulder protractor muscles (pec minor, serratus anterior), which pull the shoulders forward and down, giving a hunched posture. It's essential to stretch these before strengthening the opposing muscle group.

How to do it:
1 Stand in an open doorway and take one arm to the doorframe, with the upper arm slightly higher than horizontal to the frame. Now gently lean forward to 'open' the front of the shoulder and chest. You should feel a stretch right into the armpit area. Breathe normally and hold for 30 seconds. Swap sides.

How many?
2–4 on each side.

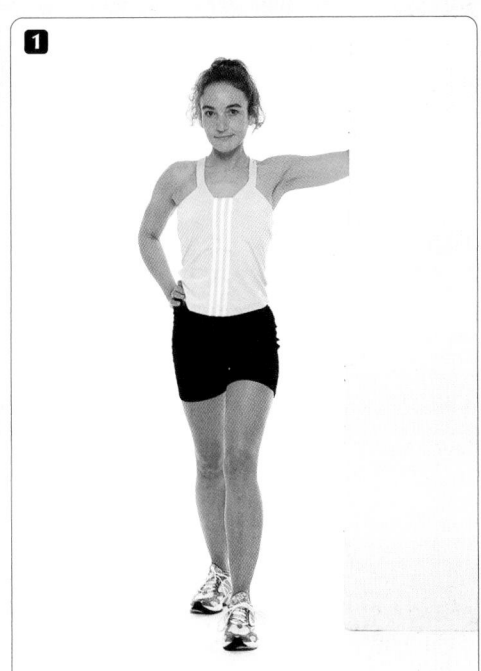

5 HIP AND THIGH STRETCH

What's the point?
The front of the hip is a classically tight area in women, particularly in those who spend a lot of time sitting down and post-pregnancy. Tight hip flexors pull the front of the pelvis down, throwing the back out of alignment and causing the tummy to protrude.

How to do it:
1 Adopt a lunge position, and drop down on to your back knee, with the foot outstretched, your torso upright and your front leg bent at a right angle. Tilt the pelvis under and lean slightly forward from the hips until you feel a deep stretch along the front of the hip and thigh of the back leg. (The back knee should be well behind the back hip.) Once you feel the stretch, hold the position for 30 seconds – if the tension eases off, take the stretch further. Swap sides.

How many?
2–4 on each side.

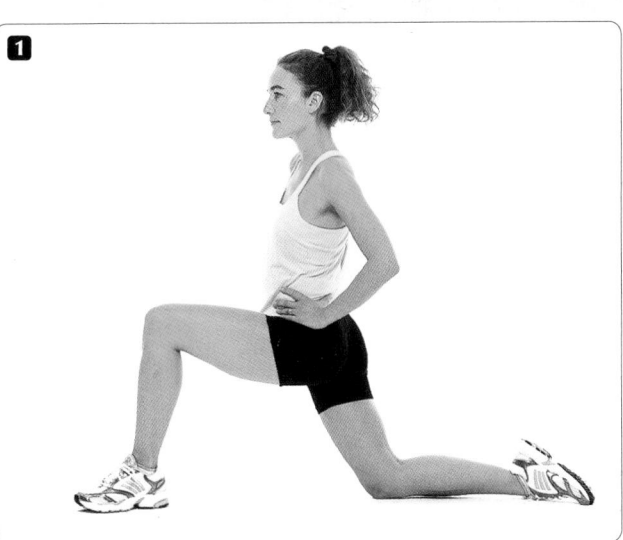

6 FACE-DOWN BUTT LIFT

What's the point?
To strengthen the gluteus muscles without aid from the hamstrings – to improve pelvic stability. This also actively stretches the hip flexors.

How to do it:
1 Lie on your tummy with your navel drawn up to your spine and your forehead resting on your hands. Bend your right leg so that the lower leg is at a right angle to the floor.

2 Squeeze your buttock cheeks gently and, pressing the hipbones into the floor, raise the thigh a few centimetres off the floor. Hold for 10 seconds then lower. Swap sides.

How many?
Do 5 lifts on each side, alternating from left to right.

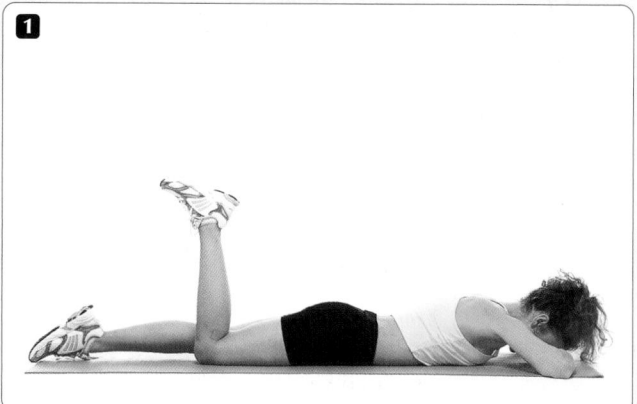

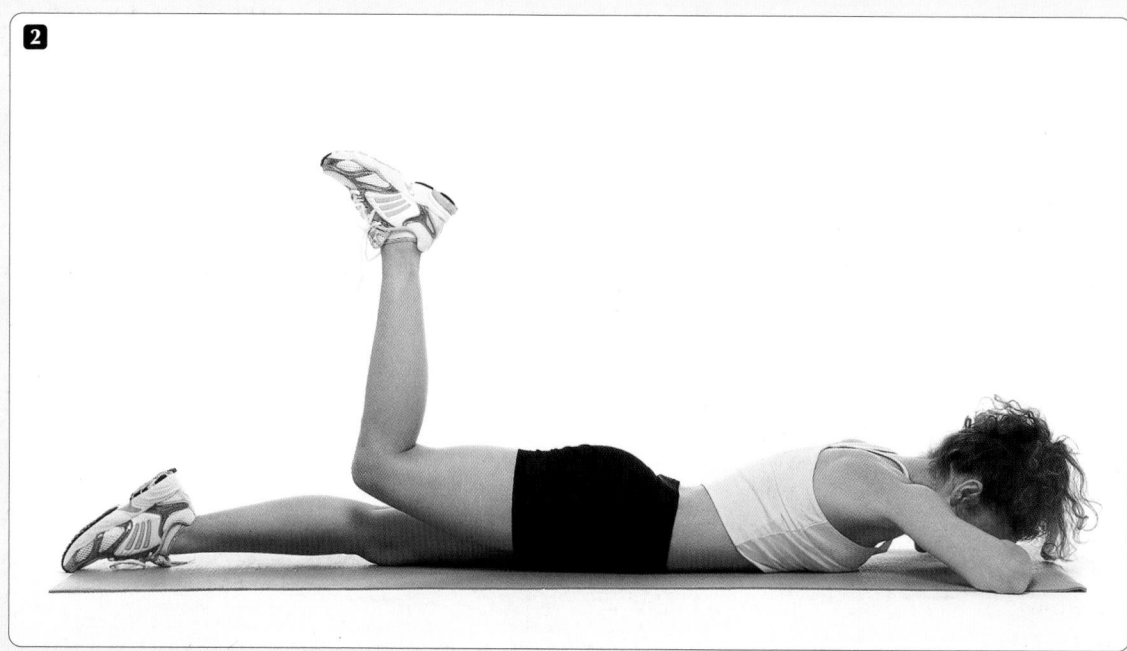

[7] SHOULDER BLADE SQUEEZE

What's the point?
To strengthen the lower half of the trapezius muscle and rhomboids, which depress and retract the scapulae and work the back of the shoulders.

How to do it:
1 Lie on your tummy with your forehead resting on the floor and your arms outstretched to the sides, bent at the elbow at a right angle.

2 Draw your arms off the floor by squeezing the shoulder blades back and down – trying to keep the hands and elbows level. Hold for 5 seconds, lower and repeat.

Once this gets easy, try doing the exercise using wrist or light weights.

How many?
2 sets of 10 reps, increase the load or the length of the hold as you get stronger.

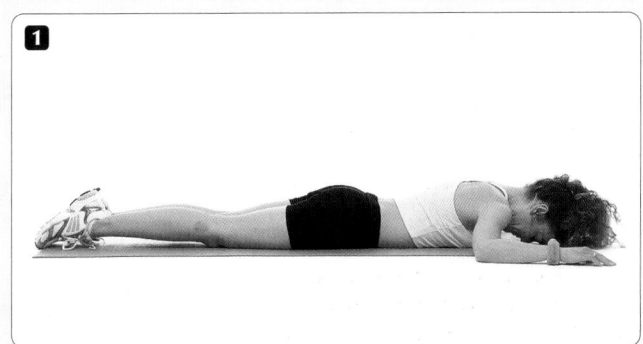

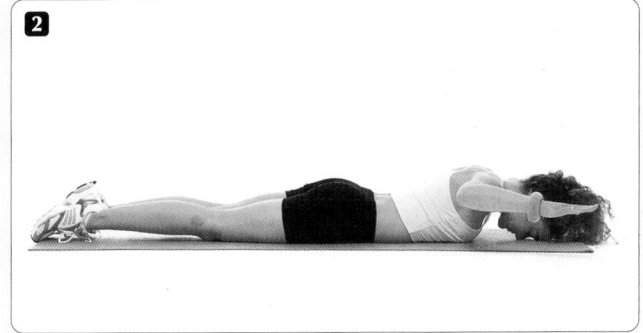

[8] ARM AND A LEG

What's the point?
It strengthens the muscles of the lower back in a functional way, because the arms and legs are moving while the back stabilises.

How to do it:
1 Lie on your tummy in a superman position, with your arms extended overhead and legs out straight. Engage the core and then lift the right arm and left leg simultaneously off the floor. Hold for 3–5 seconds, thinking of lengthening the limbs rather than aiming for height (don't hunch the shoulders), then lower and repeat on the other side.

How many?
3 sets of 10 reps.

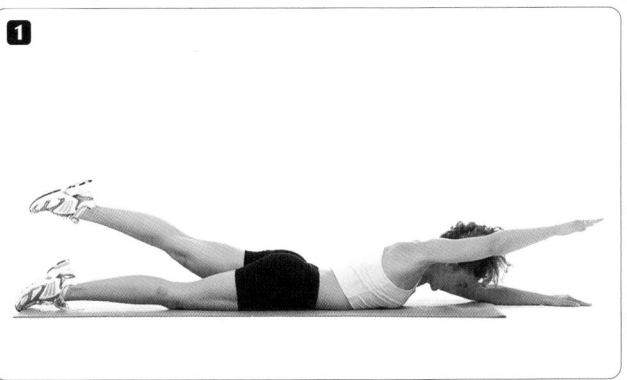

9 CORE QUARTET

What's the point?

Improving the strength and function of the 'core' is probably the most important thing you can do to ensure that you progress to weight training safely and effectively. A strong, reactive core will protect your spine whether you are picking a weight up off the floor, squatting, or lifting a weight above your head. These exercises work the transversus and rectus abdominis, obliques and pelvic floor, helping to flatten your tummy, nip in the waist and provide a base for the more challenging abdominal exercises in the main workout.

PART I NAVEL TO SPINE HOLD

1 Start on all fours, with weight evenly distributed between your hands and knees. Keep your back long and straight (neck in line with spine) and allow your tummy to relax completely.

2 Now, contract the pelvic floor and begin pulling up and back from the pubic bone to the navel. Picture most of the work being done by the sides of the tummy *below* the belly button. When the whole of the lower tummy is contracted, hold for 8–10 breaths. Rest, then repeat 2 more times. Don't worry if you have to 're-contract' halfway through – and think of using minimal force to sustain the contraction – don't grip.

When this feels easy, do the exercise exactly as above but, once you've contracted the tummy, extend one arm out in front of you, without letting the shoulders, back or hips change position. Hold for 2 breaths, then lower with control and smoothly lift the other arm. That counts as one rep. Do 3 sets of 4 reps.

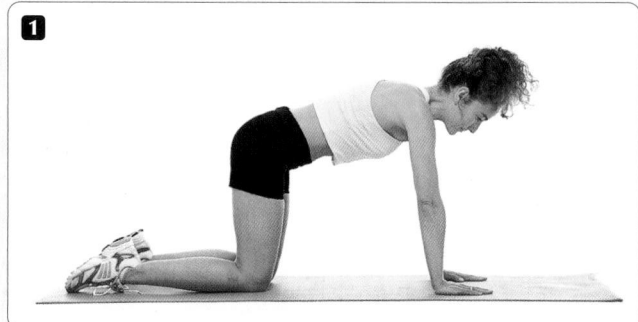

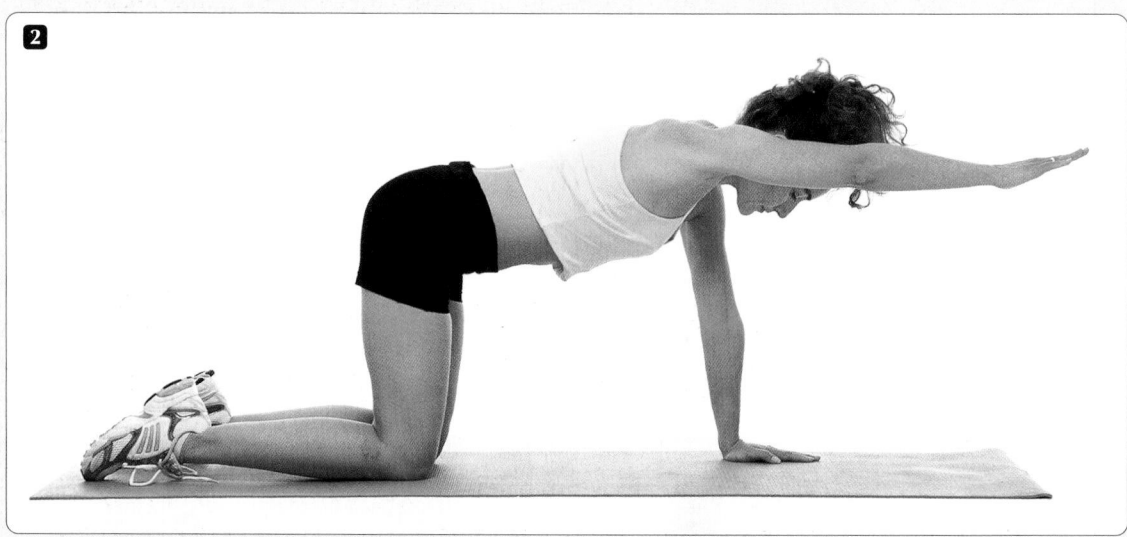

PART II BENT KNEE DROPS

1 Now lie on your back with your right leg extended straight out on the floor and your left leg bent, with the foot flat on the floor next to the right knee.

2 Engage the core and then slowly let the bent leg lower out to the side without allowing the pelvis to twist or rotate or the back to move.

How many?
Aim for 2 sets of 8–12 reps on each side.

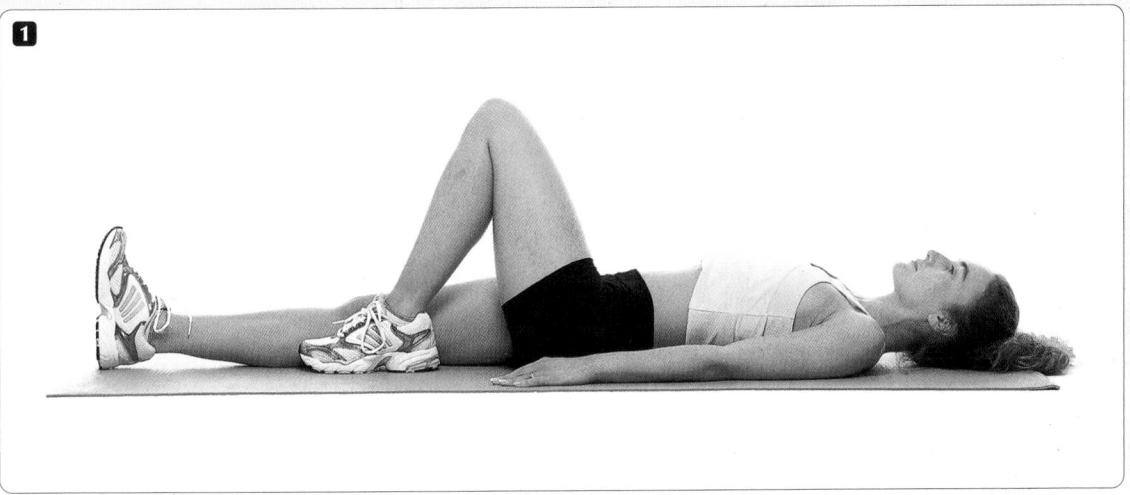

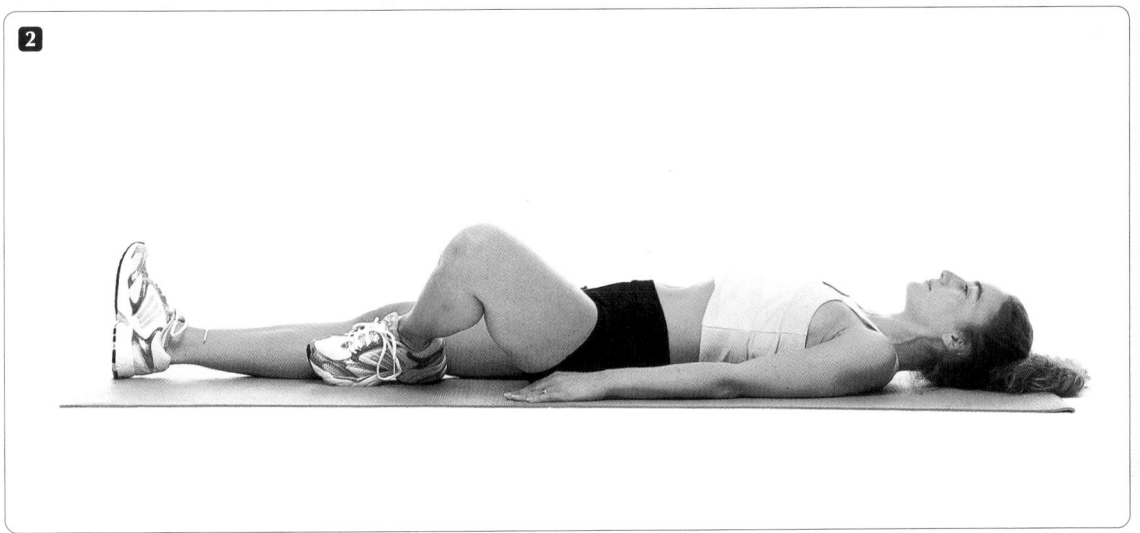

PART III TOE TOUCHDOWNS

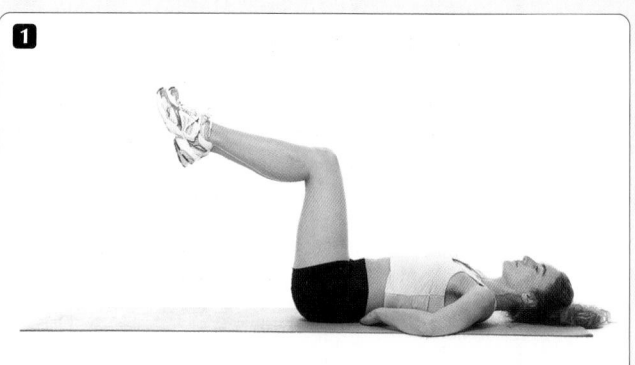

1 Still on your back, lift both feet off the floor until your knees are above your hips with the lower legs bent to 90 degrees. Engage the core to stabilise the spine.

2 Now, slowly lower one heel until it is 5cm off the floor. Pause, then raise the leg back and drop the other heel.

3 When this feels easy, once you have lowered the heel, begin to extend the leg out in front, as far as you can without allowing any flexion or extension of the spine. Draw the leg back in and repeat on the other side. To ensure the core stays engaged, you can slip your fingertips underneath your lower back throughout this exercise and ensure the pressure remains the same against the fingers throughout.

How many?
Aim for 2 sets of 8–12 reps, or stop when you can no longer maintain the neutral lower back position.

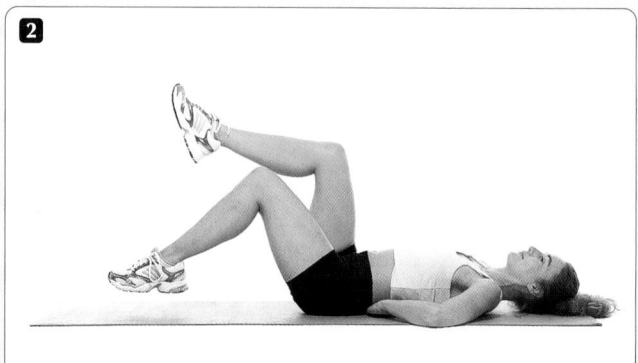

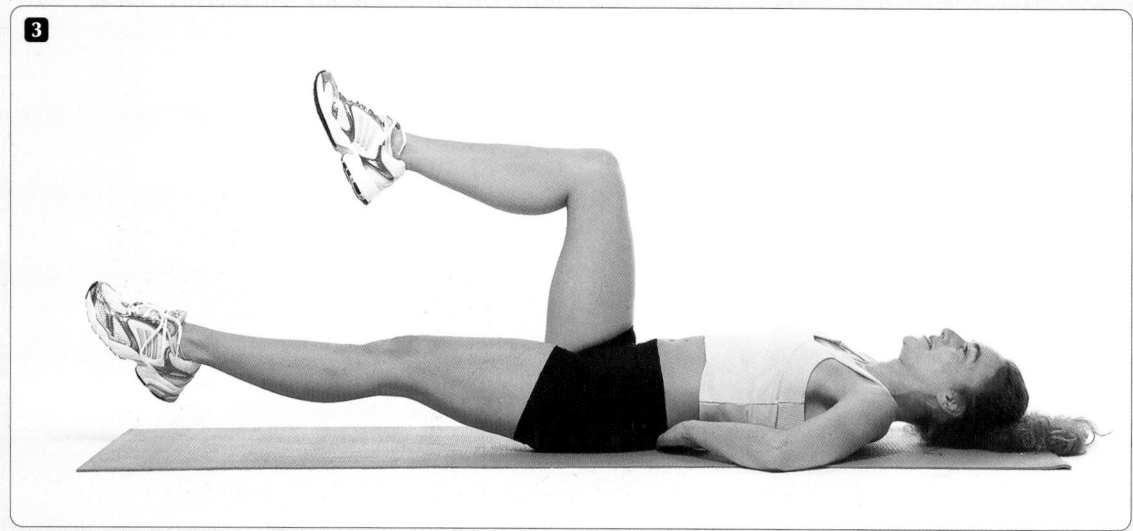

PART IV SIDE BRIDGE

1 Lie on your side with knees and hips stacked and your weight resting on the lower elbow. Bend the bottom leg to a right angle at the knee but keep the hips on top of one another.

2 Now lift your body up so that the weight is supported on the lower part of the bottom leg and the elbow only. Keeping your abdominals contracted, draw the side of the waist closest to the floor up towards the centre of the body. Don't let the bottom stick out.

How many?
Do 2 sets of 3 reps on each side, holding each rep for 5–10 seconds.

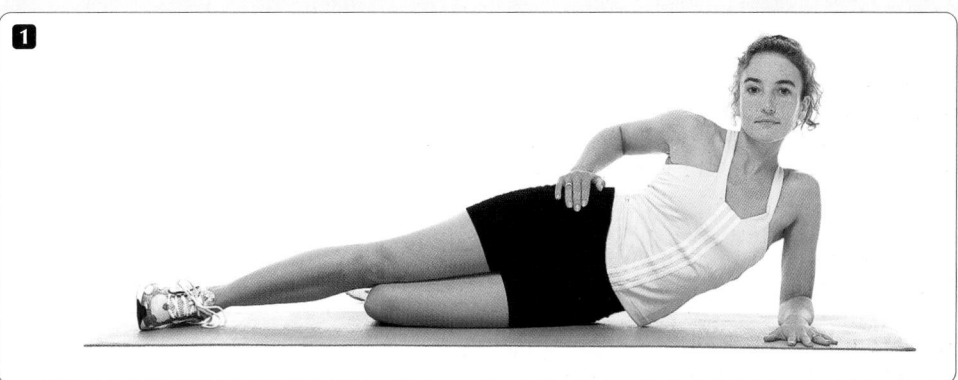

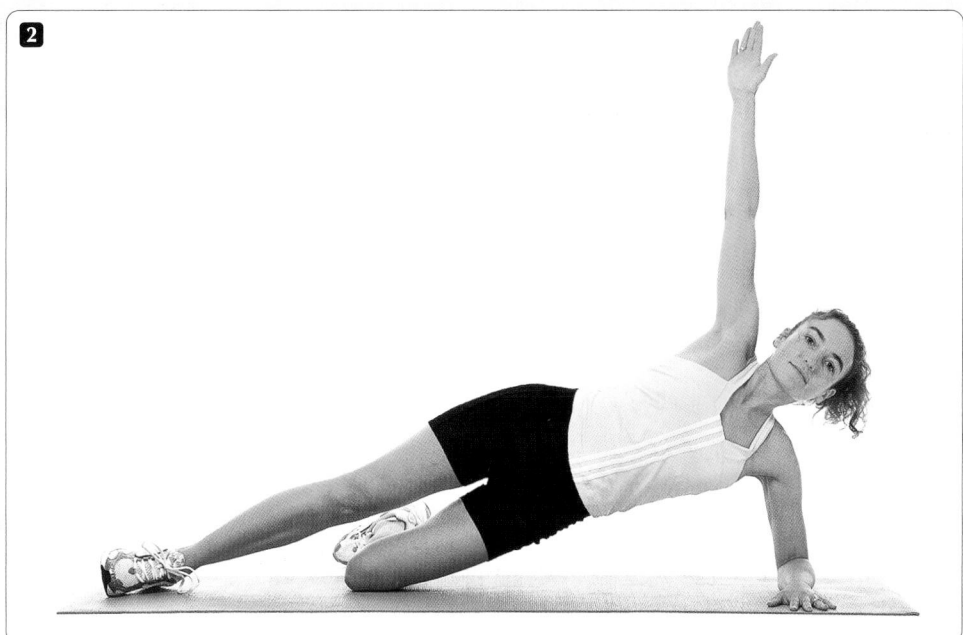

10 THE OYSTER

What's the point?
To strengthen the hip rotators and stabilisers.

How to do it:
1 Lie on your left side with your left arm outstretched, your head resting on it and both legs bent, feet in line with your bottom. Do a small pelvic tilt so that you reduce the arch in your lower back, keeping the abdominals tight.

2 Now keeping the feet glued together, open the right leg. Only go as far as you can without rolling the pelvis – and hold each raise for 2–3 seconds.

How many?
Do 2 sets of 10–12 reps on each side.

11 LEG LOCKOUT

What's the point?
This exercise helps to strengthen a muscle known as the vastus medialis obliquus (VMO), which aids alignment of the kneecap.

How to do it:
1 Sit on the floor with your left leg extended, the right leg bent and your hands slightly behind you. Place a rolled-up towel under your left knee and with your leg slightly turned out from the hip, press down on the towel firmly, locking out the knee and aiming to feel the muscle that sits just above the knee cap on the inner side of the thigh contracting. Hold for 5–8 seconds.

2 Once you can do this comfortably, press down on the towel as above and then lift the leg off the ground completely, holding it for 2–3 seconds. Swap legs.

How many?
Do 4 sets of 5 on each side.

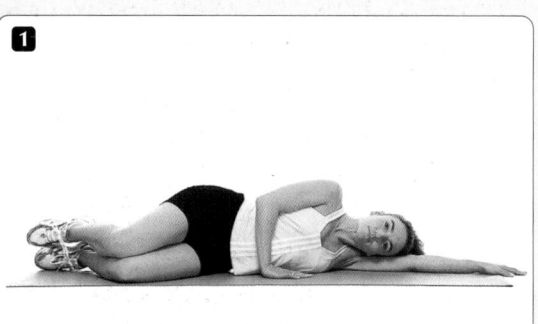

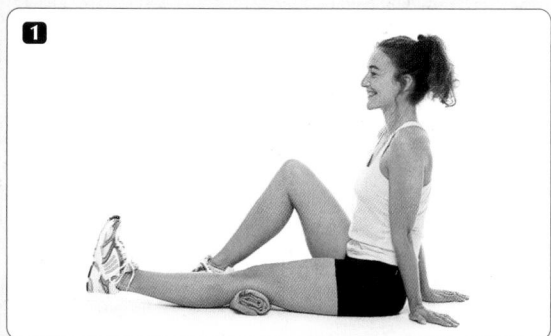

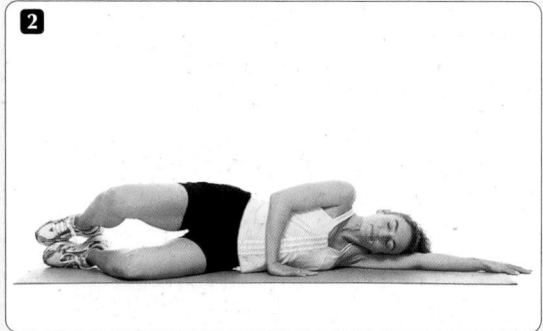

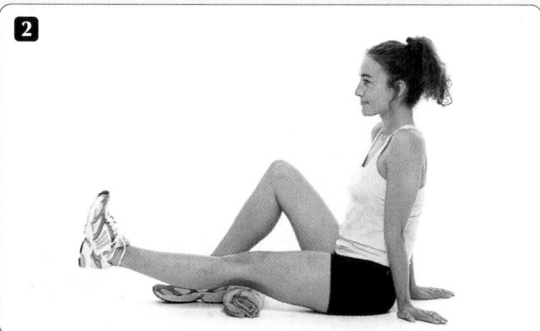

12 PELVIC BRIDGE

What's the point?
To strengthen the pelvic stabilisers, lower back and inner thighs.

How to do it:
1 Lie on the floor with the knees bent, feet flat, and a rolled-up towel or foam ball between your knees.

2 Raise the body up by rolling through the spine enough to allow the pelvis to clear the floor, squeezing the towel with your inner thighs. Visualise your knees moving away from your body. Hold for 10 seconds, then release and repeat.

How many?
Aim for 5–8 reps.

To progress:
Do the same as above, but once your pelvis is raised, alternately extend one leg and then the other, without allowing the pelvis to rock from side to side or the towel to drop. Allow 2 seconds to extend the leg and 2 seconds to bring it back. Do 10–12 reps.

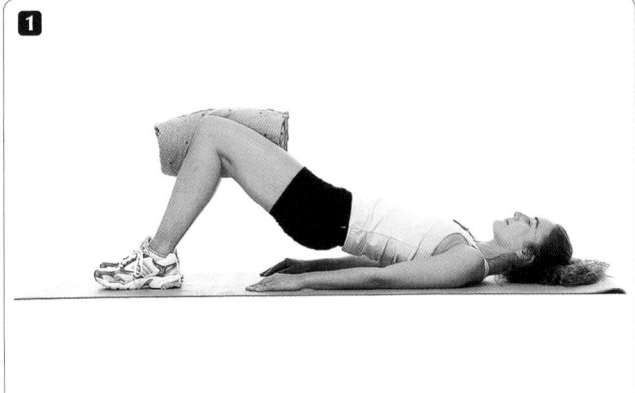

STRONG WORDS

CHANGING TIMES

If you've started training but have yet to see results, don't be discouraged. Research from Ohio and Pennsylvania State Universities has found that physiological changes begin to take place in the muscles as quickly as after four workouts – it's just you can't see them yet. Changes included an increase of testosterone and growth hormone, both involved in promoting muscle gain and fat loss. If, on the other hand, you feel as if you have seen 'too much' in the way of results, worry not. The initial 'puffing' that some people experience after beginning weight training is due to increased carbohydrate storage, which makes the body hold on to more water. Once you get into the rhythm of training, this side effect will diminish.

The weights for weight loss workout

The *Weights for Weight Loss* Workout is a simple yet challenging routine involving twelve exercises that will:
• make every muscle firmer and stronger;
• maintain the right balance between muscle groups to ensure you look longer and leaner rather than bulky and muscle-bound;
• boost your daily energy expenditure and preserve or increase your metabolic rate;
• make daily physical tasks feel effortless, improve your energy levels and – above all – help you to lose body fat and keep it off.

One workout – three ways to do it

Since not everyone has a gym on their doorstep, or wants to use one, the workout comes in three forms. Firstly, there is a free weights workout – the 'gold standard' method of training. Then there is the gym-based version, for those who enjoy the training environment of the gym and like the support and familiarity of the machines and apparatus. And finally, there is a home-based version, which uses nothing but your own body weight and a few inexpensive pieces of equipment that you can stow easily. Use 'the rules' on page 34 to ensure you do the workout safely and effectively and use the right weight and number of reps and sets – and to make sure that you keep making progress, and don't get stuck on a plateau.

Lifting safely

I know I have drummed in the importance of good technique when strength training but that goes for when you are actually picking up and putting down weights, too. NEVER bend over with straight legs to pick weights up off the floor or from a low rack. Bend your knees, engage the core and use the glutes to help you straighten up rather than your back. If necessary, pick up the weight with both hands and hold it as close to your body as possible. In lying down exercises, make sure you have a firm grip of the weight before you extend it – particularly if lifting it over your face or head. And, if the dumbbells are the type with removable plates on the ends, ensure the fixtures are secure before using them.

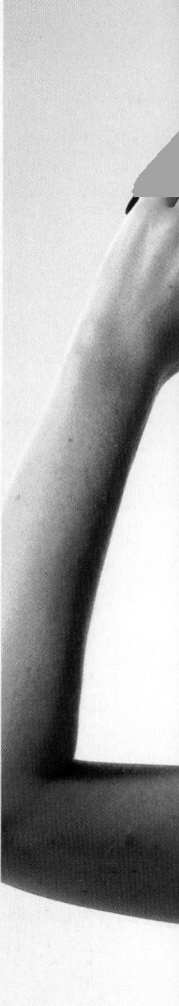

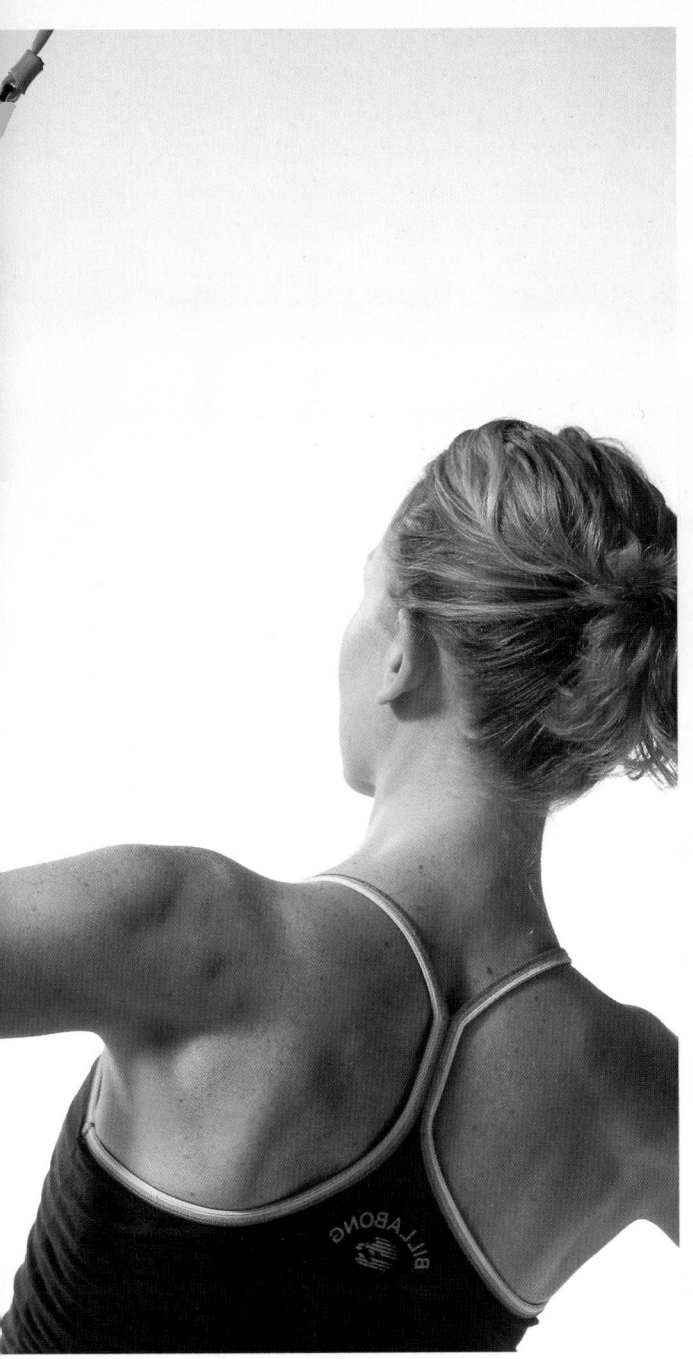

DOING THE FREE WEIGHTS WORKOUT

- Warm up first.

- Wear supportive trainers.

- Try to breathe out on the effort and in on the release – if you can't get the hang of that then breathe freely throughout.

- You will need dumbbells and barbells of varying or adjustable weight, a weights bench, a step and an exercise ball.

- Decide on your weights, reps and sets and rest (see pages 41–45). Remember, whatever weight you choose, it should feel tough by the end of each set.

- Do the exercises in the order shown.

YOU KNOW WHAT?

Research in the *European Journal of Applied Physiology* found that muscle in the upper body responds to strength training more quickly than the lower body. So you'll be getting compliments on your sculpted shoulders before you get them about your streamlined thighs!

Free weights

1 DEAD LIFT

What it works:
It emphasises the glutes, hamstrings, quads, back and the core stabilisers.

How to do it:
1 Place a barbell on the floor – with feet below the hips and toes underneath the bar. Squat down, keeping the back long and straight, the core engaged and not allowing the knees to roll in.

2 Grasp the bar, hands wider than your knees, in an overhand grip, and straighten up fully. Exhale forcefully as you straighten. Use the back muscles to keep the shoulder blades retracted and the chest open and focus your gaze forward to avoid crunching the back of the neck.

3 Lower back into a squat until the bar is just below the knees, then straighten up and repeat.

To progress:
Increase the weight

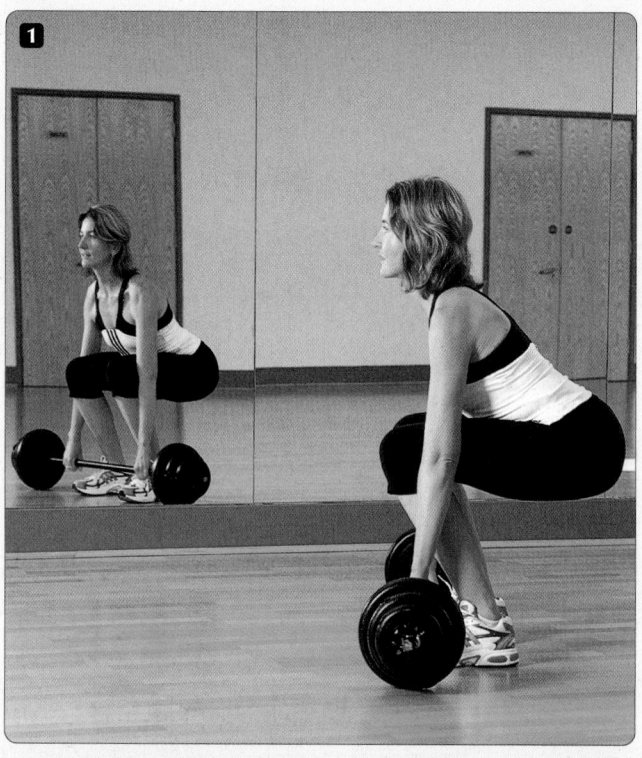

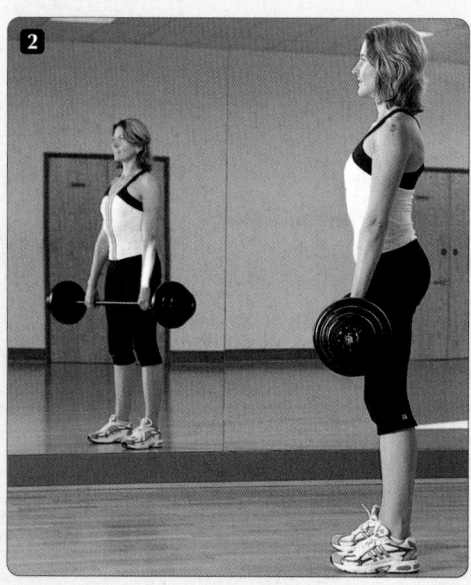

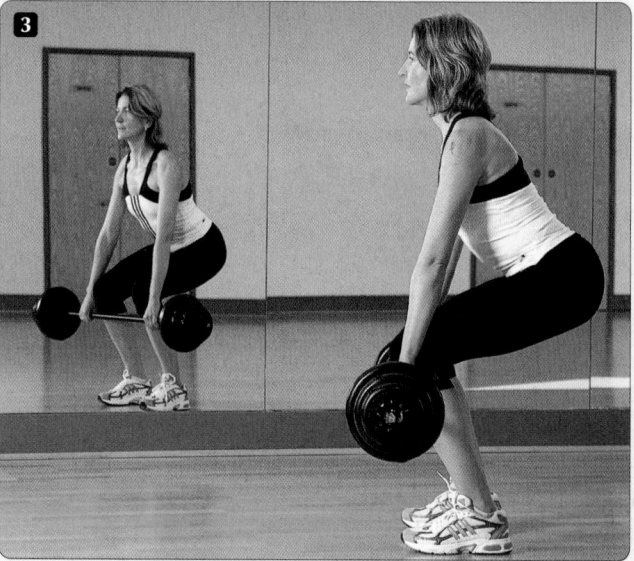

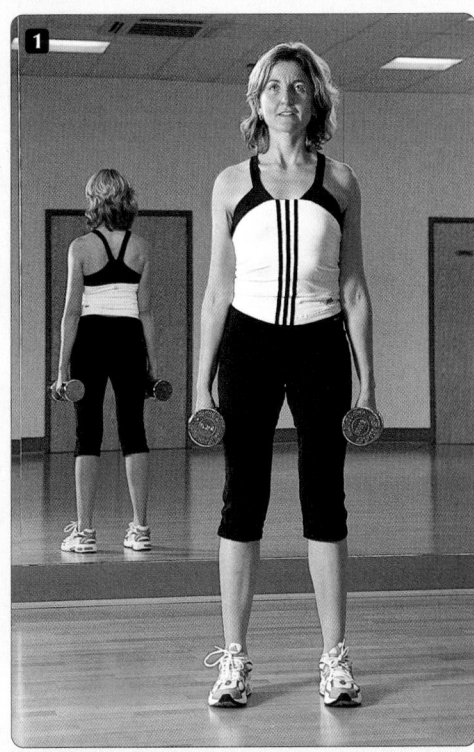

2 SQUAT

What it works:
Glutes, quads, hamstrings and calves.

How to do it:
1 Stand with your feet below your hipbones and a dumbbell in each hand.

2 Engage the core and inhale as you lower your bottom back and down (as if you were going to sit on a stool). Keep your knees tracking directly over your feet – don't let them roll in or out. When your thighs are parallel to the floor – or as close as is comfortable for you – pause and straighten up, pressing up through the heels as you push back up to a standing position.

To progress:
3 As your strength improves, it will be more comfortable to use a barbell, resting across the fleshy part of your shoulders, rather than dumbbells. Keep your torso as upright as possible without overarching the back.

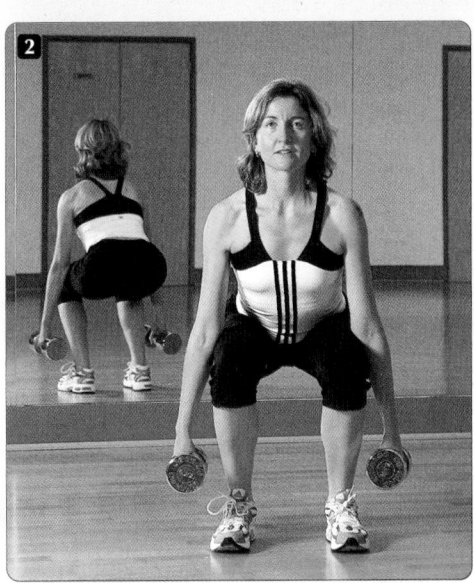

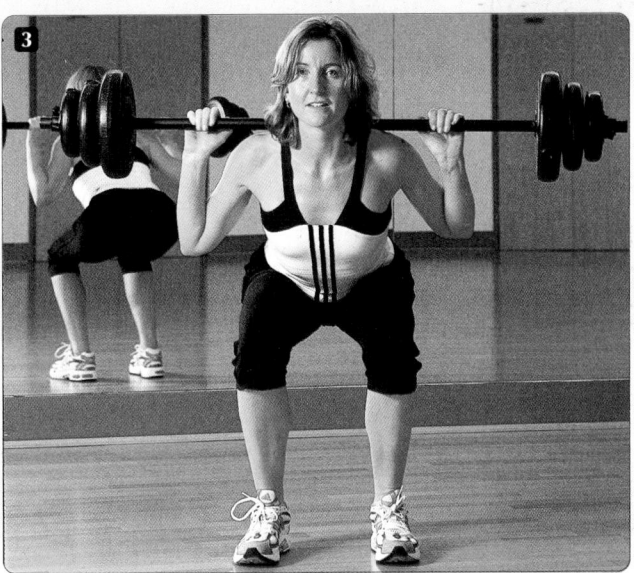

3 LUNGE

What it works:
Quads, glutes, hamstrings – the adductors and abductors also work hard to stabilise you.

How to do it:
1 Take a dumbbell in each hand and take a big step forward with the right leg, so that the left heel comes off the floor.

2 Ensure you are balanced and then bend both legs, lowering yourself towards the floor without allowing the body to rock forward (make sure your right knee doesn't extend in front of your foot). Pause when the back knee is almost touching the floor and then push back up and repeat. Focus on the front leg during the lunge exercise, as this is the one you are working hardest. Finish the set, then swap sides.

To progress:
Rather than starting in the lunge position, a forward lunge requires you to start with feet together and actually step straight into the lunge, bending both knees and ensuring your front foot remains in line with the toes.

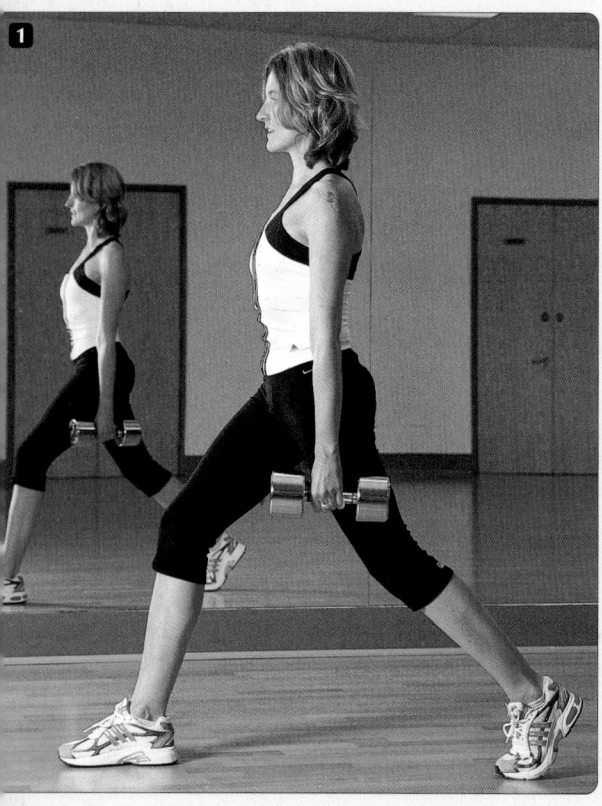 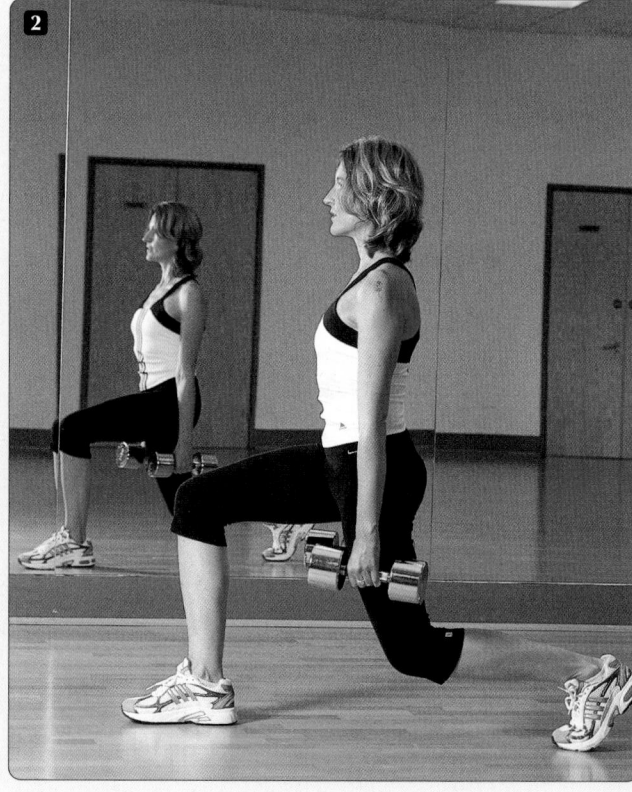

4 STEP UP

What it works:
Quads, glutes, hip flexors, hamstrings and calves.

How to do it:
1 Stand in front of a step high enough to allow your knee to bend to a 90-degree angle when your foot is on it. Take a dumbbell in each hand and step up with your right foot, ensuring the whole foot goes on to the step.

2 Bring the left foot up on to the step, then down with the right and down with the left. Continue leading with the right foot until the end of the set. Begin the next set starting with the left foot.

To progress:
Increase the weight.

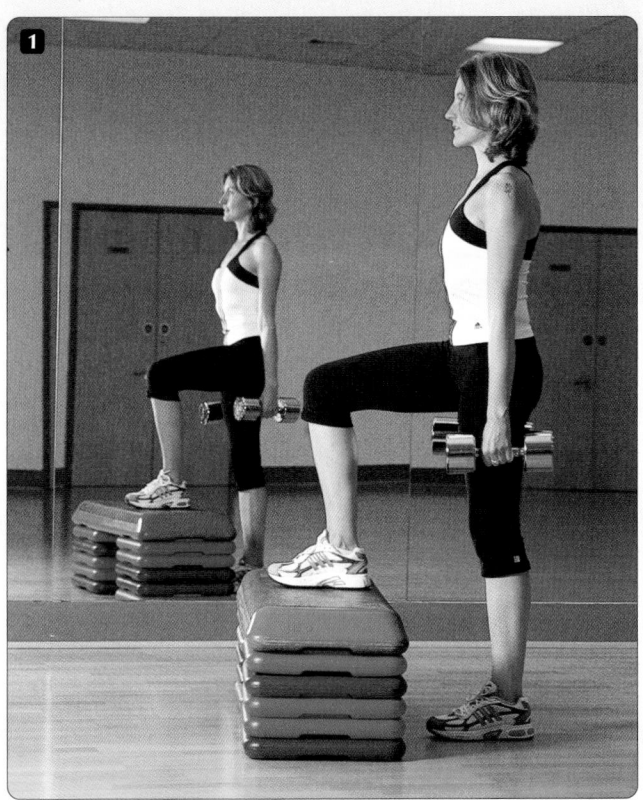

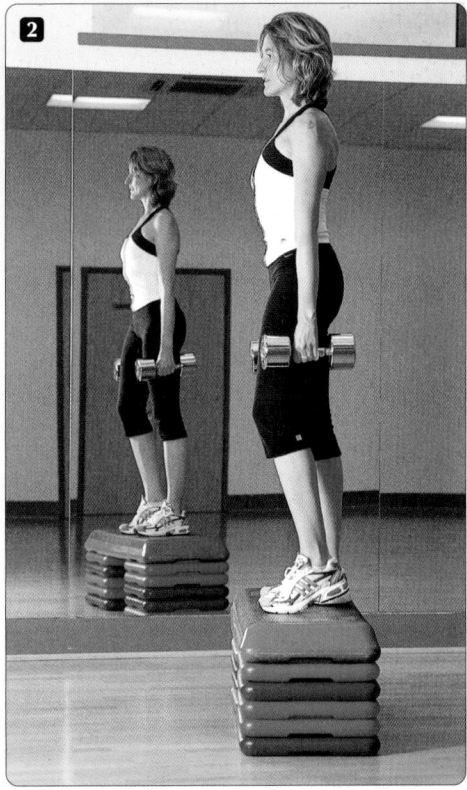

5 SINGLE ARM ROW

What it works:
Lats, rhomboids, trapezius, biceps and the back of the shoulder.

How to do it:
1 Stand side on to a weights bench with your hand and knee on the support, back parallel to the floor (neck in line) and a weight in your other hand, arm hanging straight down.

2 Bend the arm to bring the weight up to the front of the shoulder – focusing on using the back to lift the weight. Keep the core engaged and don't twist the body around or move anything other than the working arm. Repeat on the other side when you have finished the set.

To progress:
Increase the weight.

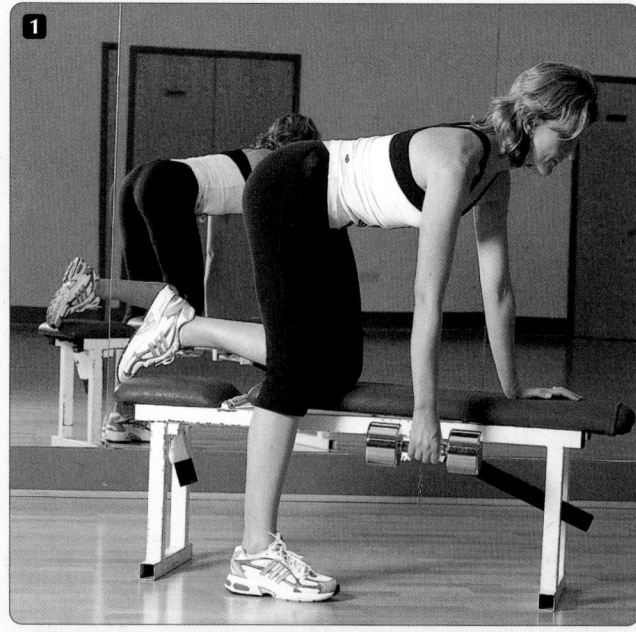

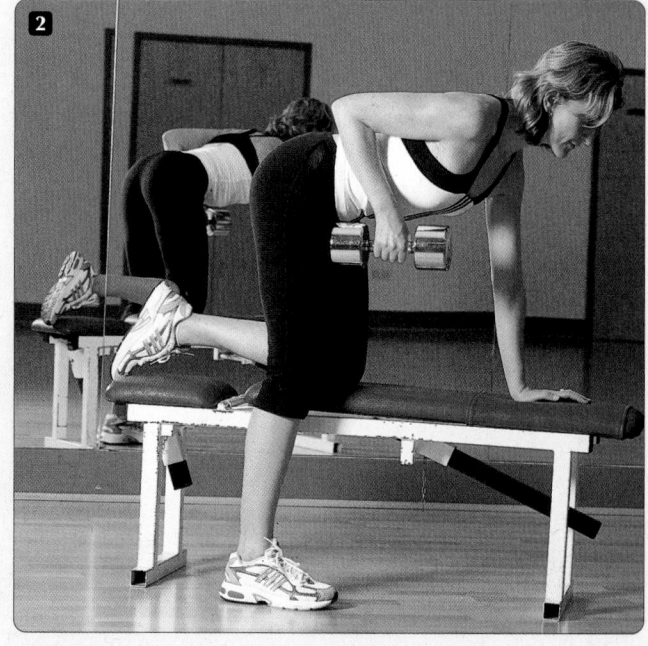

6 BENCH PRESS

What it works:
The chest, shoulders and the back of the arms.

How to do it:
1 Lie on a weights bench with your core engaged and feet on the floor or, if you feel more comfortable, on the end of the bench, knees bent. Take a barbell and hold it level with the nipple line, arms straight and palms facing upwards.

2 Exhale as you extend your arms to press the barbell up, inhale as you lower the bar to the chest. Don't lock the elbow joints out and don't bring the shoulders forward to aid extending the bar – simply bend and straighten the arms.

To progress:
A chest press using dumbbells is more challenging than a barbell, as you'll need to stabilise the arms through the arc of movement. To make it harder still, press each dumbbell alternately – this requires greater core stabilisation.

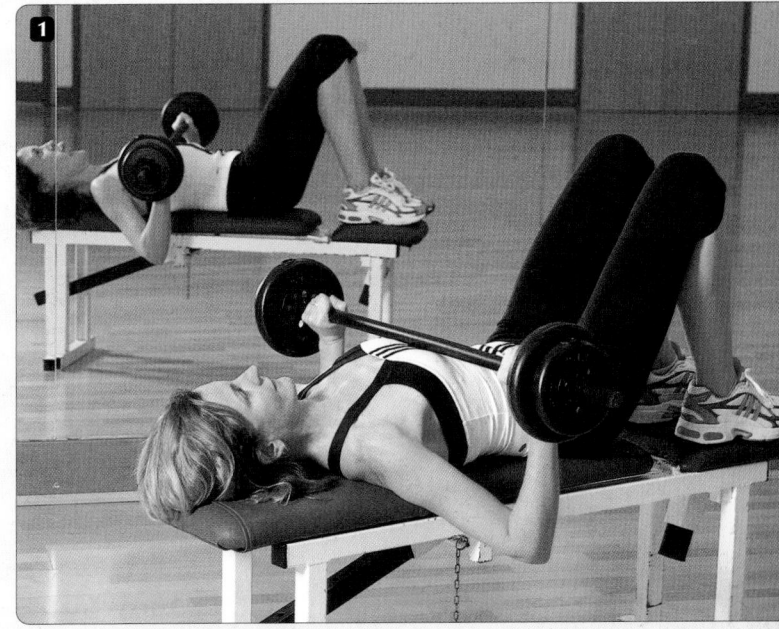

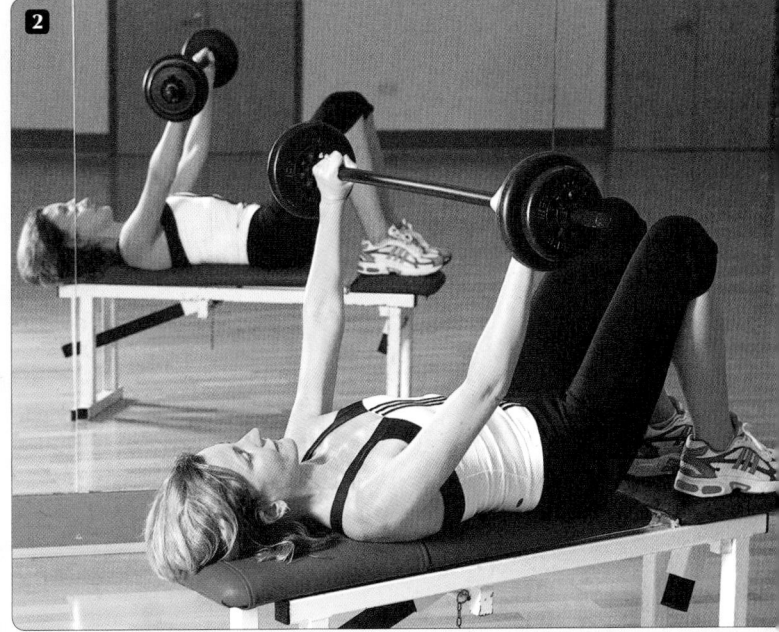

⑦ PEC FLY

What it works:
The chest and front of the shoulders. It also uses the biceps isometrically, as they are used to keep the arm almost straight.

How to do it:
1 Lie on a bench with a dumbbell in each hand, arms almost straight above the chest, palms facing each other and wrists in line with the forearms.

YOU KNOW WHAT?
One study found that for optimal training of the chest, the dumbbell and barbell bench press can be used interchangeably for variety but flys activate the pectoralis major less and should only be used as an auxiliary – not a main – lift.

2 Open the arms out to the sides, as far as is comfortable, then bring them back to the start position.

To progress:
Increase the weight.

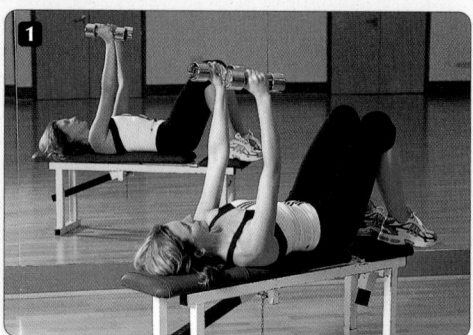

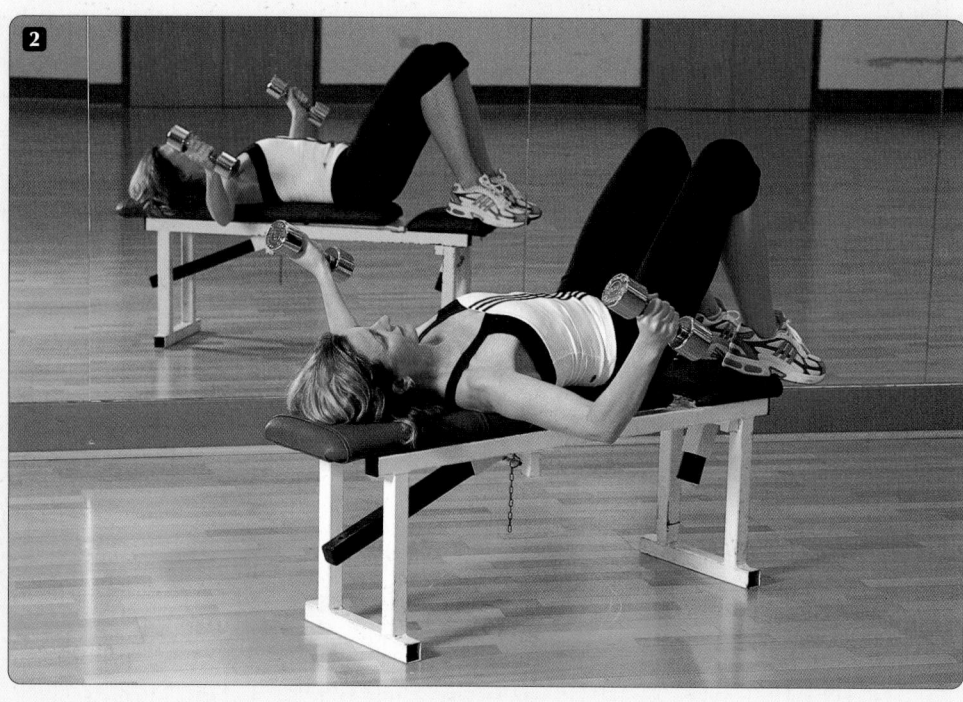

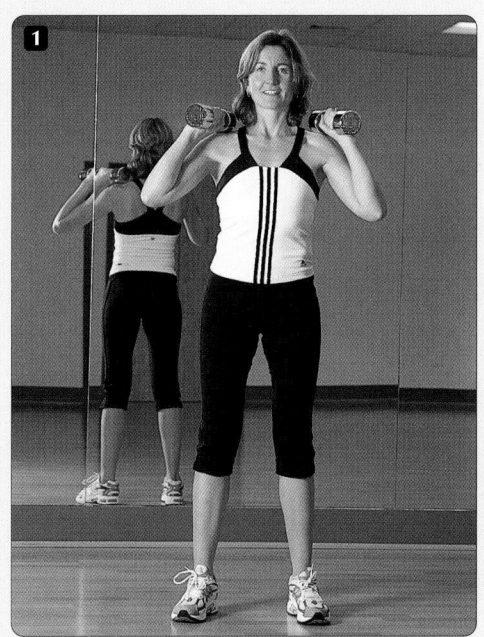

8 OVERHEAD PRESS

What it works:
The shoulders, triceps, chest, trapezius and shoulder girdle rotators.

How to do it:
1 Stand with your back straight and core engaged, with a dumbbell in each hand, resting on the shoulders with palms facing each other.

2 Extend the arms over the head, allowing them to rotate so that when the arms are straight, your palms are facing the front. Keep your trunk tight and don't allow the torso to tip back to assist you. You should be able to see your arms in your peripheral vision as they are raised – don't take the arms behind the line of the head. Pause, then lower and repeat.

To progress:
3 & 4 Using a barbell makes the exercise harder, as you aren't able to rotate the arms as the bar lifts. Also, try performing the exercise with dumbbells but sitting down, and see how much 'back' you unwittingly put into the move when you are standing.

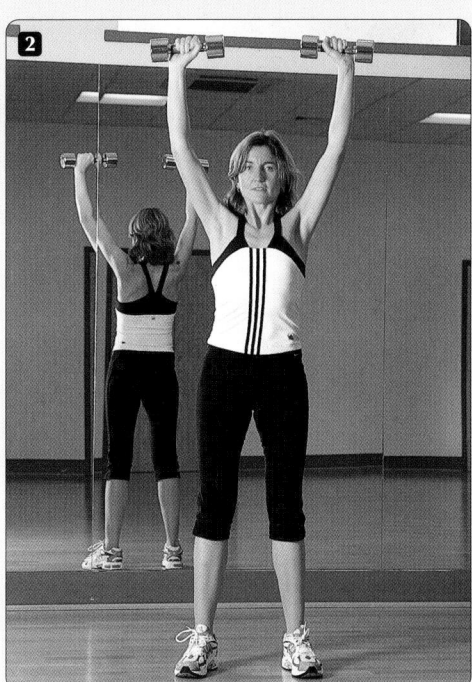

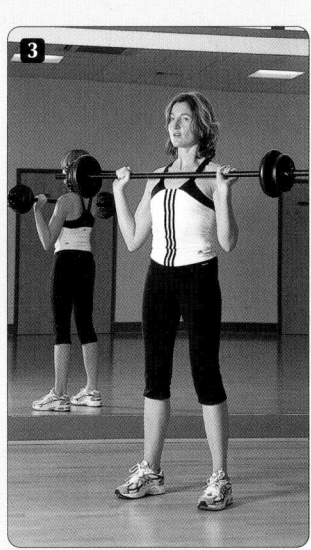

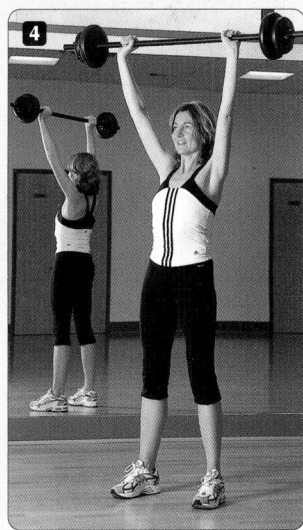

9 REVERSE FLY

What it works:
The middle and upper back and back of the shoulders. A good exercise to counteract that rounded front shoulder look caused by too much chest work or a forward posture.

How to do it:
1 Lie face down on a weights bench with a dumbbell in each hand and your chin just off the end of the bench, to keep the neck in line with the spine.

2 Take your arms out to the sides, with arms almost straight and, squeezing the shoulder blades together, lift the weights until they are level with your shoulders. Lower and repeat.

To progress:
Increase the weight.

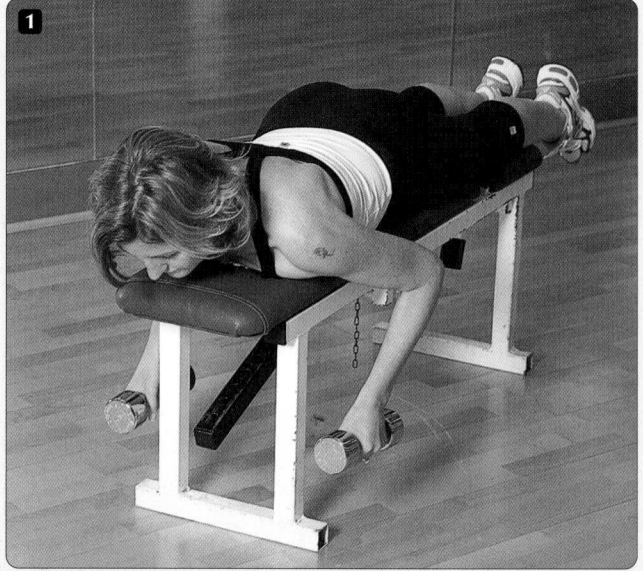

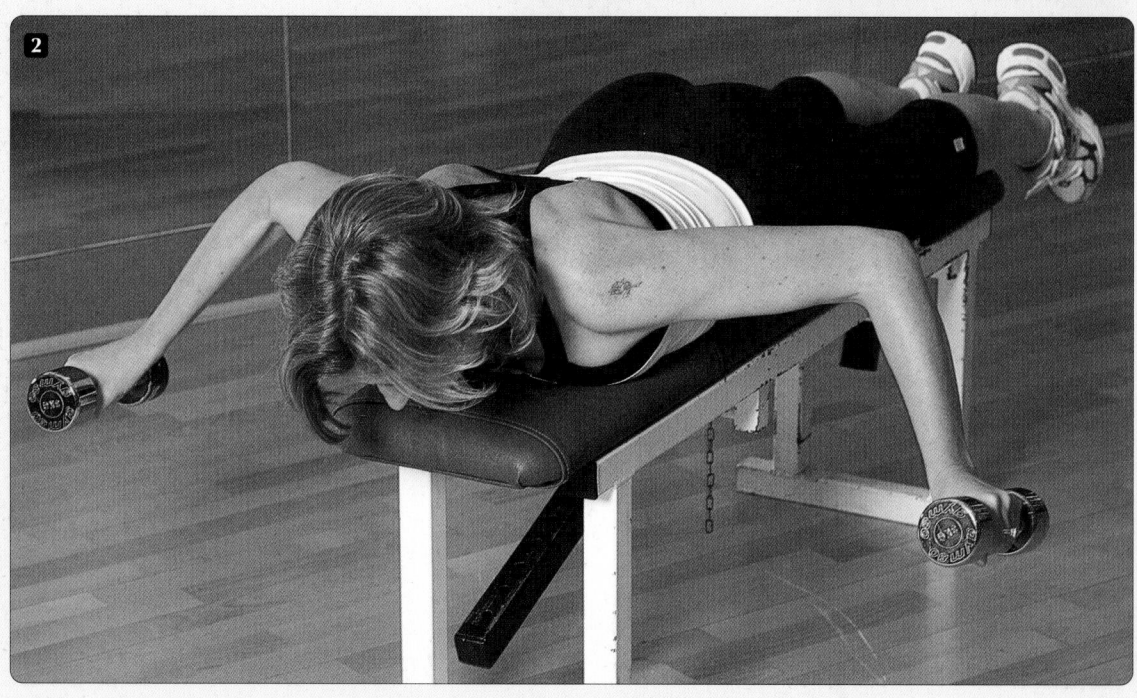

10 BICEPS CURL

What it works:
The biceps in the front of the upper arm.

How to do it:
1 Sit with a weight in each hand, your arms relaxed down by your sides, palms facing inwards.

2 Either simultaneously or alternately, bend the elbows and rotate the arms, to bring the weight up to the front of the shoulder with the palm facing the shoulder. Pause, lower and repeat.

To progress:
Increase the weight.

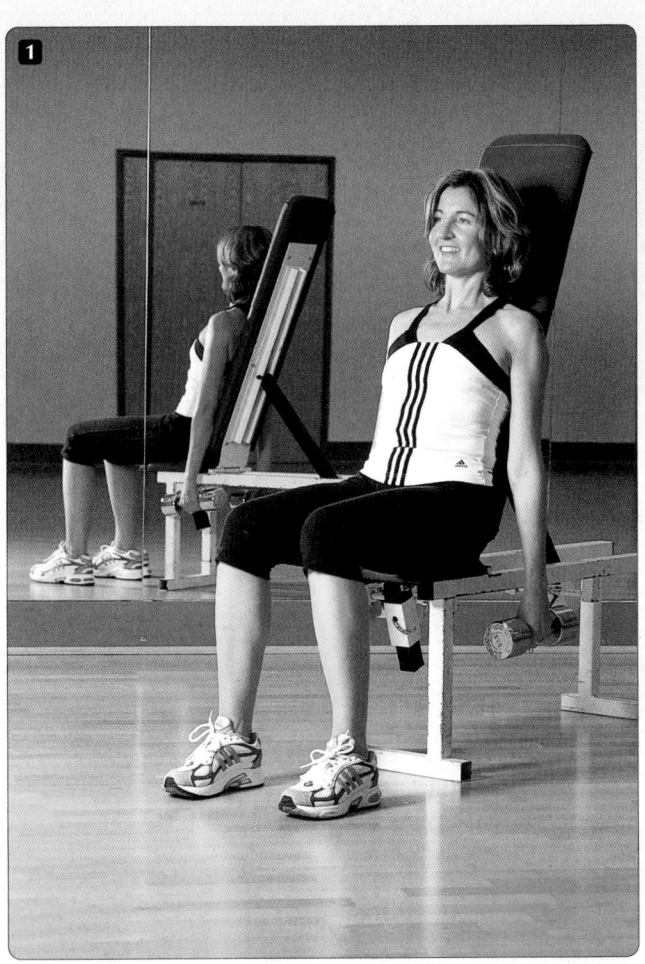

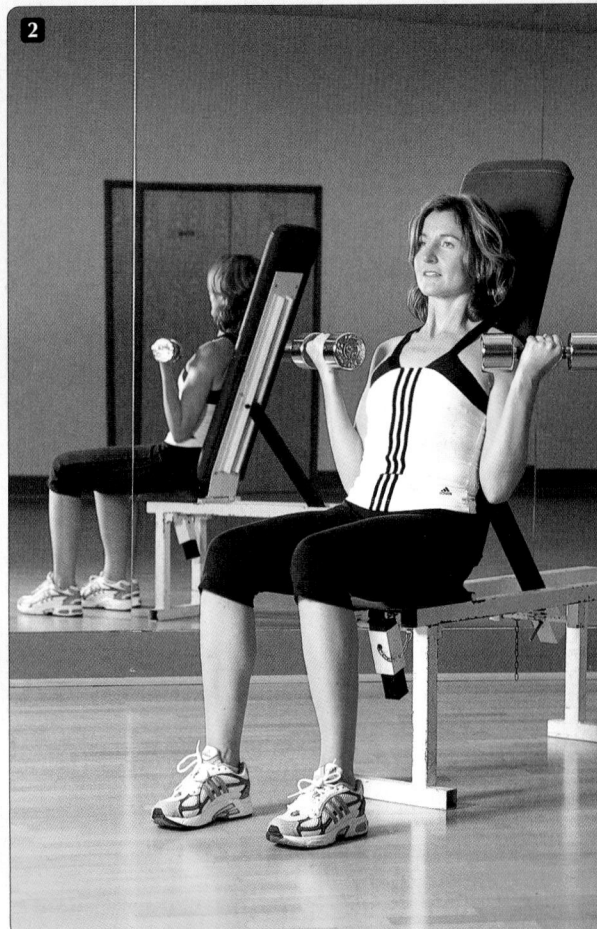

[11] TRICEPS KICKBACK

What it works:
The back of the upper arm and rear shoulder.

How to do it:
1 Stand right-side on to a weights bench with your right hand and knee on the bench, back parallel to the floor and a weight in your left hand. Start with the upper arm parallel to the body, elbow at a right angle.

2 Keeping the upper arm still, straighten the arm, taking the dumbbell past your thigh. At the end of the range, try to extend the shoulder slightly (allow the arm to go beyond the line of the body). Bend the arm back to the start position and repeat. Swap sides.

To progress:
Increase the weight.

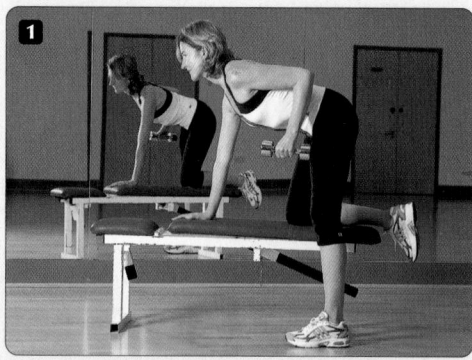

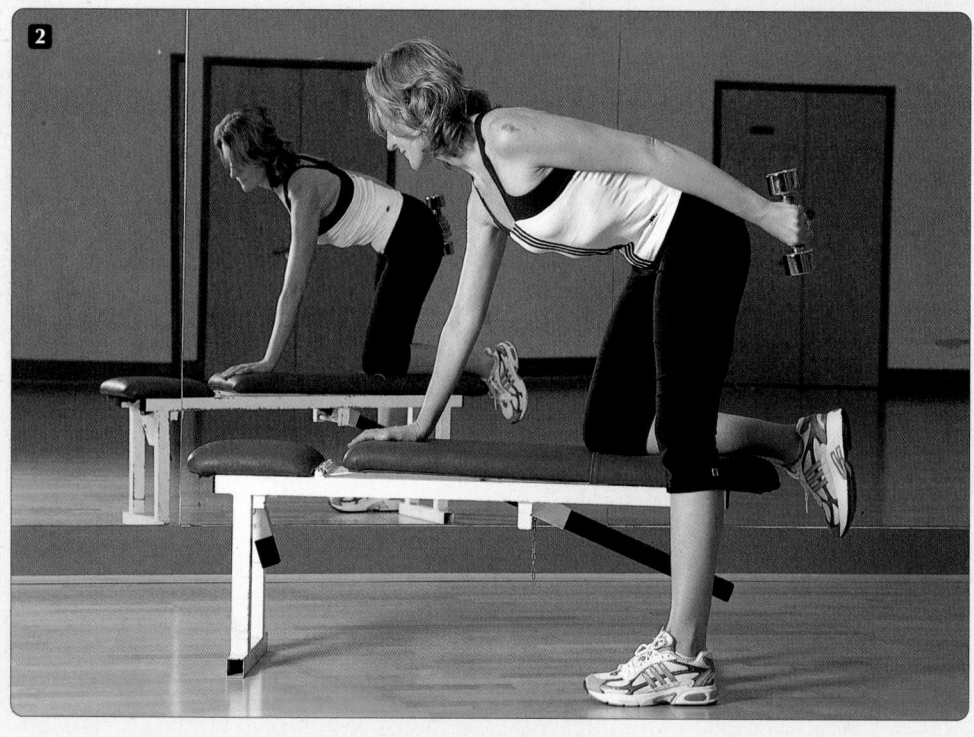

12 BALL SIT UP

What it works:
The rectus abdominis (sixpack muscle), obliques and core stabilisers.

How to do it:
1 Lie back on an exercise ball with your feet resting against the join between the wall and the floor for support. Adjust yourself so that your bottom is just off the front of the ball, with buttocks unclenched and your hands either beside your head or crossed over your chest.

2 Contracting the abdominals, raise and flex the upper torso as far as you can without moving the ball underneath you. Pause, then lower and repeat.

To progress:
Increase reps and sets.

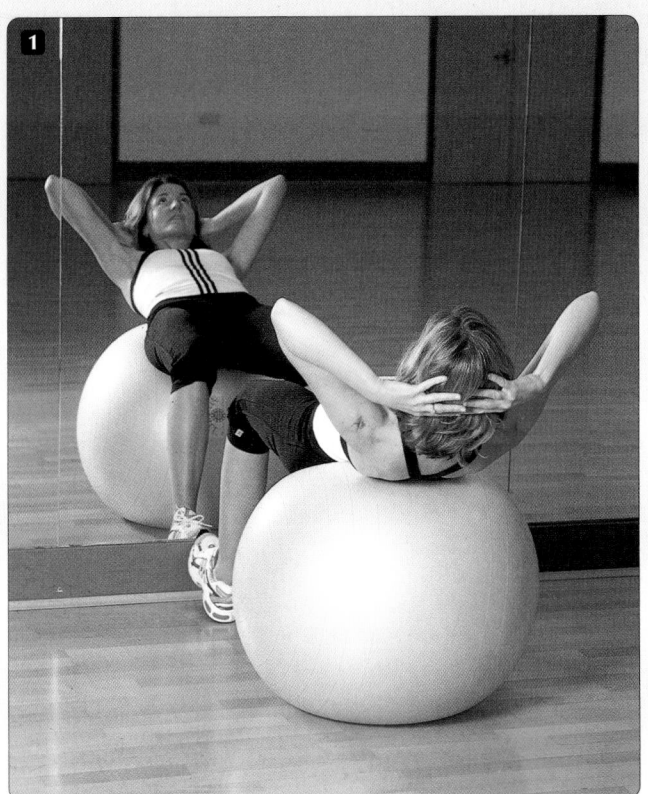

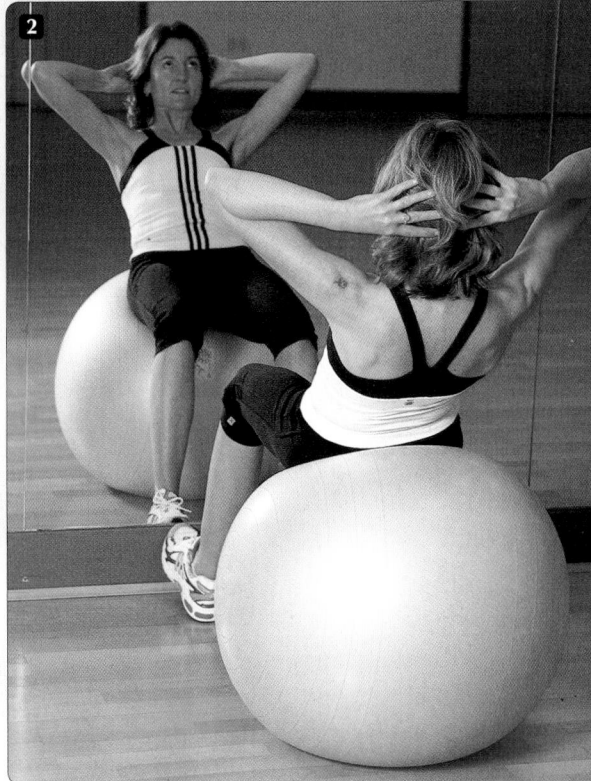

Gym workout

DOING THE GYM MACHINE WORKOUT

- Warm up first.

- Wear supportive trainers.

- Try to breathe out on the effort and in on the release – if you can't get the hang of that, then breathe freely throughout.

- Remember to keep your core engaged. Although the machine is supporting you, don't use this as an excuse to let it all hang out!

- Decide on your weights, reps and sets and rest (see pages 41–45). Remember, whatever weight you choose, it should feel *tough* by the end of each set.

- Do the exercises in the order shown.

- Remember to adjust the seat height, pad height and lever length of each machine where necessary.

- Gym machines are fairly self-explanatory and different brands vary in their set-up. For these reasons, exercise instructions are not given but there are some useful technique pointers to follow.

1 LEG PRESS MACHINE

What it works:
Quads, glutes, hamstrings and calves.

Technique pointers:
Make sure your feet are the same distance apart as your hipbones and that your feet are pointing directly forward. As you bend the legs, don't allow the knees to roll in and get as close to 90 degrees as you can.

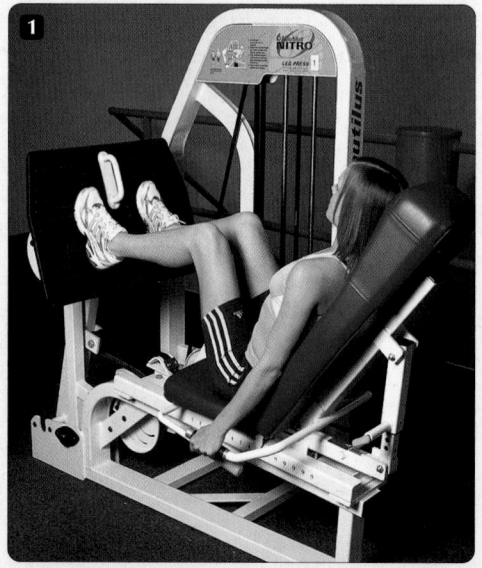

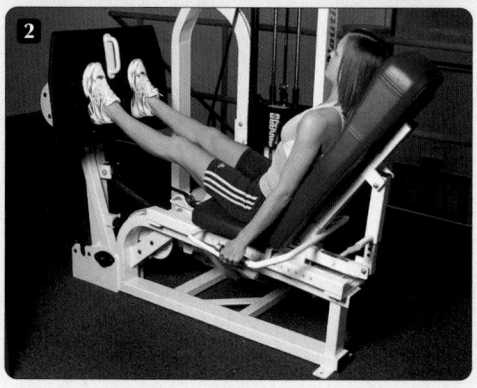

2 SEATED LEG CURL

What it works:
Hamstrings.

Technique pointers:
Maintain the curve in your lower back and don't slump in the chair, so that you get maximum range in the hamstrings. The face down lying leg curl is an acceptable alternative: if you use this machine, don't allow the bottom to lift up as the legs bend.

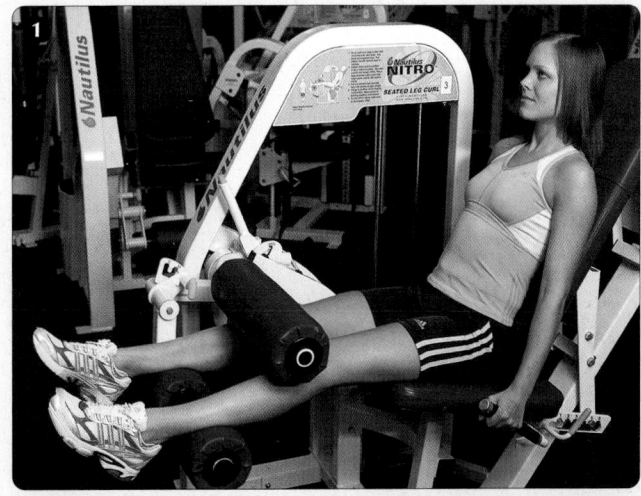

YOU KNOW WHAT?

A whole muscle is always active but the mechanical emphasis differs according to the body's position, which changes the 'line of pull' – the relation of where the body is moving compared to the line in which the fibres travel. That's why a chest press on a flat surface is slightly different from one on an incline or decline bench.

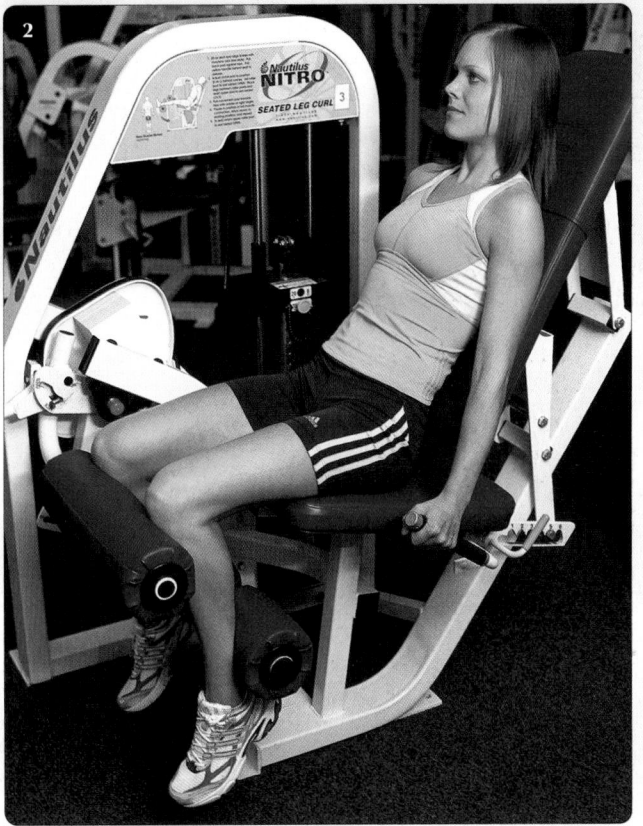

3 CLOCKFACE LUNGE

What it works:
Quads, glutes, hamstrings, adductors and abductors. (This is included instead of the classic thigh exercise – the leg extension, which can cause excessive force on the knee joint.)

How to do it:
1 Imagine you are standing in the middle of a clockface. With a dumbbell in each hand, take a big step forward (to 12 o'clock) with the right leg, so that the left heel comes off the floor and the knee travels towards the floor. The right knee should bend to approximately 90 degrees but make sure your knee doesn't extend in front of your foot. Pause when the back knee is almost touching the floor and then push back up.

2 Now lunge to 2 o'clock with the right leg, following the same technique pointers as above.

3 Push back up and then lunge to 11 o'clock. Swap legs.

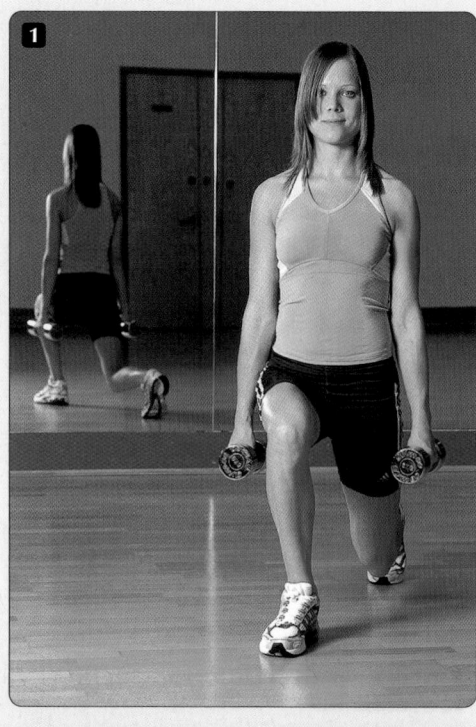

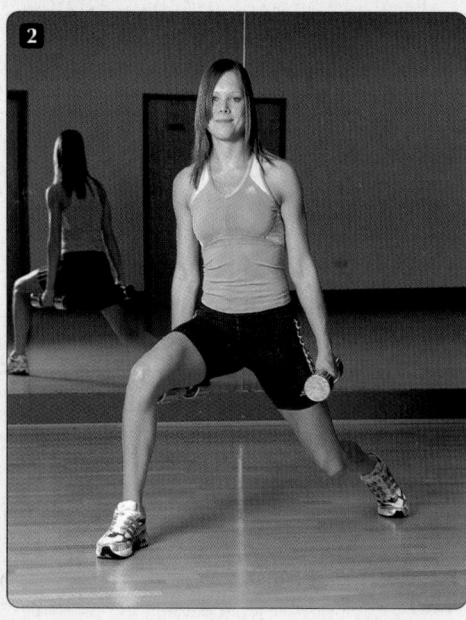

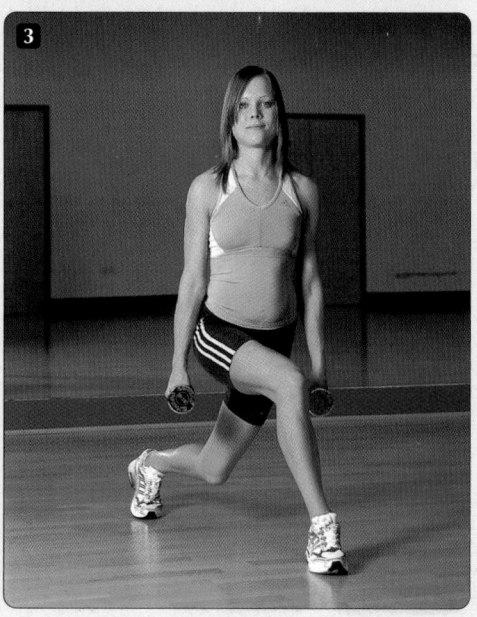

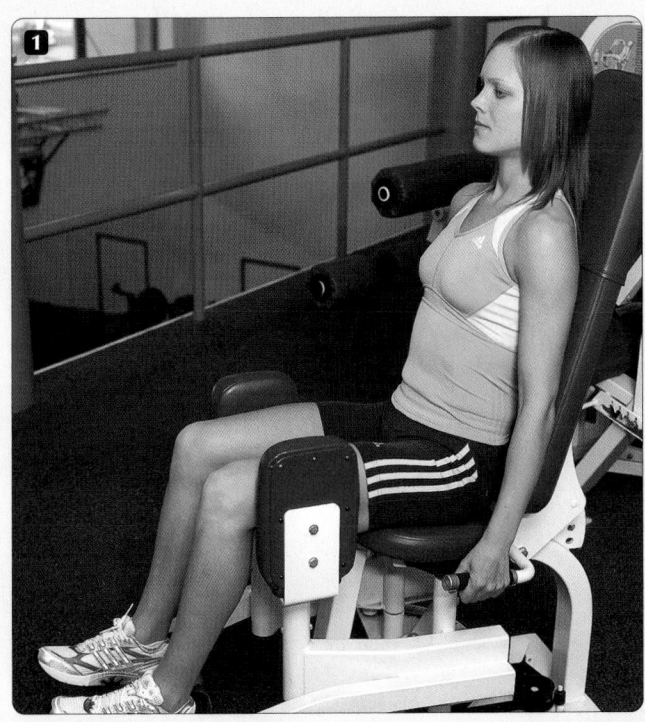

4 ABDUCTOR MACHINE

What it works:
Opening the legs against resistance works the outer thighs.

5 ADDUCTOR MACHINE

What it works:
Closing the legs against resistance works the inner thighs.

Technique pointers:
Use the fullest range of motion you can and use smooth movements – do NOT swing or 'pulse' the legs open and closed.

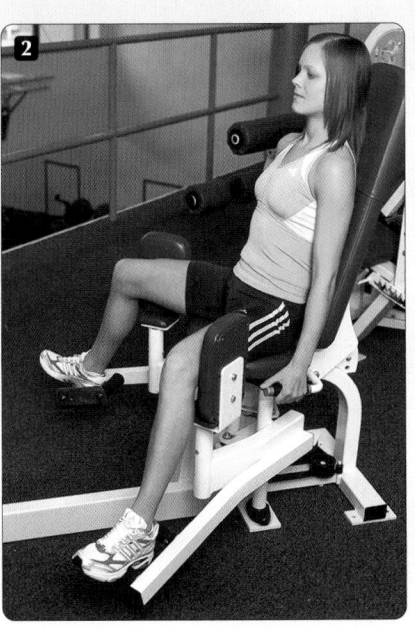

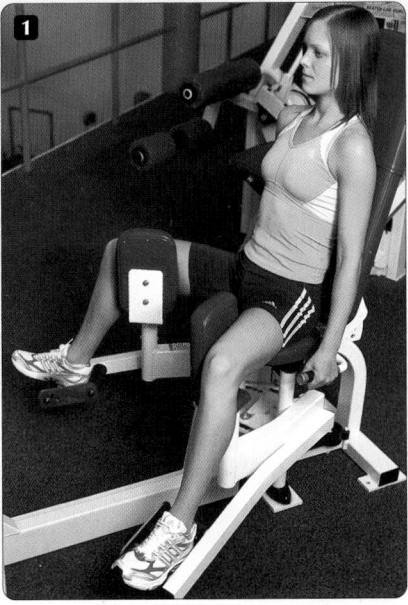

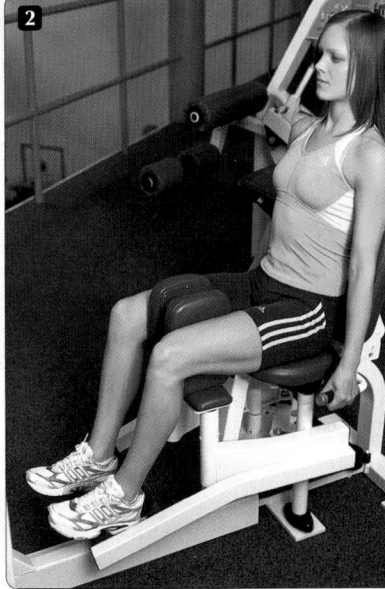

6 CHEST PRESS MACHINE

What it works:
The chest, shoulders and the back of the arms.

Technique pointers:
Whether you are using a seated or lying chest press, ensure that the handles are level with your nipple line and your elbows and wrists are in line with each other. Don't protract the shoulder blades as you straighten the arms, keep them drawn back.

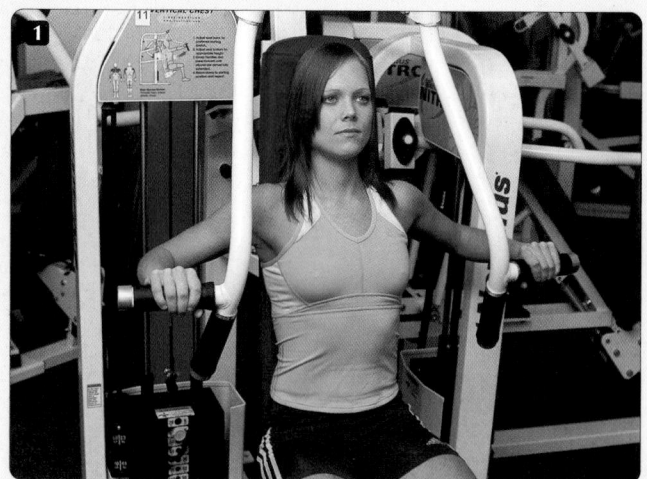

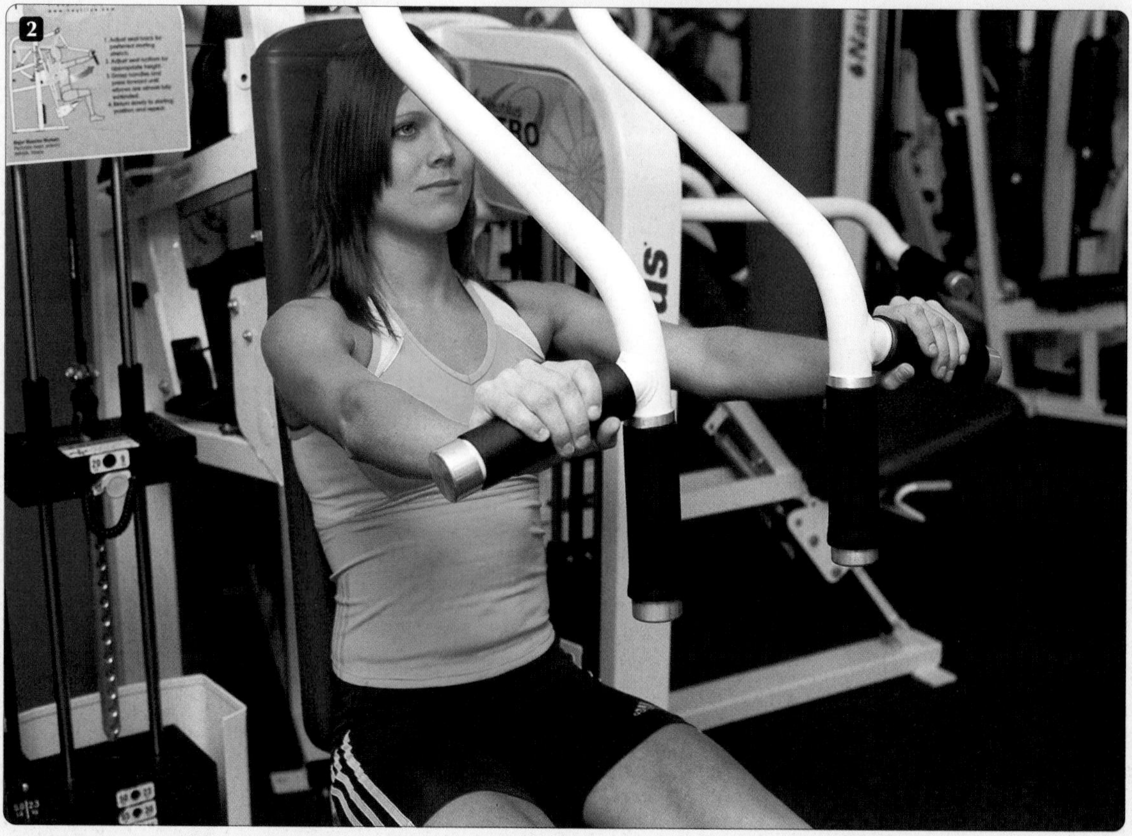

⑦ LAT PULLDOWN

What it works:
Lats, rhomboids and biceps

Technique pointers:
Use a wide, overhand grip to focus most on the lats. Think of squeezing the shoulder blades together as you lower the bar and don't allow the shoulders to ride up as you straighten the arms. You can bring the bar to the back of the neck or the front of the chest – but taking it to the back requires good shoulder flexibility. In general, the front position is preferable.

⑦ ALTERNATIVE: ASSISTED PULL-UP

Technique pointers:
The design of this machine means that the higher the weight you select, the easier the exercise. This is because the weight counterbalances your own body weight. This is an excellent exercise not just for the lats but also for the chest, shoulders, upper back and biceps. Remember to squeeze the shoulder blades together as you pull yourself up. The wide overhand grip best mimics the lat pulldown but you can experiment with a narrow 'palms up' grip to emphasise the biceps.

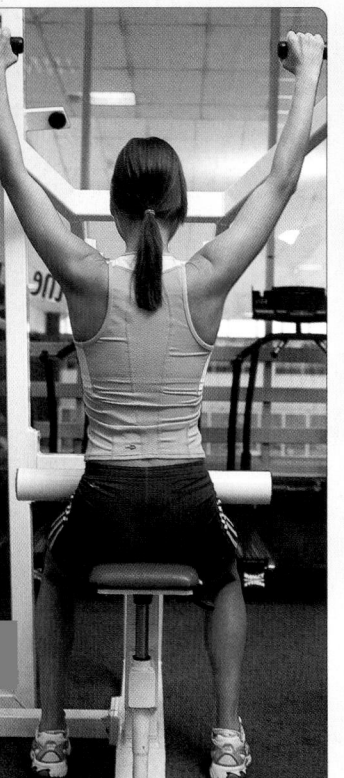

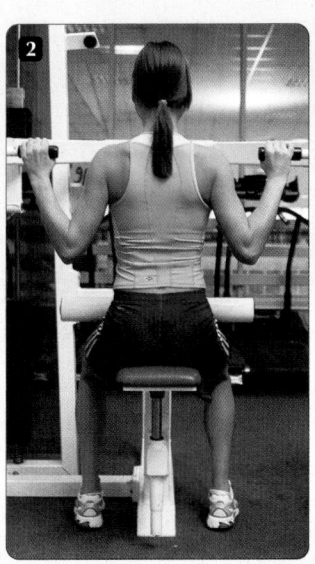

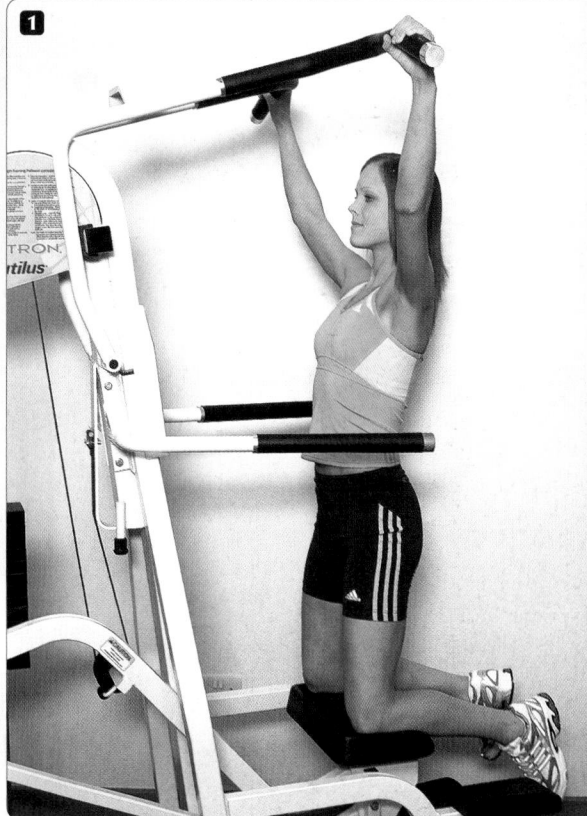

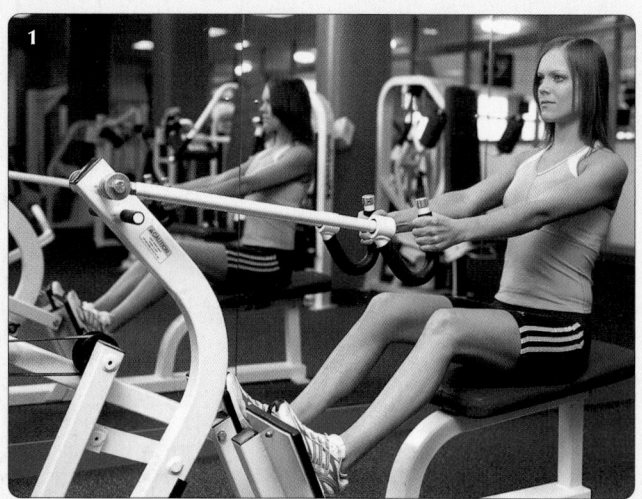

8 SEATED ROW

What it works:
The upper and middle back, the back of the shoulders and biceps.

Technique pointers:
To focus on the back muscles, use a 'palms facing' grip; to focus on the back of the shoulders, use a 'palms down' grip and bear in mind that you will need to use a lower weight for this smaller muscle group. Don't allow the back to arch or move backwards as you bend the arms. Instead, focus on opening the chest and squeezing the shoulder blades together.

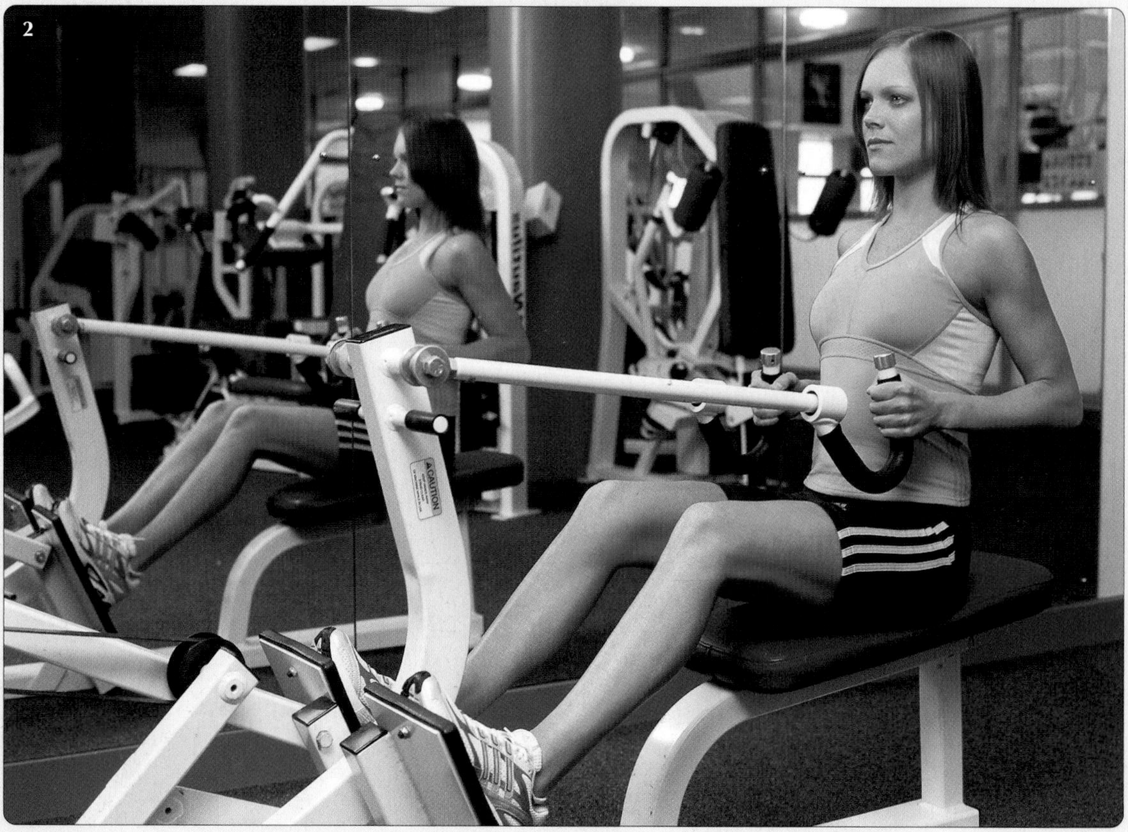

9 SHOULDER PRESS MACHINE

What it works:
The shoulders, triceps and chest.

Technique pointers:
Sit tall and engage your core while you do this exercise. Don't over-arch the back to help you straighten the arms.

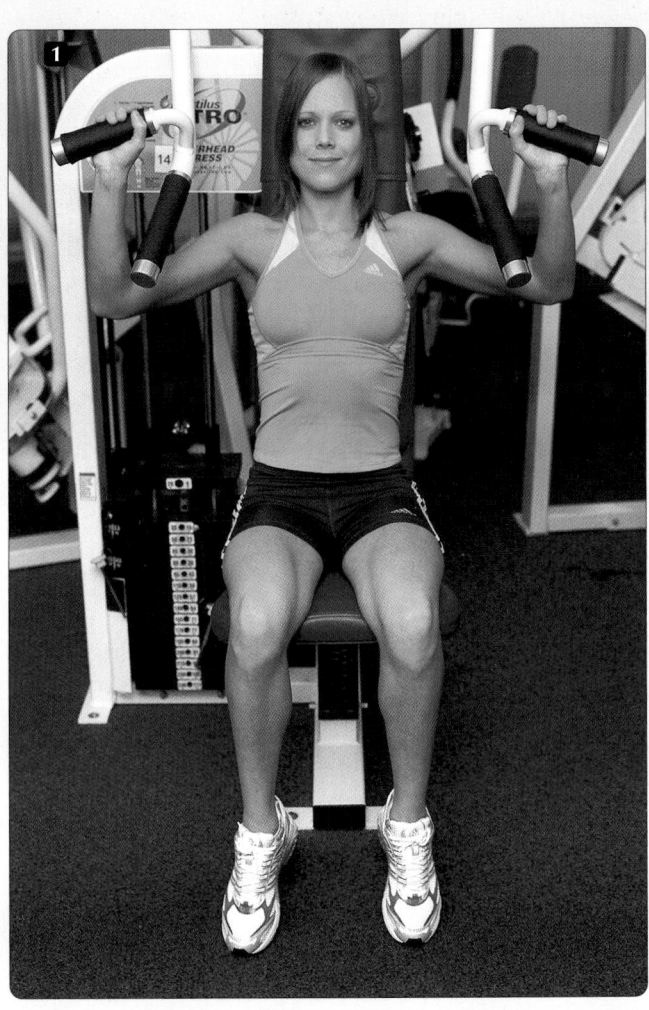

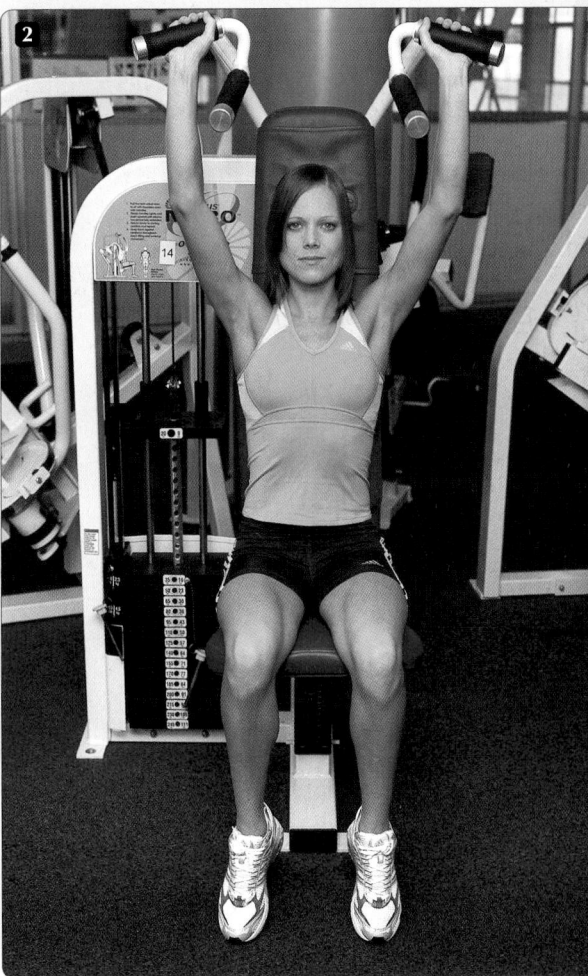

⑩ TRICEPS PUSHDOWN

What it works:
Triceps.

Technique pointers:
You can use a straight bar, angled bar or rope to perform a pushdown. Start with your elbows close into your sides, forearms perpendicular to the floor and wrists in line with forearms. Come back to this position between each rep – don't allow the arms to bend further than 90 degrees.

⑩ ALTERNATIVE: ASSISTED DIP MACHINE

Technique pointers:
As with the assisted pull-up, the higher the weight you select the easier the exercise. Don't 'sink' into the shoulders as you bend the arms – keep them back and down, and only lower until you reach a 90-degree angle at the elbow. Keep the body properly aligned and core engaged.

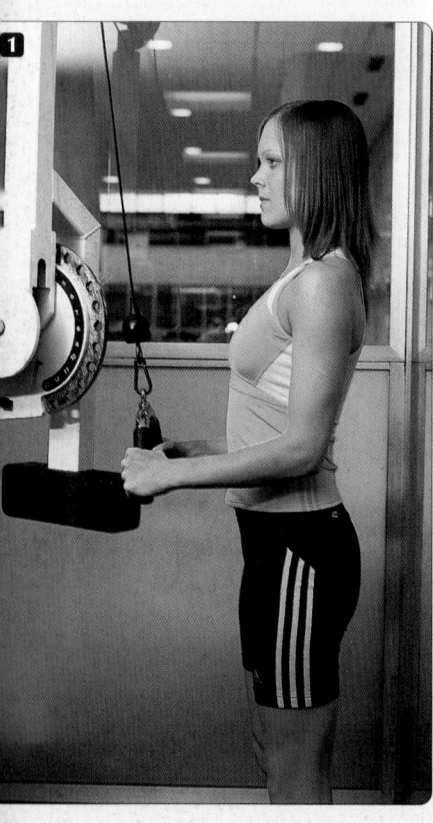
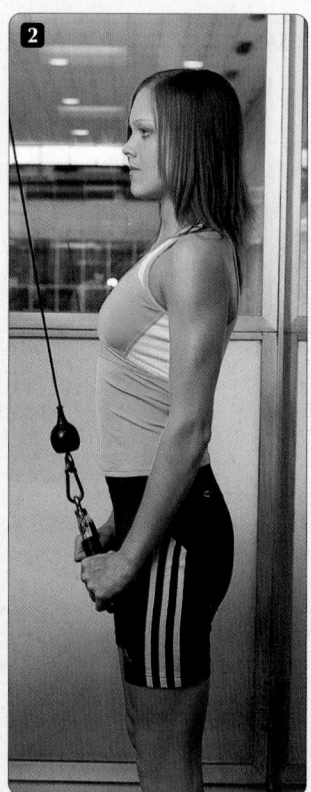
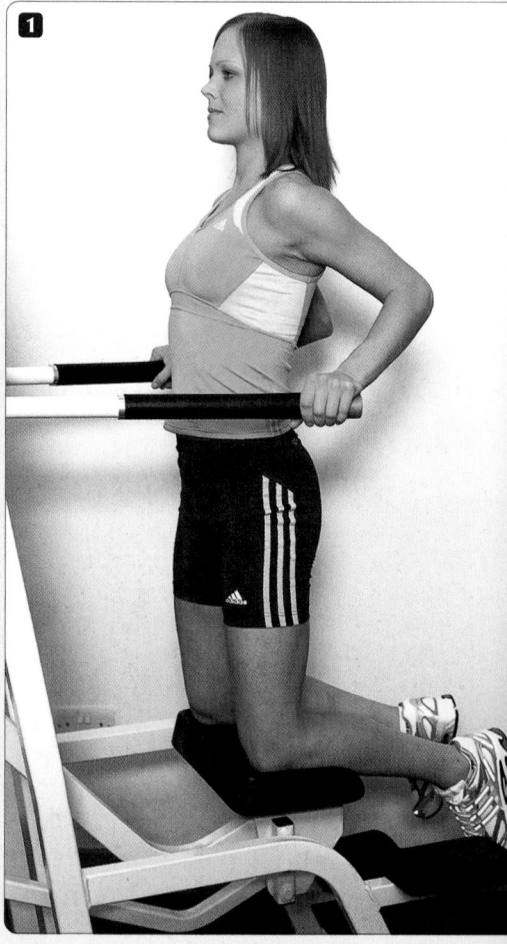

11 BICEPS CURL

What it works:
The biceps in the front of the upper arm. (This free-weights version of this exercise is more effective than using a biceps curl machine.)

How to do it:
1 Stand with a weight in each hand, your arms relaxed down by your sides, palms facing each other.

2 Either simultaneously or alternately, bend the elbows and rotate the arms, to bring the weight up to the front of the shoulder with the palm facing the shoulder. Pause, lower and repeat.

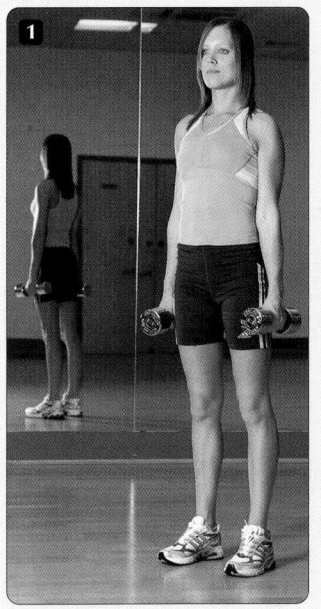
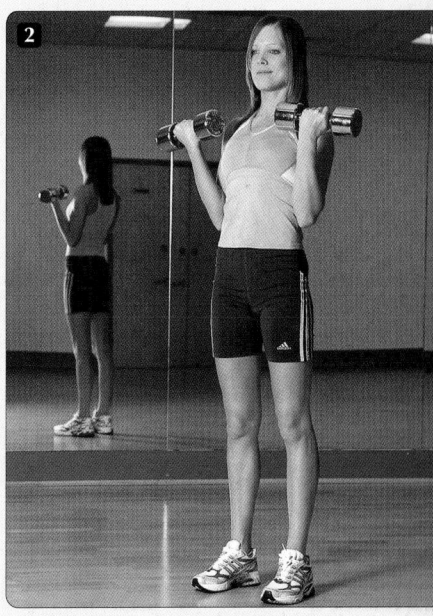

12 AB CURL MACHINE

What it works:
Rectus abdominis and obliques.

Technique pointers:
It's really important to get your position correct in this exercise, so experiment with the seat height and pad position. Don't 'lead' with the head as you curl the torso forward and remember to engage the core. If you don't feel you 'fit' the machine properly, then substitute this move with one of the ab exercises from the Targeted Toning sequence on page 106.

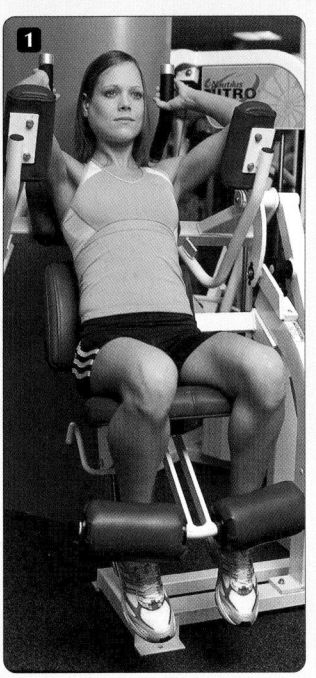
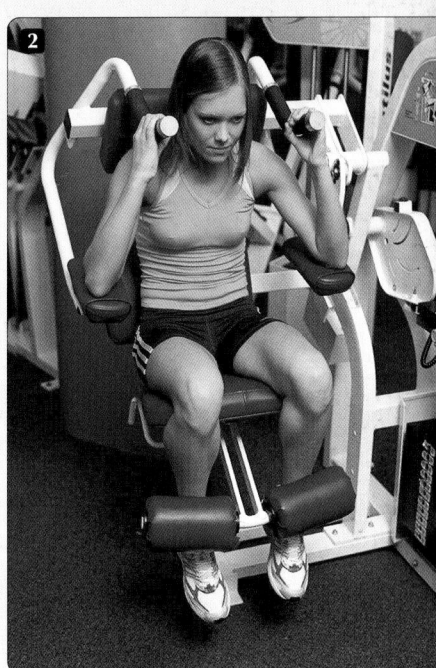

Home workout

DOING THE HOME WORKOUT

- Warm up first and wear supportive trainers.

- Clear some space before you begin your workout and gather all the equipment you'll need. Have a mirror in the room so that you can monitor your technique and body position.

- You will need an exercise ball, a resistance tube, a chair, an exercise mat, a medicine ball, a balance pad or wobble board and some dumbbells.

- Do the exercises in the order shown.

- Try to breathe out on the effort and in on the release – if you can't get the hang of that, then breathe freely throughout.

- Some of these exercises use no weight but a change in body position can make the exercise easier or harder.

1 KNEE DRIVE WITH DUMBBELLS

What it works:
Glutes, quads, hamstrings, calves, adductors and abductors.

How to do it:
1 Stand with your feet under your hipbones with a dumbbell in each hand. Drive up with the right knee, bringing it up to the chest...

2 Then swing it back into a lunge position and immediately drive back up from the lunge into the next repetition. Then swap sides.

To progress:
3 Stand in front of a step between shin and knee height (the higher, the tougher) with a dumbbell in each hand.

4 Place your right foot fully on the step and then drive up, bringing the left knee to the chest as you straighten the right leg. Pause, then lower and repeat until the end of the set.

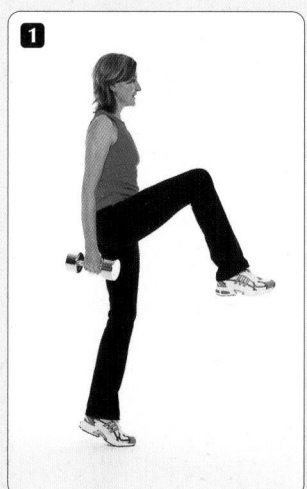
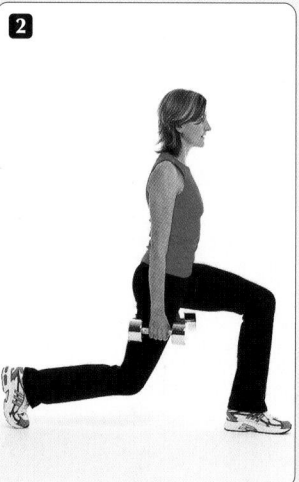
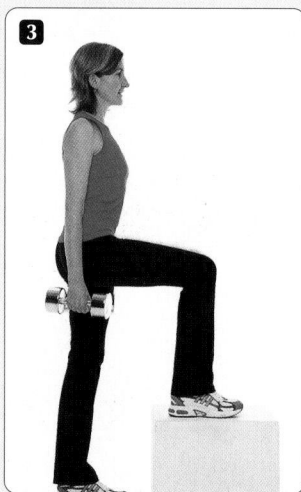
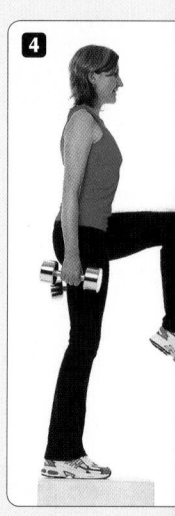

2 SQUAT WITH MEDICINE BALL

What it works:
Glutes, quads and hamstrings.

How to do it:
1 Stand with your feet below your hipbones and a medicine ball clasped to your chest.

2 Engage the core and inhale as you lower your bottom back and down (as if you were going to sit on a stool). Keep your knees directly over your feet – don't let them roll in or out. When your thighs are parallel to the floor – or as close as is comfortable for you – pause and straighten up, pressing up through the heels as you push back up to a standing position.

To progress:
3 Perform the squat on a balance pad, wobble board or core board to add an element of instability. Alternatively, use a heavier ball or swap the ball for dumbbells, held at your sides.

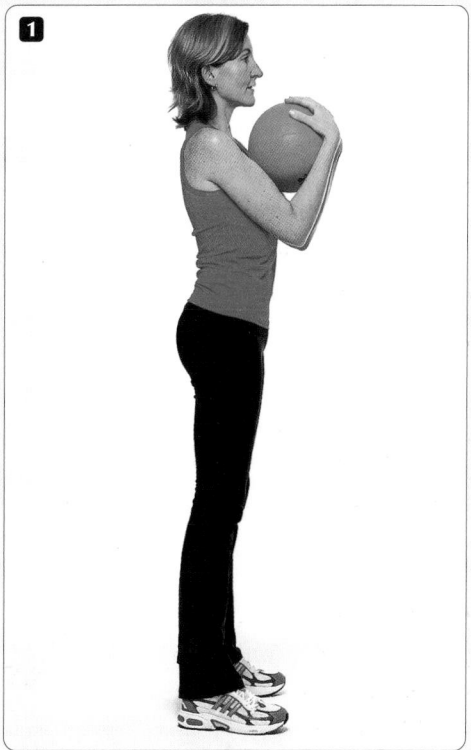

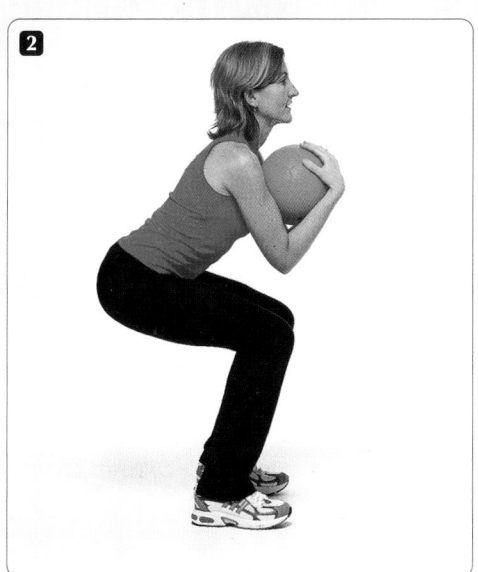

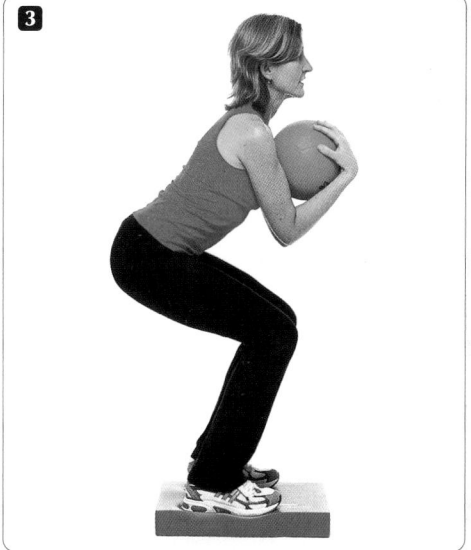

3 SINGLE LEG SQUAT

What it works:
Quads, glutes and hamstrings.

How to do it:
1 Stand tall, next to a support and take the foot furthest from the support off the floor.

2 On one leg, slowly lower your bottom back and down, keeping your weight on the mid-point of the foot, at the back of the arch, and ensuring the knee bends directly over the fourth toe. Allow the torso to tip forward as you bend but keep the back long and straight. This is a tough exercise and no weight is necessary. Swap sides.

To progress:
Increase the reps or slow the movement down.

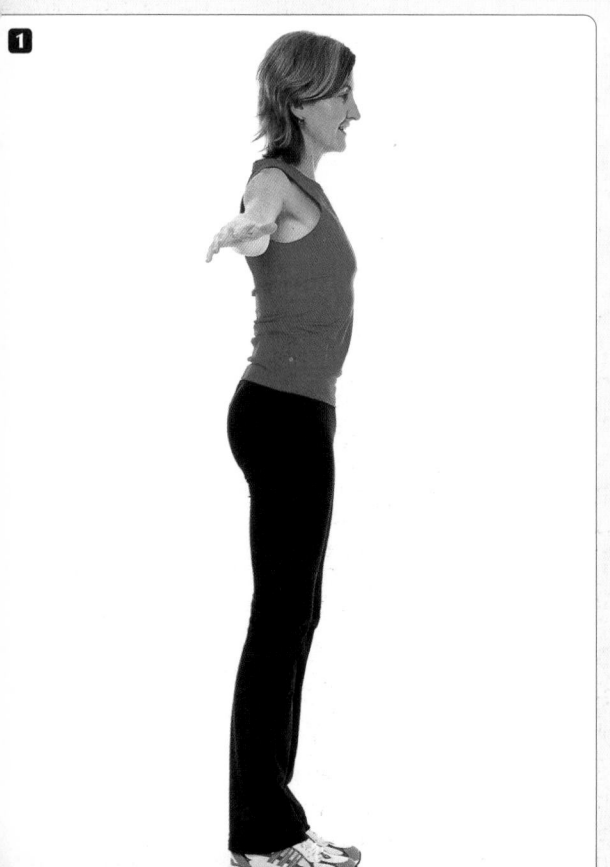

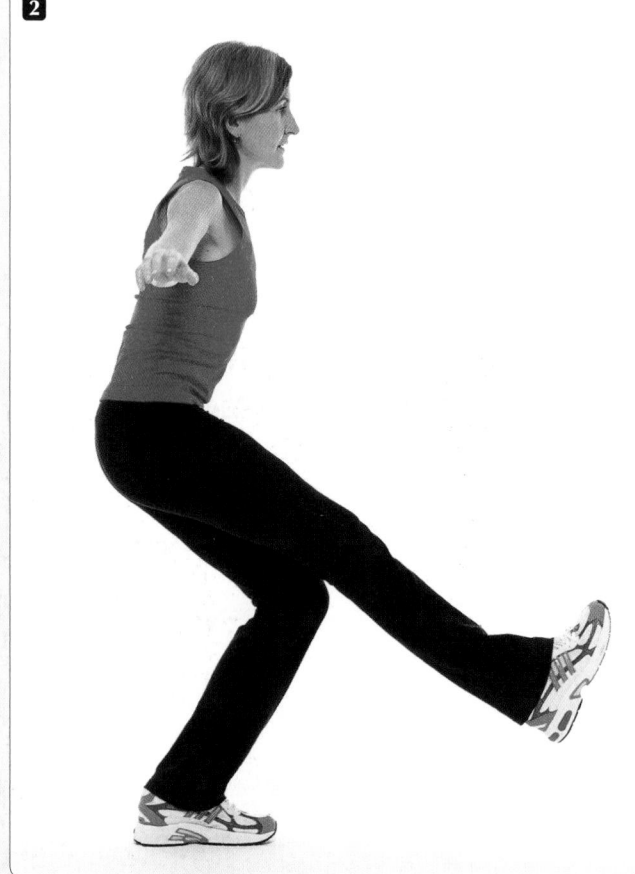

4 SIDE STEP-UP

What it works:
The hips, thighs, hamstrings and glutes.

How to do it
1 Stand side on to a step, quite close to it, with a weight in each hand. Step up with the foot closest to the step…

2 …following with the other foot. Then step down with that foot and follow with the first foot. Make sure the knee is aligned over the toes and keep the body centred as you step up. Repeat on the other side.

To progress:
Increase the weight.

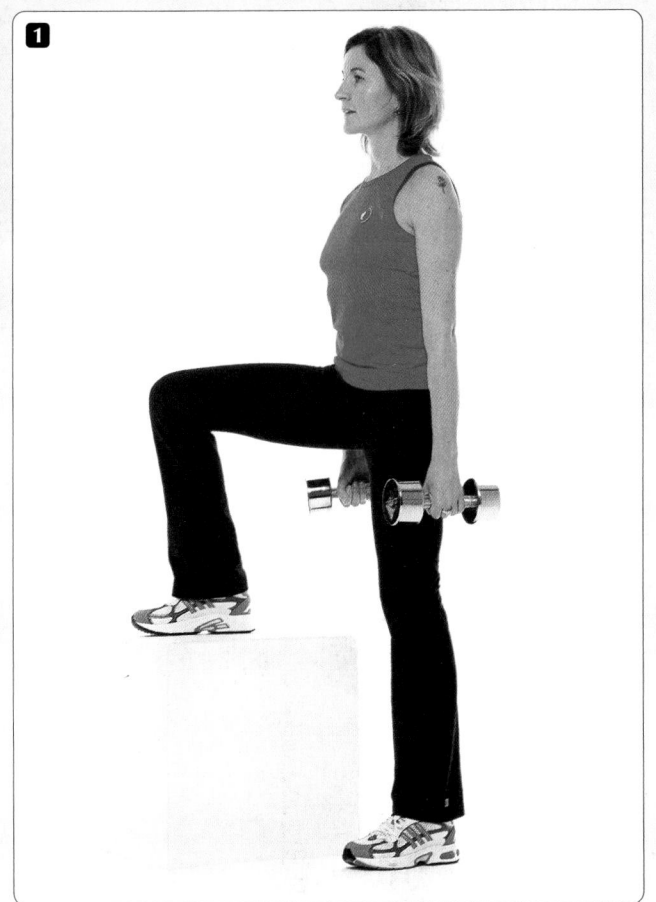

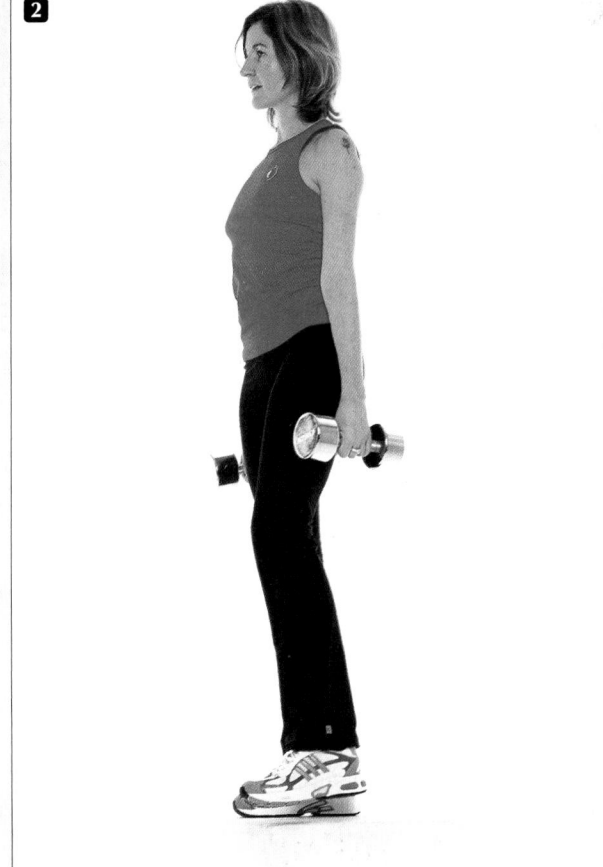

5 HAMSTRING CURL ON BALL

What it works:
Hamstrings, glutes and lower back.

How to do it:
1 Lie face up with your heels on an exercise ball, legs straight and arms by your sides.

2 Lift yourself up so that your body forms a straight line from head to heels and then, bending your knees, roll the ball in towards your bottom. Pause, then slowly extend it again.

To progress:
3 First, try doing the exercise with your arms crossed over your chest to challenge stability. Then progress to rolling one leg in at a time.

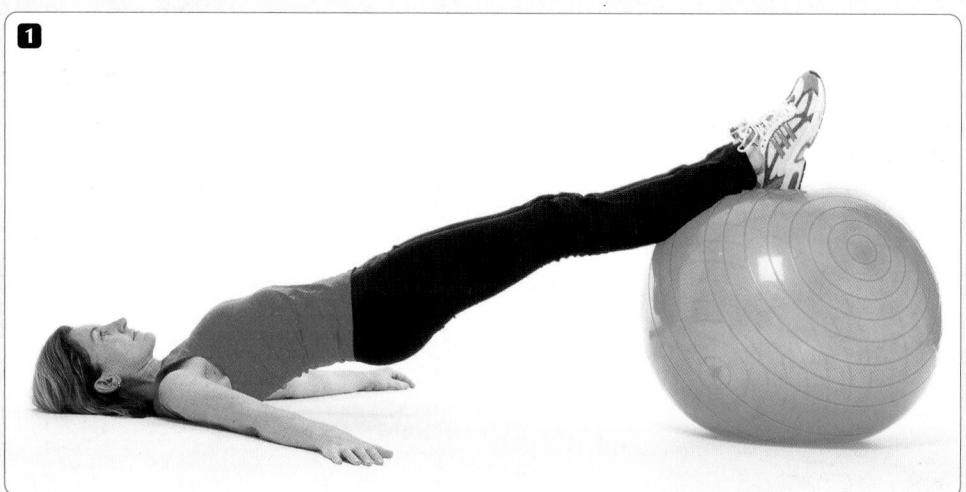

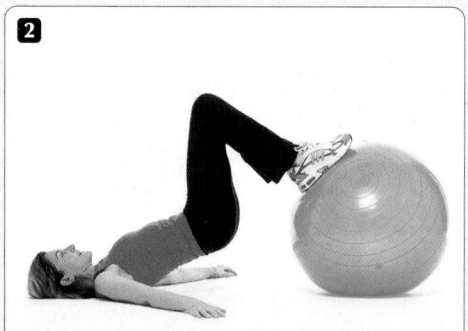

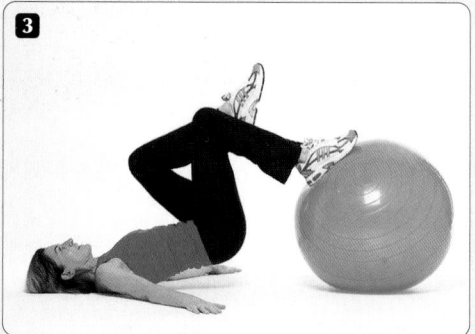

6 PUSH UP

What it works:
The chest, shoulders, triceps and abdominals.

How to do it:
1 Stand in front of a surface somewhere between waist and knee height (the higher, the easier) and place your hands on the support. Form a straight line from head to toe, with your arms straight and shoulder-width apart or a little wider, abdominals contracted and head in line with the spine. Lower the body towards the support by bending the arms. When your arms reach a right angle, pause and straighten to repeat.

To progress:
2 Try full push-ups on the floor or place your lower legs on an exercise ball.

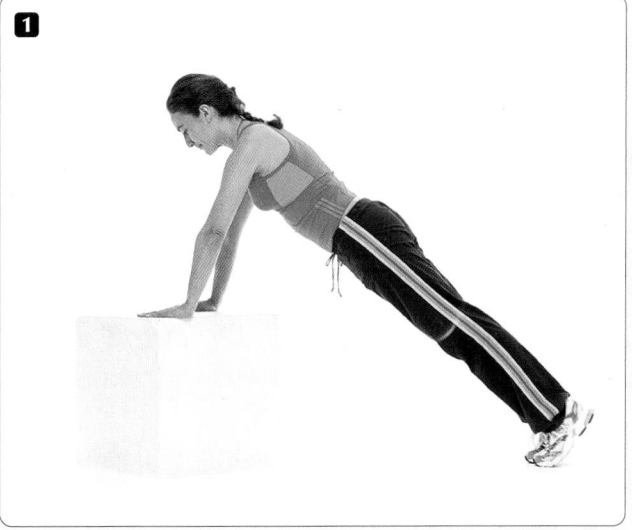

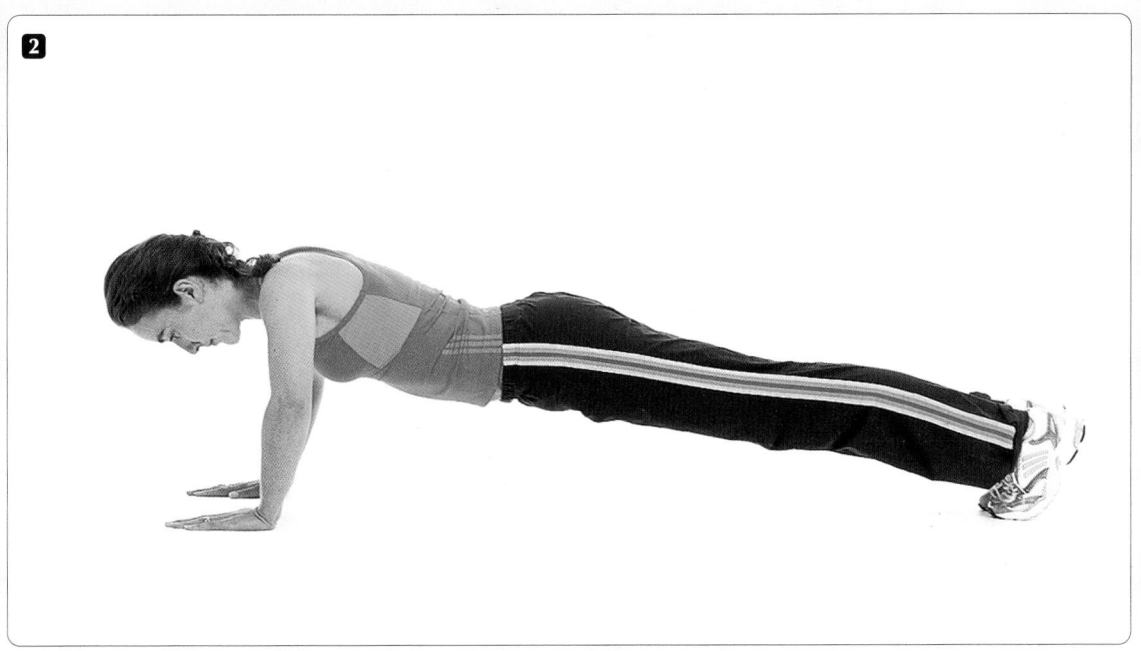

7 ANGLED PULL-UP

What it works:
Lats, rhomboids, shoulders and biceps.

How to do it:
1 Find a sturdy surface that you can get underneath and hold on to (one of those bike parking rails is ideal). Shift underneath the surface and place your feet flat on the floor, legs slightly bent.

2 Grip the surface with an underhand grip and pull yourself up towards it by bending the arms and drawing the shoulder blades back. Pause then lower.

To progress:
Use a lower support.

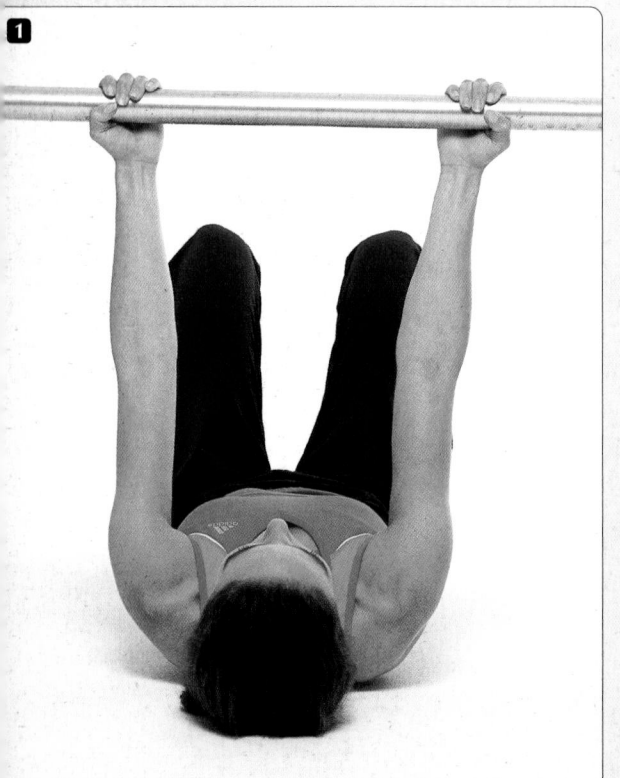

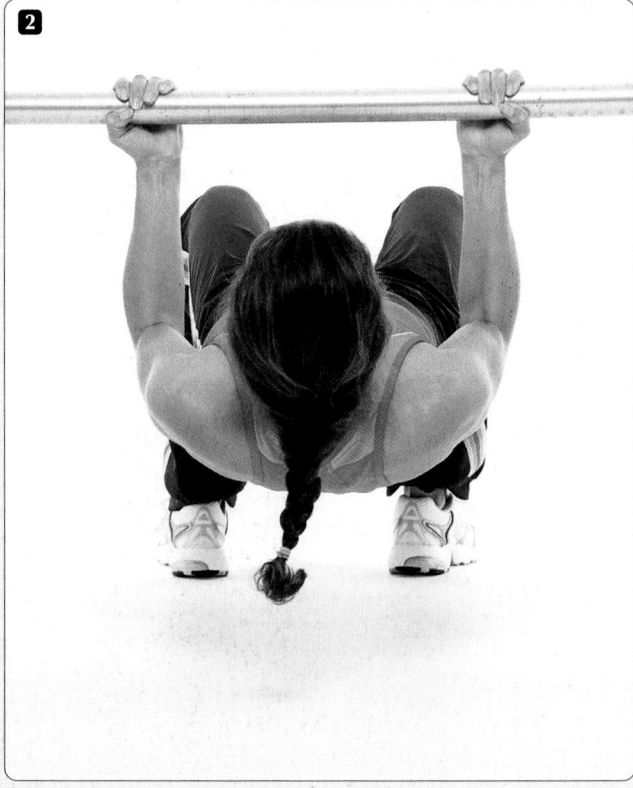

8 OVERHEAD PRESS

What it works:
The shoulders, triceps and chest.

How to do it:
1 Sit on an upright bench or chair with your back straight and a weight or an end of resistance tubing in each hand, resting on the shoulders with palms facing each other.

2 Extend the arms over the head, allowing them to rotate so that when the arms are straight, the palms are facing the front. You should be able to see your arms in your peripheral vision as they are raised – don't take the arms behind the line of the head.

To progress:
Increase the resistance or use a heavier weight.

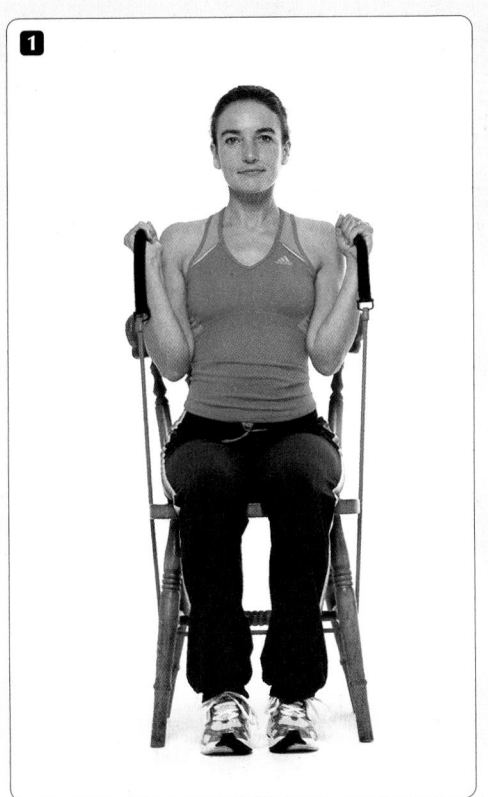

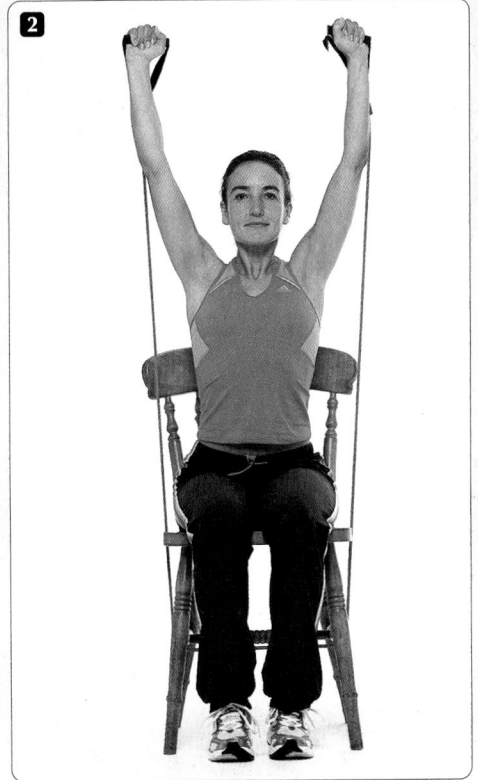

9 BICEPS CURL

What it works:
The biceps in the front of the upper arm.

How to do it:
1 Sit with a weight or an end of resistance tubing (thread the tube under the chair) in each hand, your arms relaxed down by your sides, palms facing each other.

2 Bend the elbows and rotate the arms, to bring the weight up to the front of the shoulder with the palm facing the shoulder. Pause, lower and repeat.

To progress:
Increase the resistance or use a heavier weight.

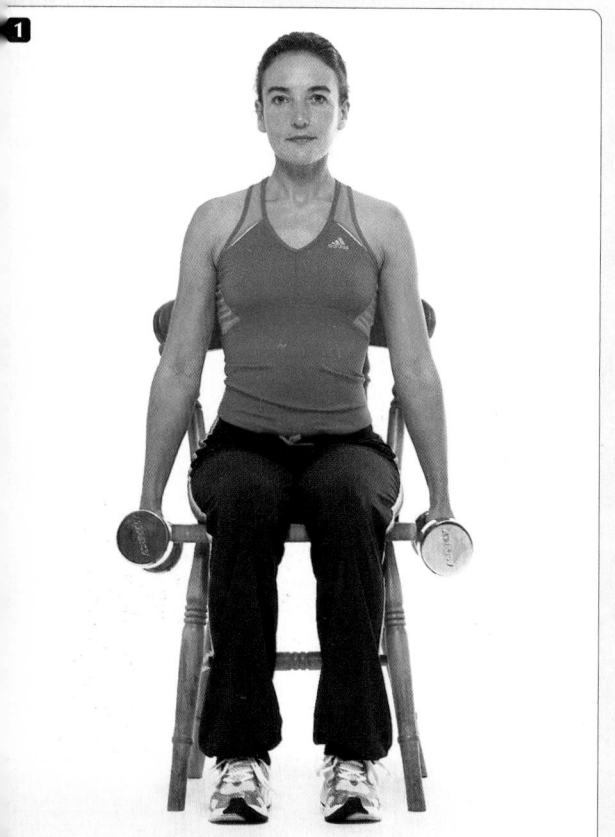

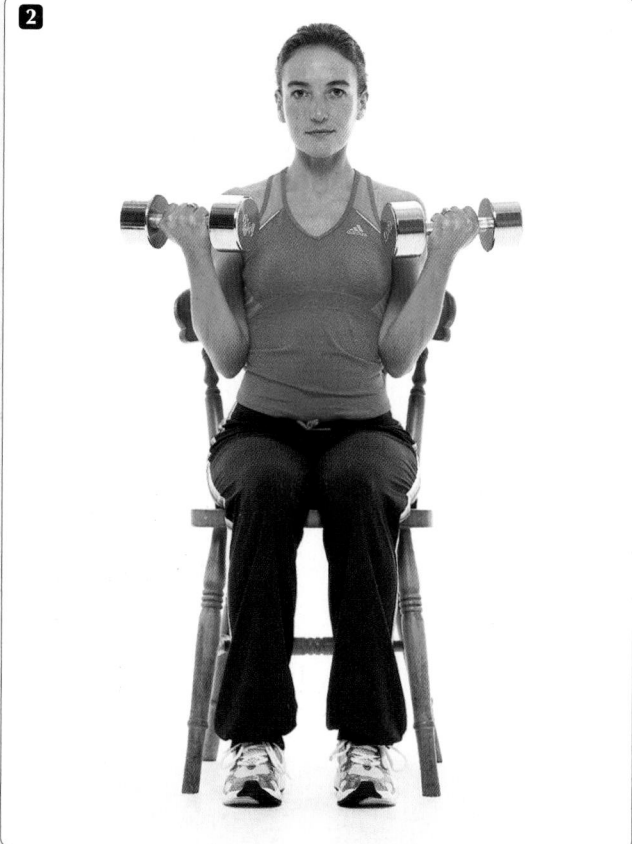

10 DIPS

What it works:
Triceps, chest and shoulder blade retractors.

How to do it:
1 Sit at the front of a sturdy chair with hands on the edge, fingers facing forward. Before you start, depress and retract the shoulder blades.

2 Now shift your bottom off the front of the chair so that your weight is supported by your arms. With your knees bent and feet flat on the floor, lower your bottom by bending the arms. Don't go beyond 90 degrees, and stop when your shoulders start to hunch up or roll forward. Pause and straighten.

To progress:
You can do this exercise with a medicine ball or weight over your thighs.

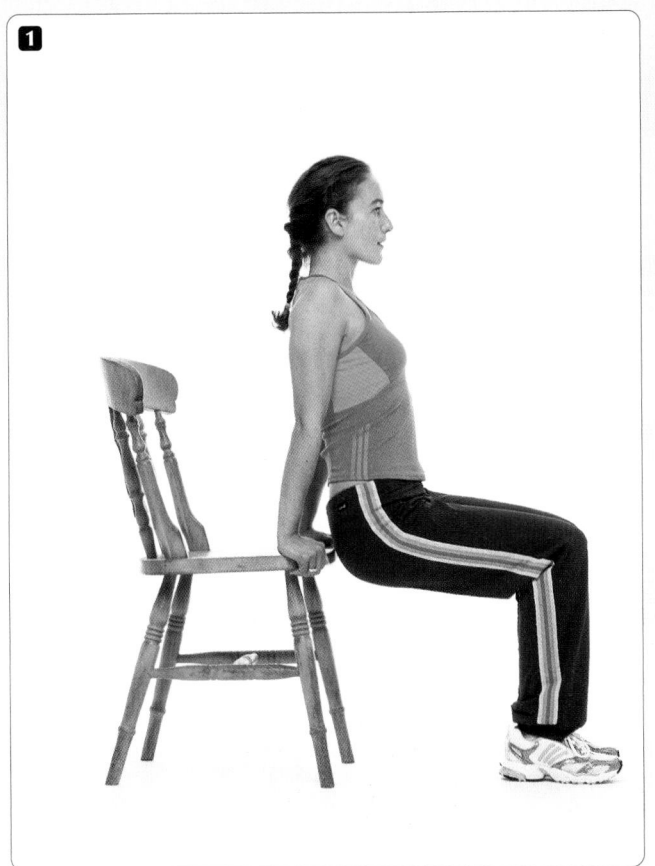

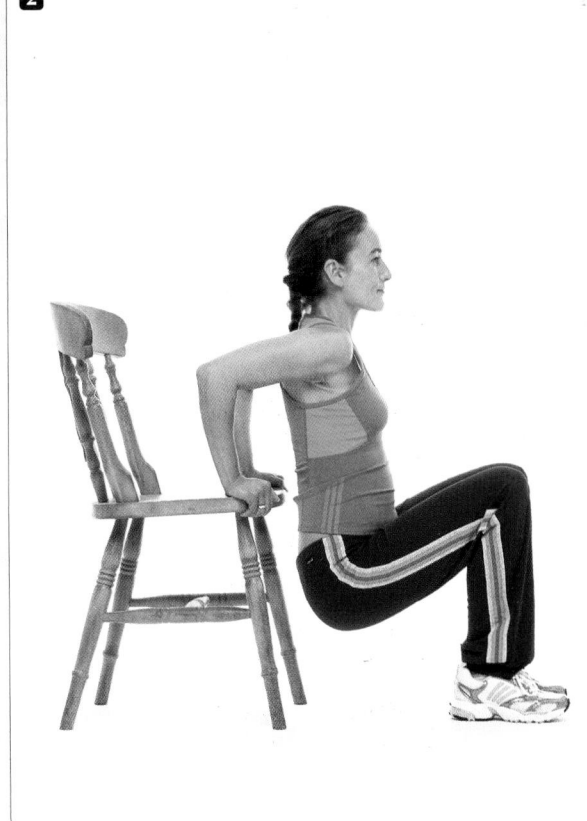

11 BACK EXTENSION ON BALL

What it works:
The lower and middle back and glutes.

How to do it:
1 Lie face down on an exercise ball with your feet anchored against the join of the wall and the floor. Adjust your position until your torso is lower than your hips, and put your hands beside your head.

2 Now, using the back and butt muscles, raise the torso up until it is just beyond forming a straight line with the legs. Hold, then lower and repeat.

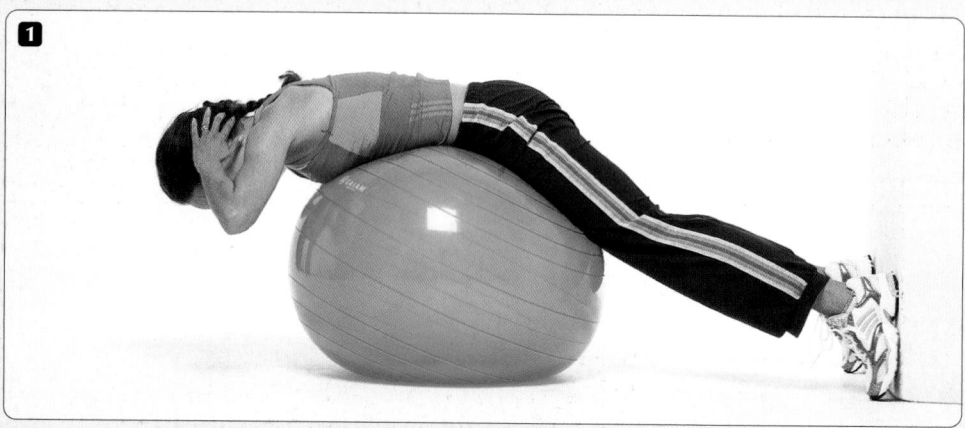

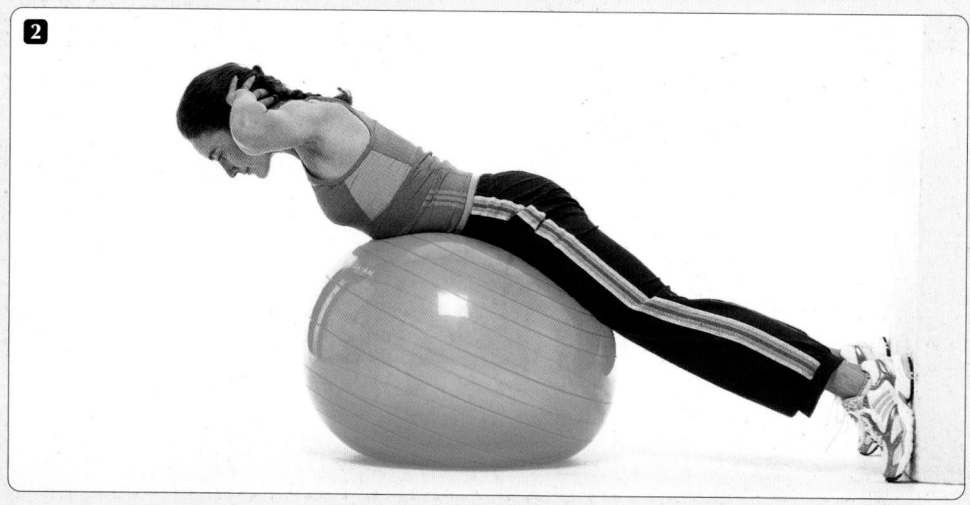

12 BALL ROLL-IN

What it works:
The core stabilisers, abdominals, chest, front of shoulders, upper arms and hip flexors.

How to do it:
1 Lie face down over an exercise ball, and shunt forwards until just your shins are on the ball, and your weight is supported on your hands, arms shoulder width apart. Contract the abdominals and tilt the pelvis so your back is in a straight line with your legs.

2 Now curl the ball in towards your chest by contracting the abs and rolling the ball towards your torso with your lower legs. Hips should never be below shoulder height – keep your

shoulders drawn back. The movement should be slow and controlled, taking 4–5 seconds each way.

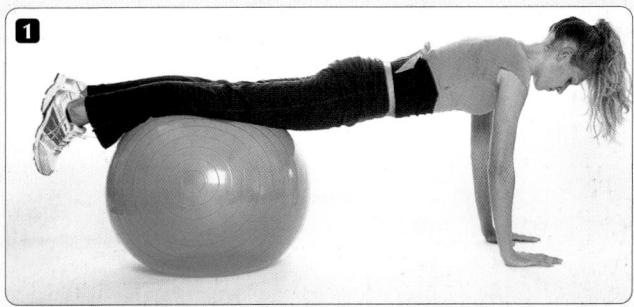

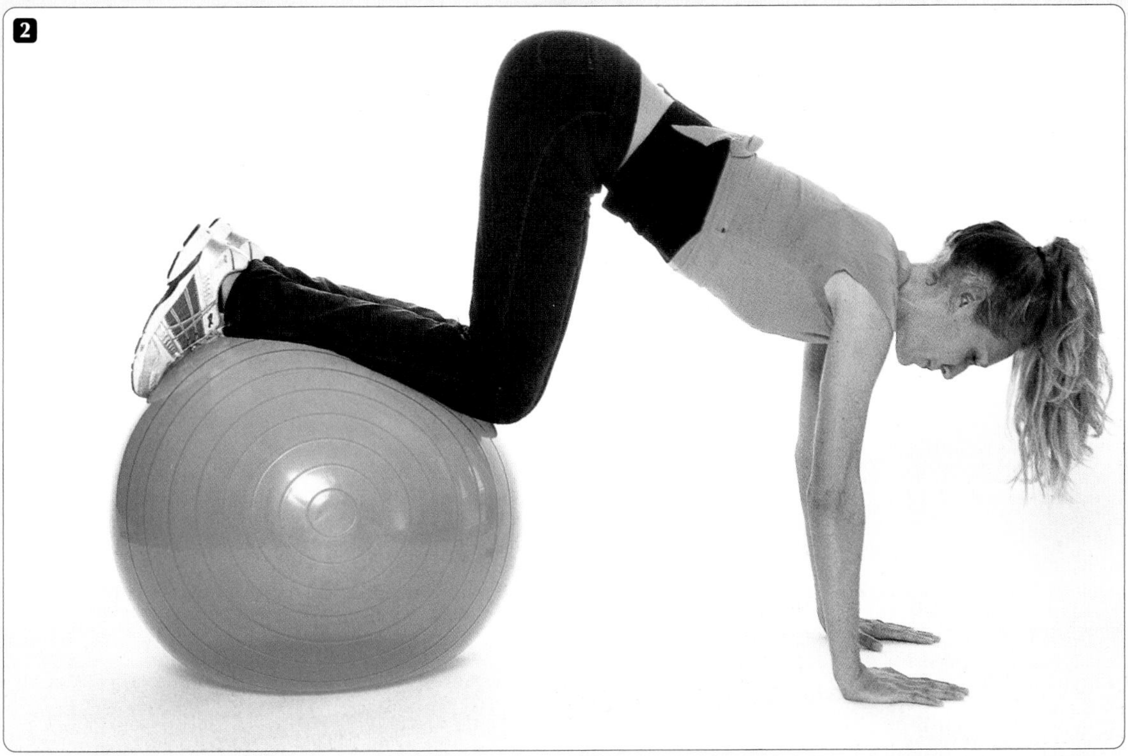

1

2

Targeted toning

Any of the exercises below can be substituted for those in the preceding workouts for variety, or in case you don't have the relevant equipment. Alternatively, if you want to home in on a particular muscle group, you can add some or all the targeted toning exercises for that area to your workout.

ABS

1 BALL SIDE RAISE

1 Anchor your feet against the join between the wall and the floor and lie sideways over an exercise ball. The top foot should be in front of the bottom foot and the legs a little bent. Ensure your body is in a straight line.

2 Place your hands beside your ears and, using the muscles at the side of the waist, raise the torso up. It doesn't need to go very far.

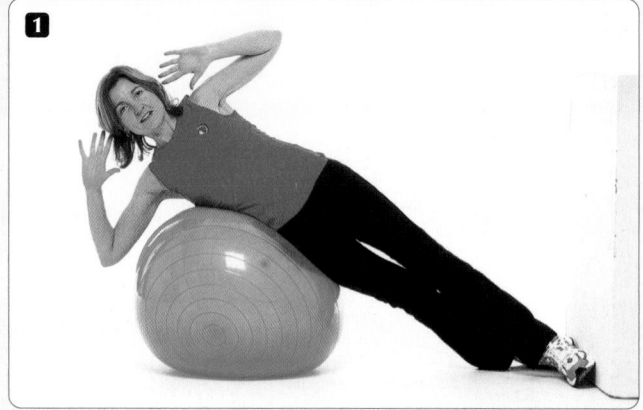

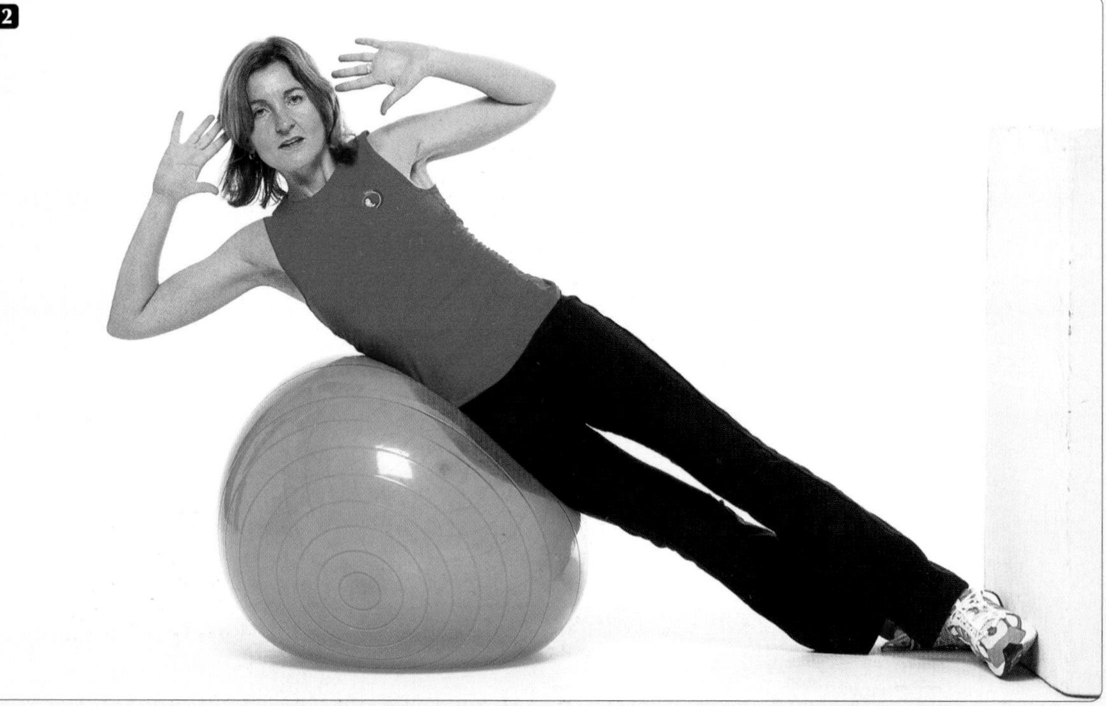

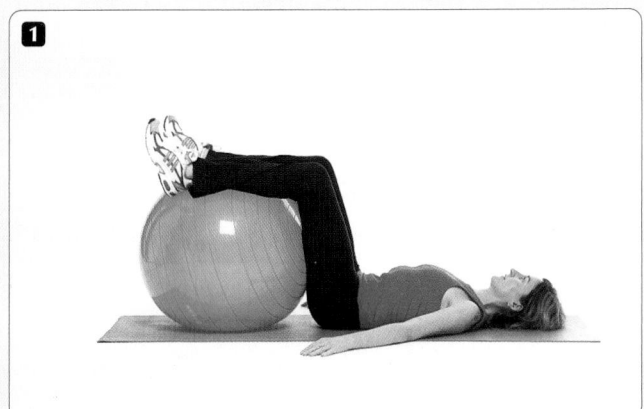

1

2 BALL REVERSE CURL

1 Lie on a mat with an exercise ball between your calves and the back of your thighs.

2 Engage the core and, gripping the ball with your legs, roll the ball off the floor and towards your chest. Do not use momentum to raise the ball – keep the movements slow and controlled.

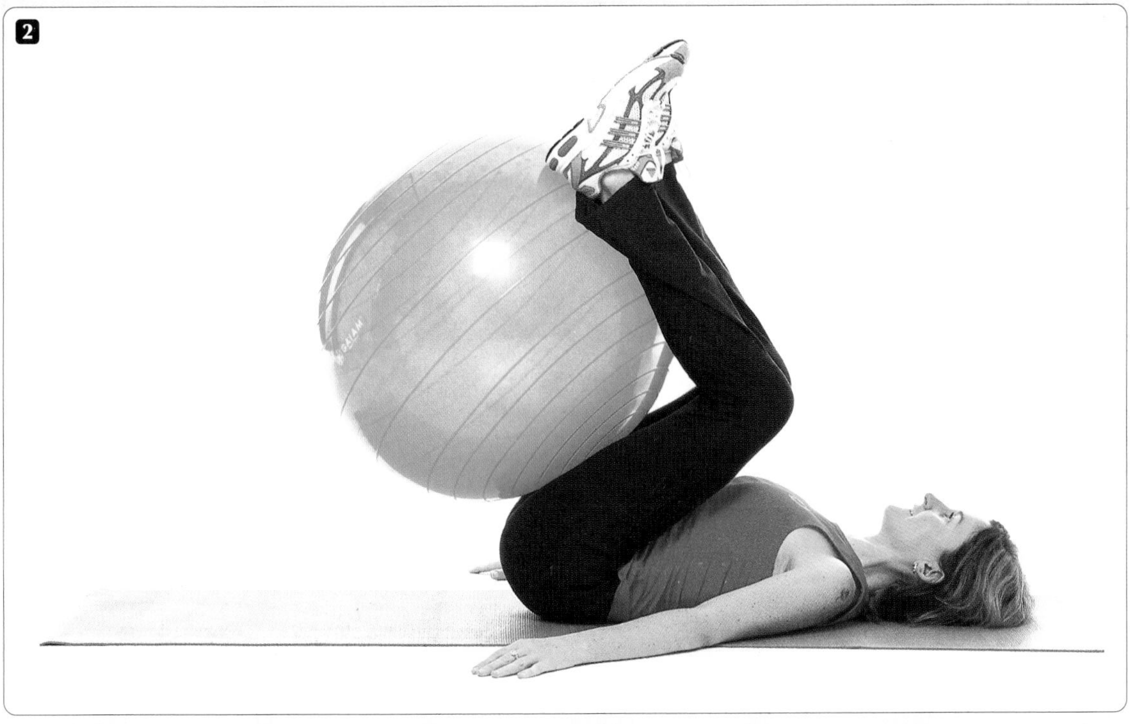

2

3 LEG LOWERING

1 Lie on your back with both legs extended straight up in the air. Engage the core.

2 Slowly lower the legs away from the torso, only as far as you can without arching the back. As soon as that happens, draw the legs back to the start, focusing on using the lower tummy to do so, and repeat. You can do this with your legs 30–50cm from a wall, to prevent yourself going too far. If you like, put your fingertips (palms down) under your lower back and use the point at which the back begins to peel away from the fingers as your cue to raise the legs back up.

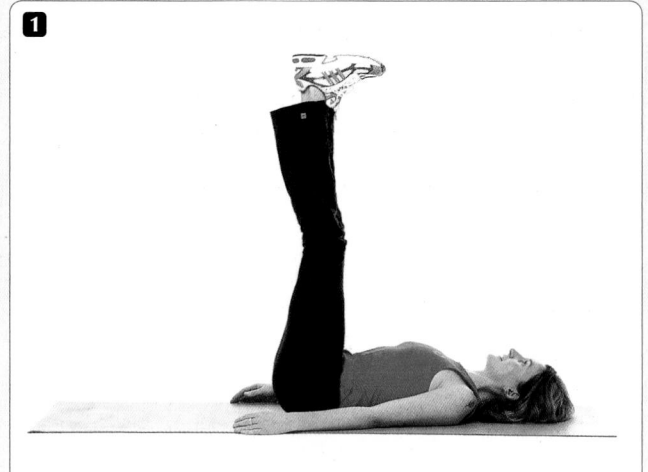

1

2

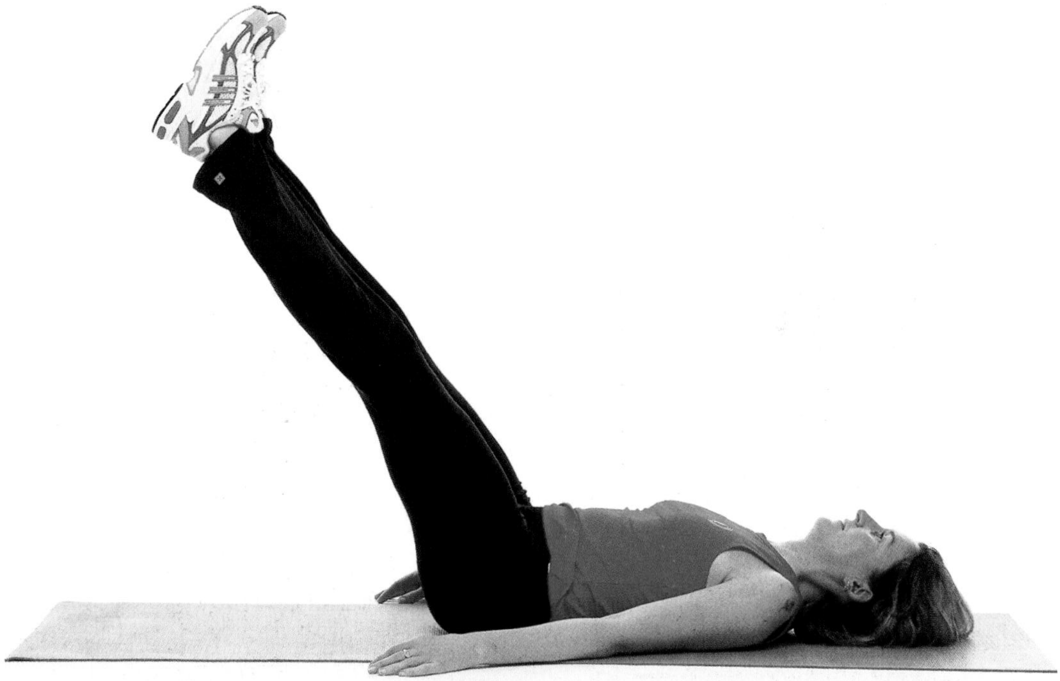

4 BALL KNEELING BALANCE

1 Stand in front of an exercise ball. If you are new to this exercise, either get a friend to stand on the opposite side of the ball to help you balance, or have a wall the other side of the ball which you can hold on to if necessary.

2 In a swift movement, put your hands on the ball and rock your body forward to place both knees simultaneously on the ball. Then roll the pelvis forward so that you are in a kneeling up position and take your hands away. You need to constantly adjust your body position to stay balanced – really focus on using the abs, pelvic floor muscles and glutes to help you.

To progress:
Once you can hold the pose for 30 seconds or so try making tiny figures of eight with the ball, using your core muscles to initiate the movement. When that's easy, try balancing with your eyes shut!

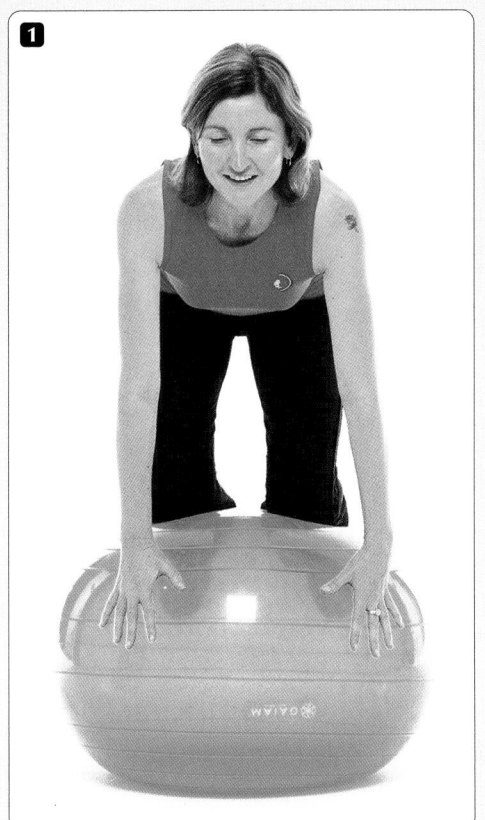

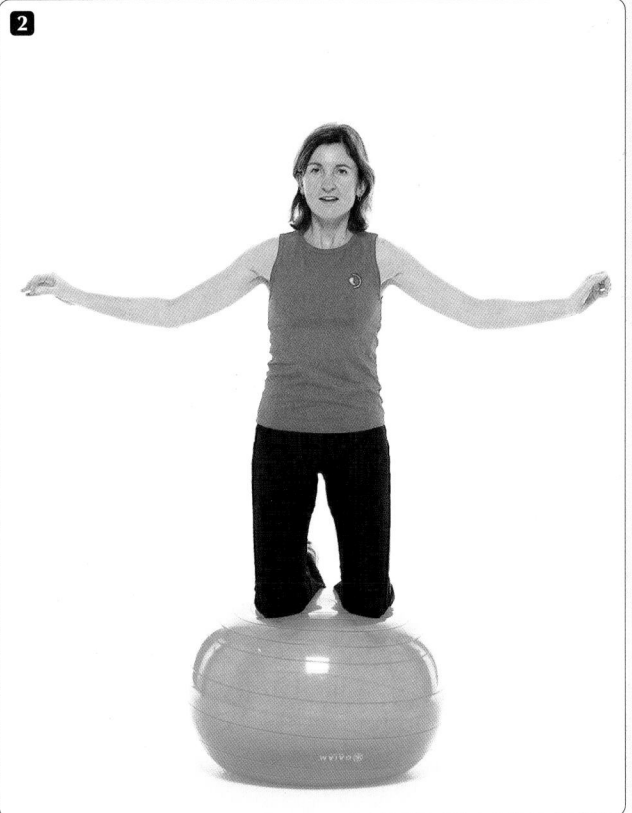

INNER THIGHS

1 SUMO SQUAT

1 Stand with your feet together.

2 Take a large step to the side with knees and hips opening out over the toes. Step back to the start position and repeat on the other side.

To progress:
3 Add a weighted bar across the shoulders or hold a dumbbell in each hand.

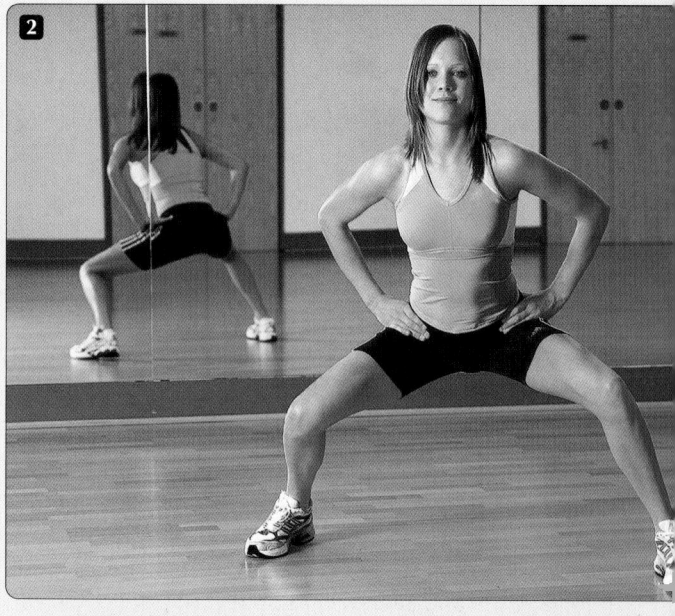

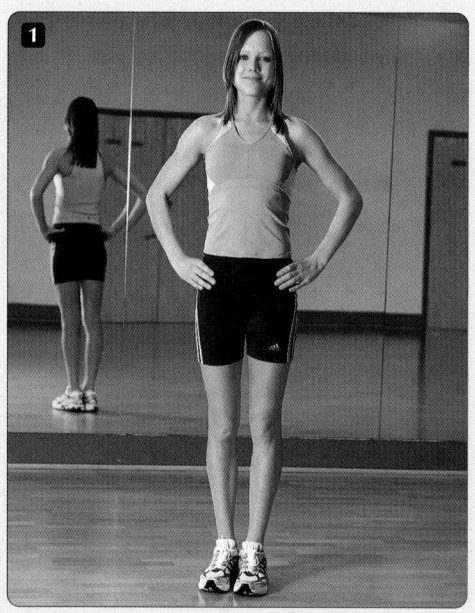

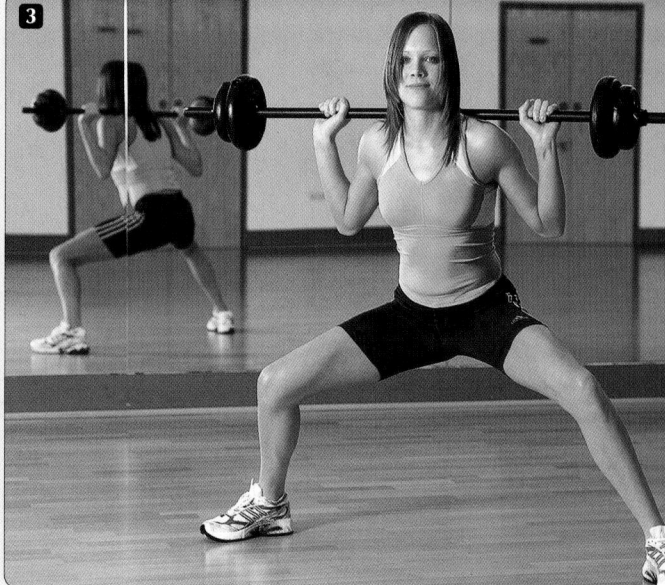

2 LEG CROSSOVER

1 Hook one end of a resistance band around something sturdy and loop the other end around your left leg. Shuffle away from the attachment point until there is enough tension in the band, and your left leg is lifted out to the side.

2 Now bring your left leg in towards the centre, taking it just across the front of the right leg, toes facing directly forward. Do not allow the hip of the supporting leg to 'dip' and keep the core engaged. Release the leg back to the start position and repeat.

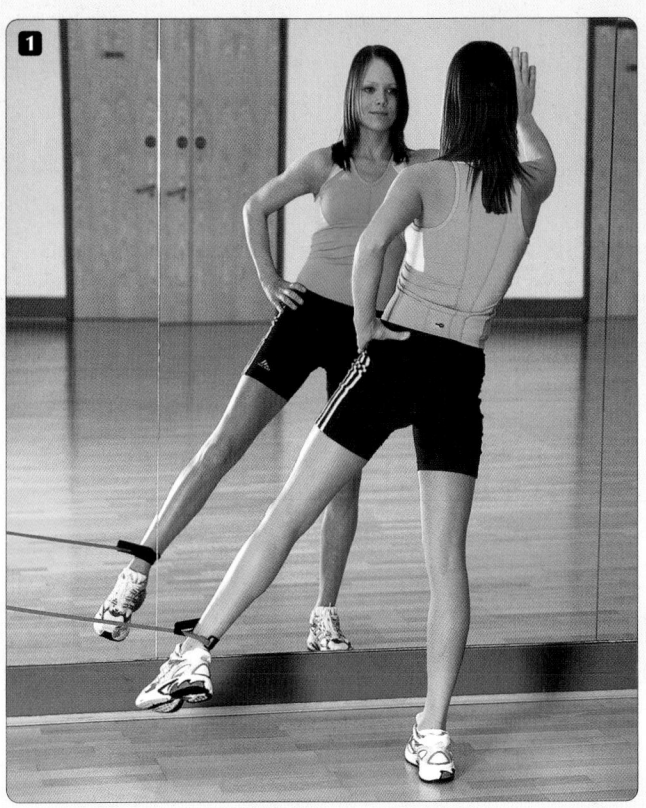

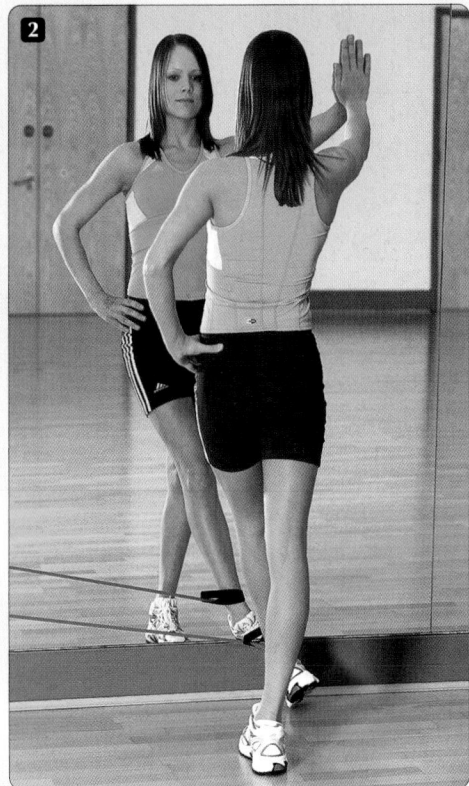

3 CUSHION SQUEEZE

1 This is one you can do anywhere, anytime! Simply place a cushion, rolled-up towel or foam ball between your thighs.

2 Keeping the feet flat on the floor, squeeze your knees together for a count of 5. Then slowly release the tension over a count of 5 and repeat.

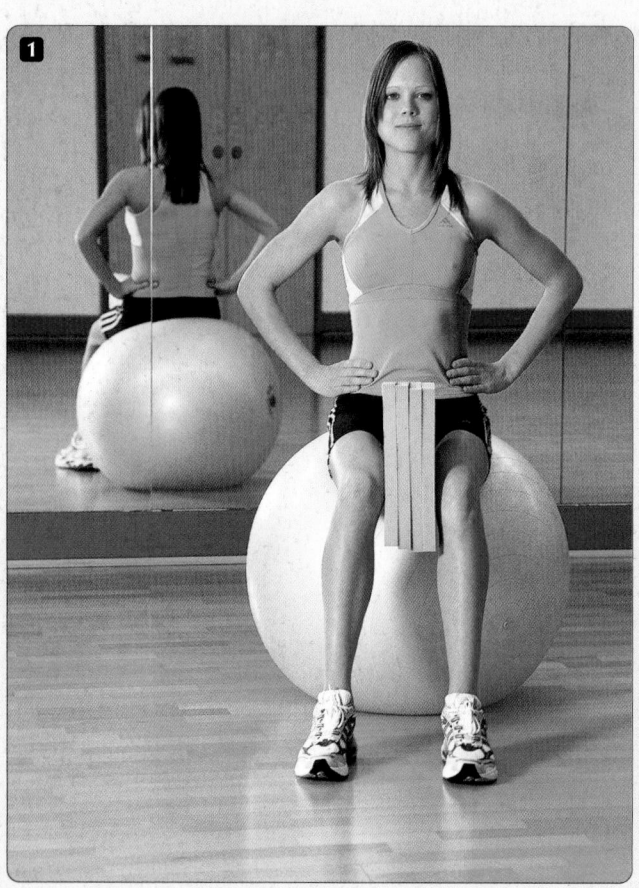
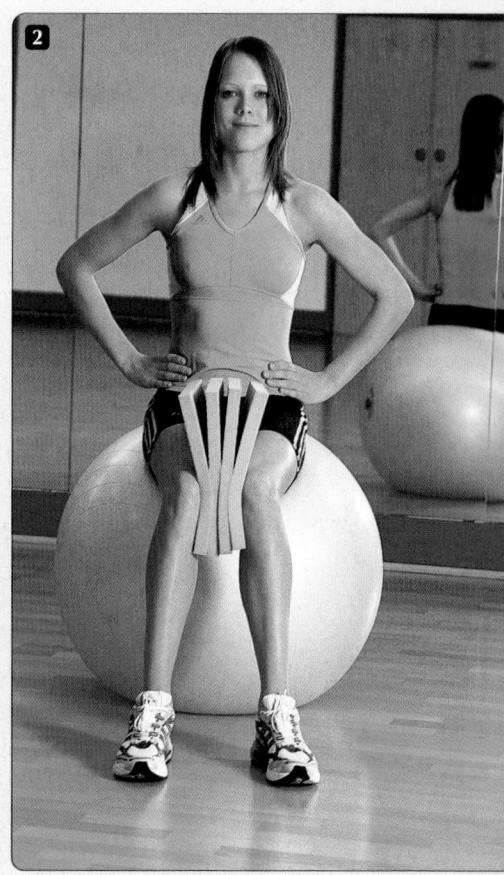

4 BALL LIFT

1 Lie on a mat with your legs bent and astride an exercise ball.

2 Squeezing the ball between the knees and feet, extend the legs, lifting the ball up, and then lower. This is also a great core stability exercise.

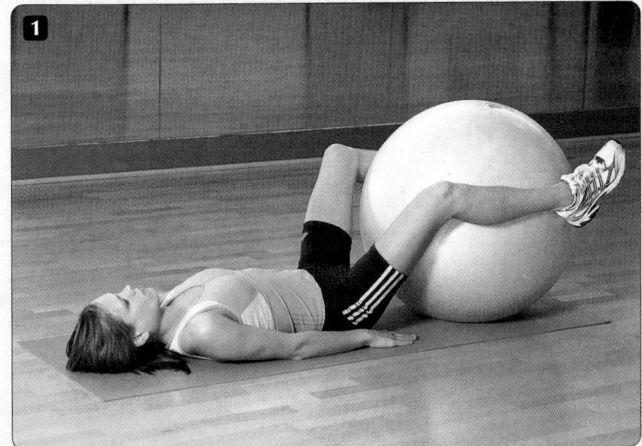

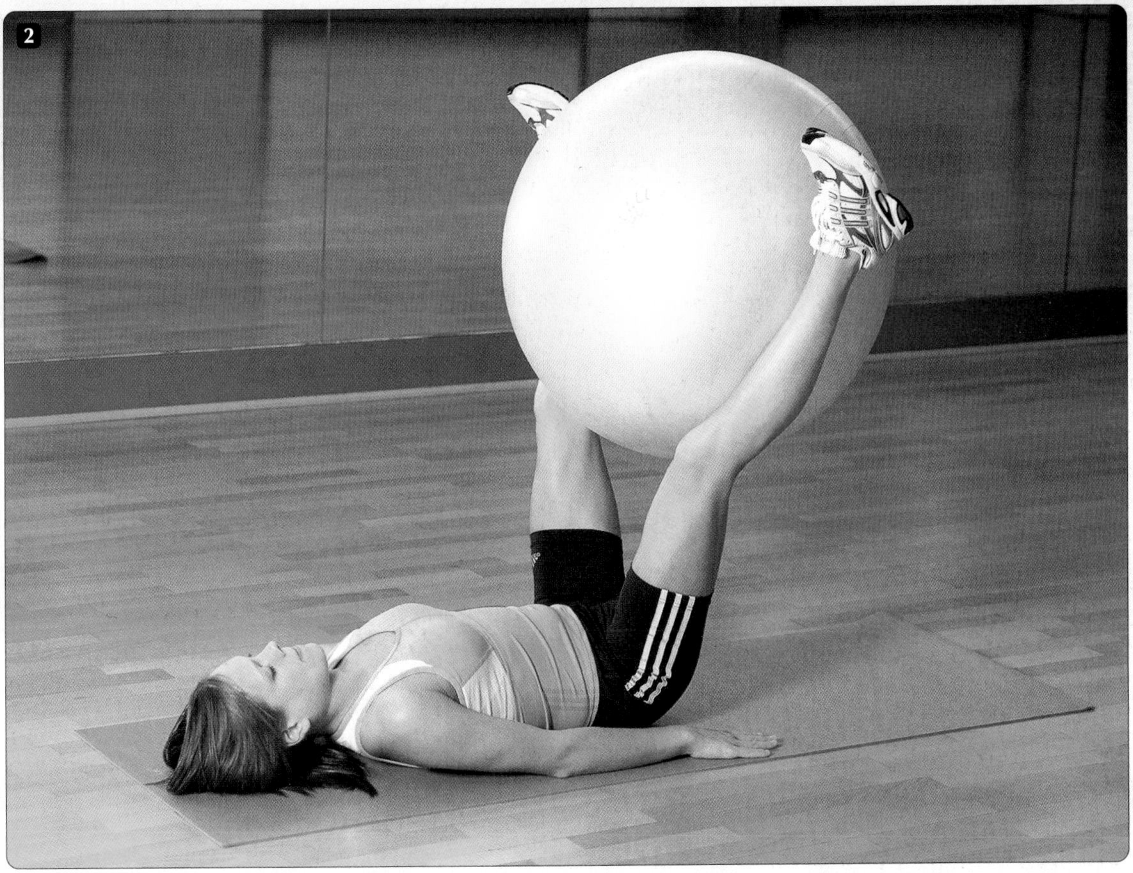

UPPER ARMS

1 NARROW PUSH UP

1 Start on all fours on a mat with your knees behind your hips and your hands below your shoulders, about 15cm apart, elbows close into your sides.

2 Keeping your neck in line with your spine, bend the arms to lower the chest towards the floor, ensuring the elbows don't 'splay out' but remain close to your sides. Pause, straighten the arms and repeat.

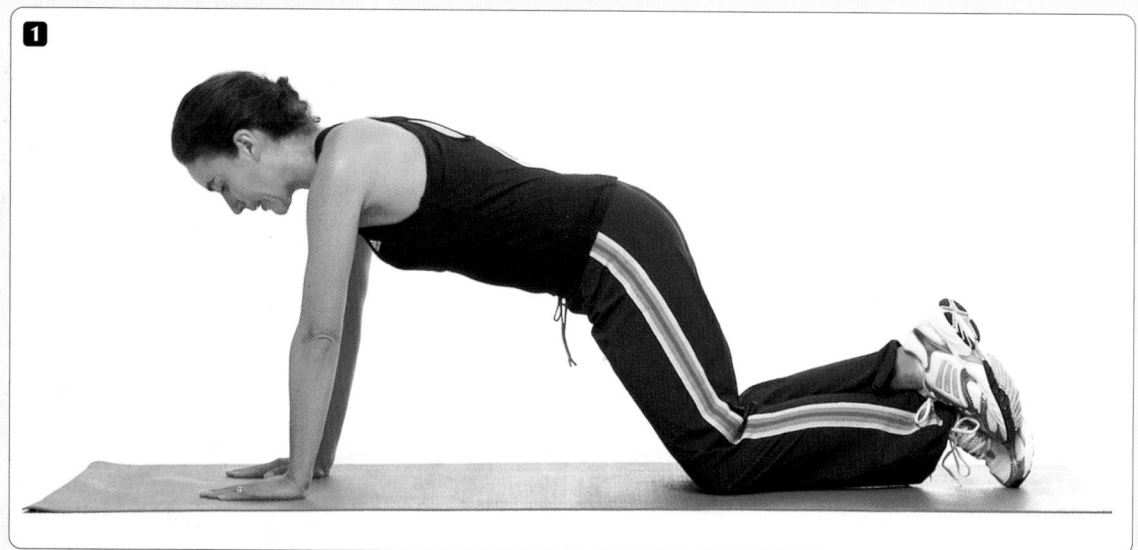

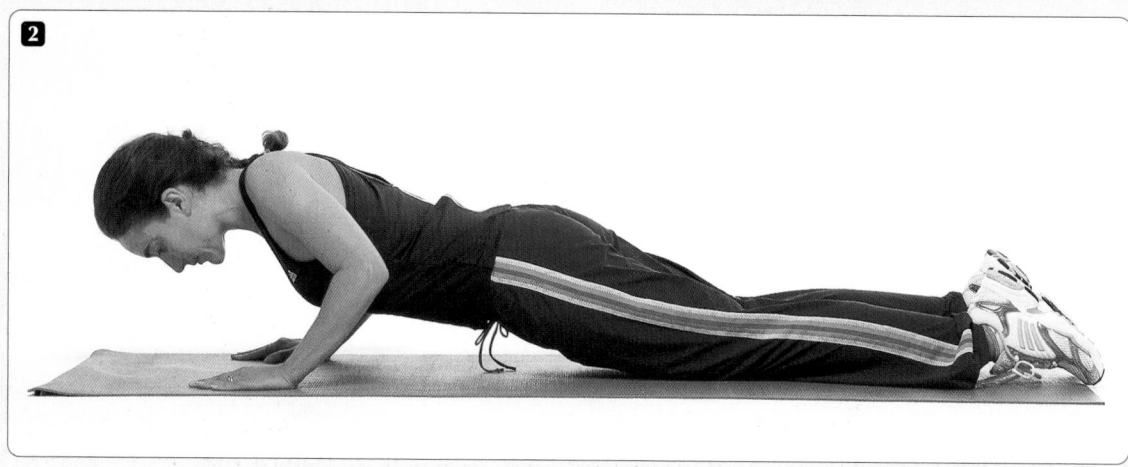

[2] MEDICINE BALL OVERHEAD PRESS

1 Hold the medicine ball in both hands above your head. Stand tall and engage the core.

2 Now keeping the upper arms vertical, lower the ball behind your head by bending the elbows. Only go as far as 90 degrees and then straighten the arms and repeat.

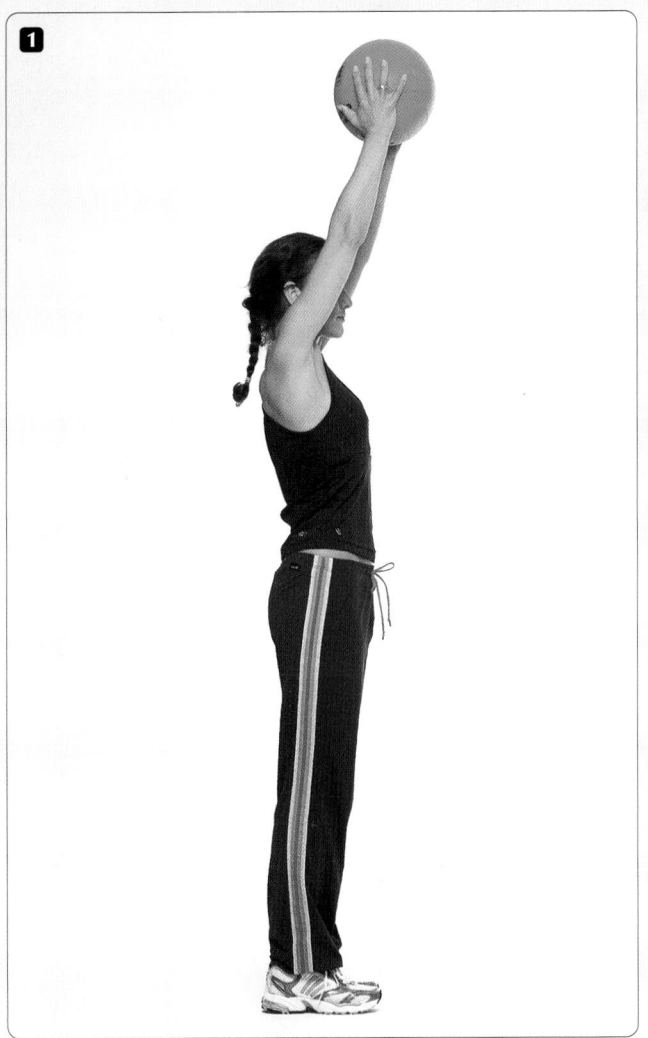

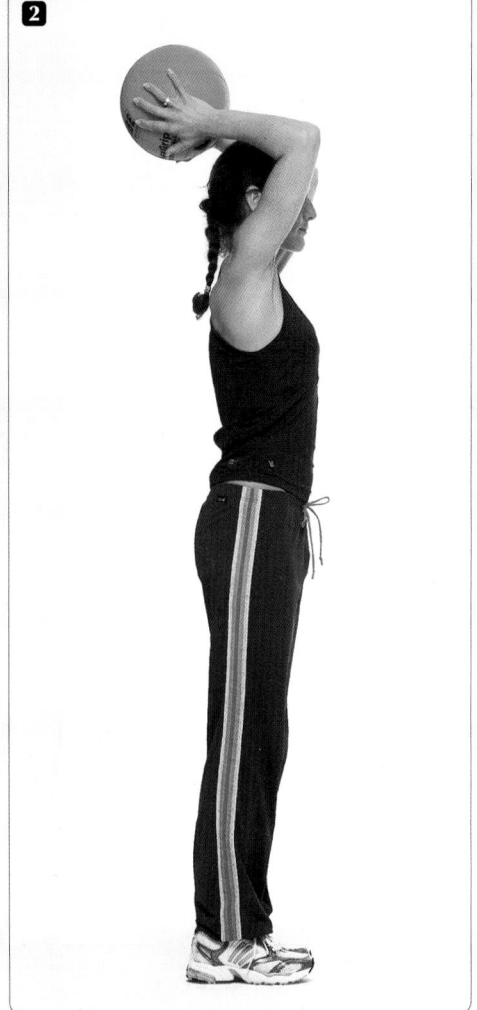

3 RESISTANCE TUBE PUSHDOWN

1 Hook a resistance tube over a sturdy hook or use a door attachment and take an end in each hand, with the elbows close to your sides and arms bent to a right angle.

2 Keeping the shoulder blades pulling together and the chest lifted, straighten the arms, allowing them to go slightly beyond the midline of the body. Pause, then return to the 90-degree position and repeat.

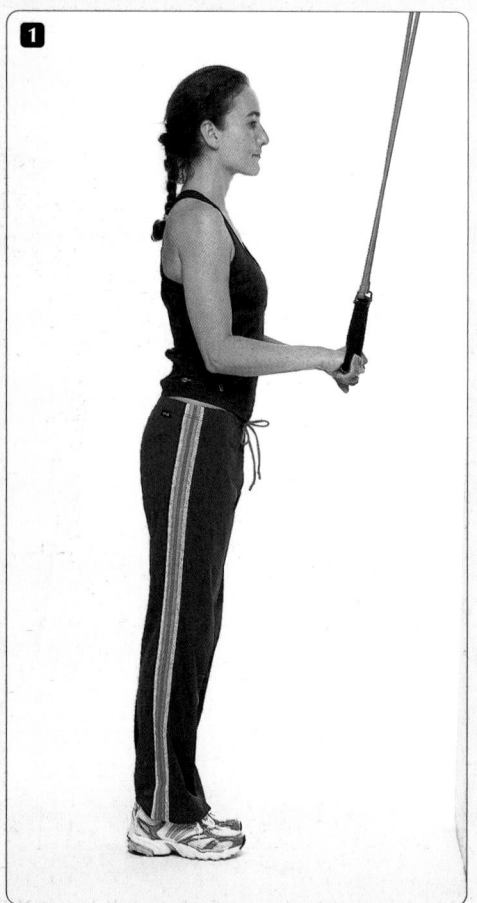

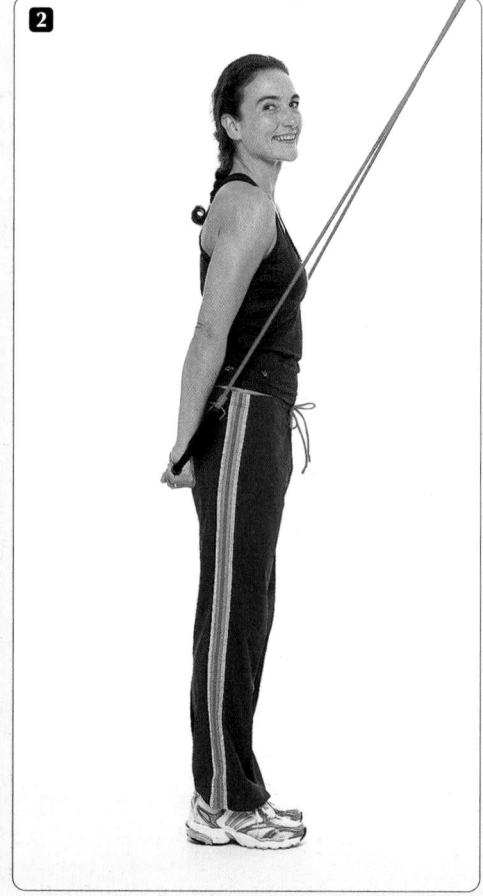

4 TRICEPS KICKBACK

1 Stand side on to a bench, with your left knee and hand supported on it, your back parallel to the floor and one end of a resistance band (or a weight) in your right hand – the other end of the band can be secured with the resting hand. Start with the upper arm parallel to the body, elbow at a right angle.

2 Keeping the upper arm still, straighten the arm, taking the forearm past your thigh. At the end of the range, try to extend the shoulder slightly (allow the arm to go beyond the line of the body). Bend the arm back to the start position and repeat. Swap sides.

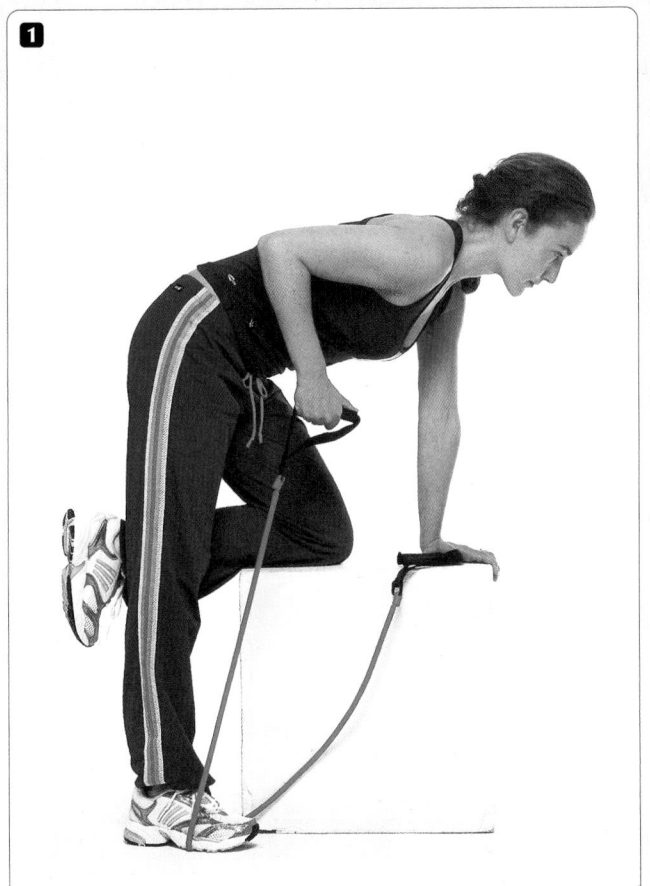

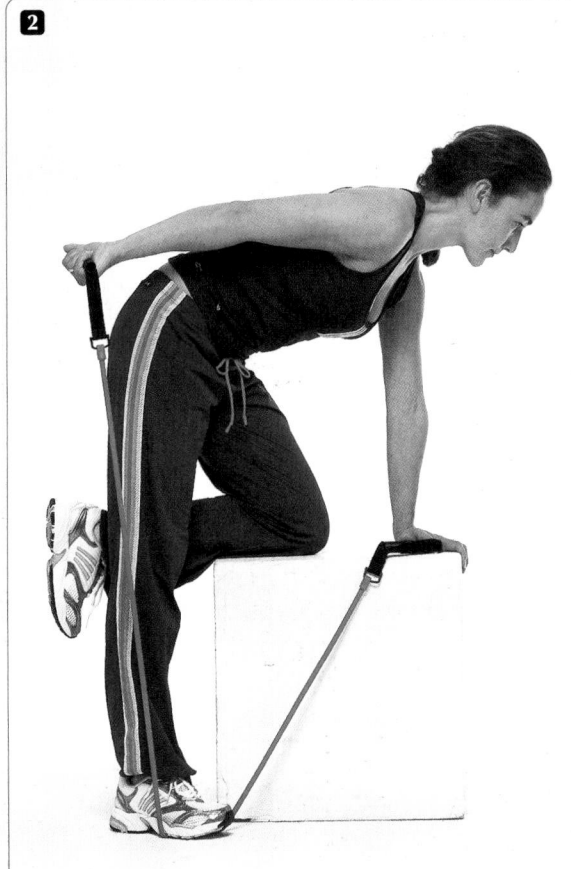

HIPS AND BUM

1 SIDE LYING LEG RAISE ON FLOOR

1 Lie on your side with your legs 'stacked' from ankle to hip (directly on top of one another) and your weight supported on your elbow – don't let the body sink into the supporting arm.

2 Raise the top leg a few centimetres from the supporting one, keeping the toes facing directly forwards. Lengthen the leg out of the hip socket as you extend it. Lower, repeat and swap sides.

To progress:
Tie a resistance tube around both ankles to create extra resistance (other than gravity) as you lift the leg, or use an ankle weight.

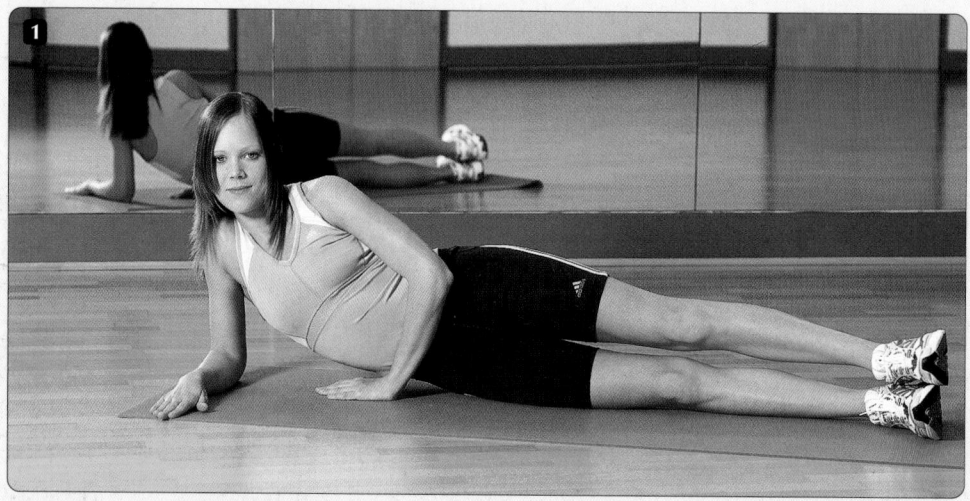

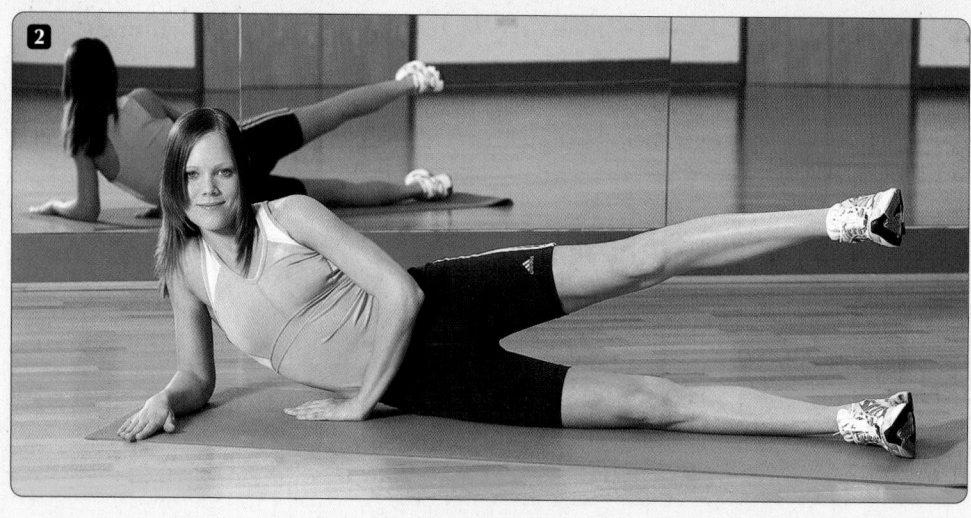

2 BALL LEG RAISES

1 Lie face up on your mat, with your feet resting on the ball and hands beside you on the floor. Lift the body off the mat, so that you are in a straight line from shoulders to feet.

2 Get your balance and then lift one foot off the ball, without allowing the pelvis to tilt to the other side. Pause, then lower and repeat with the other leg.

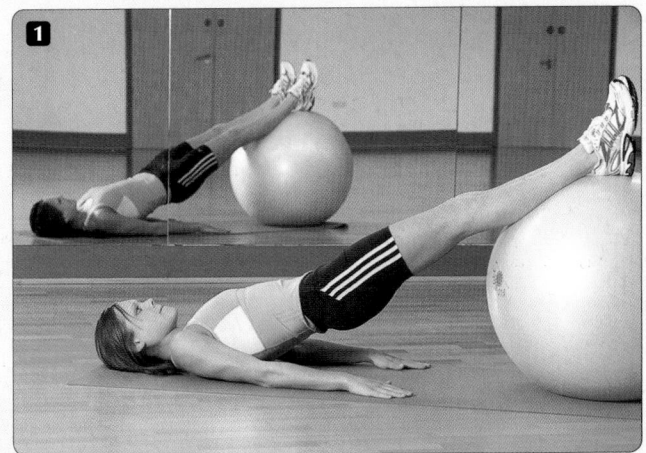

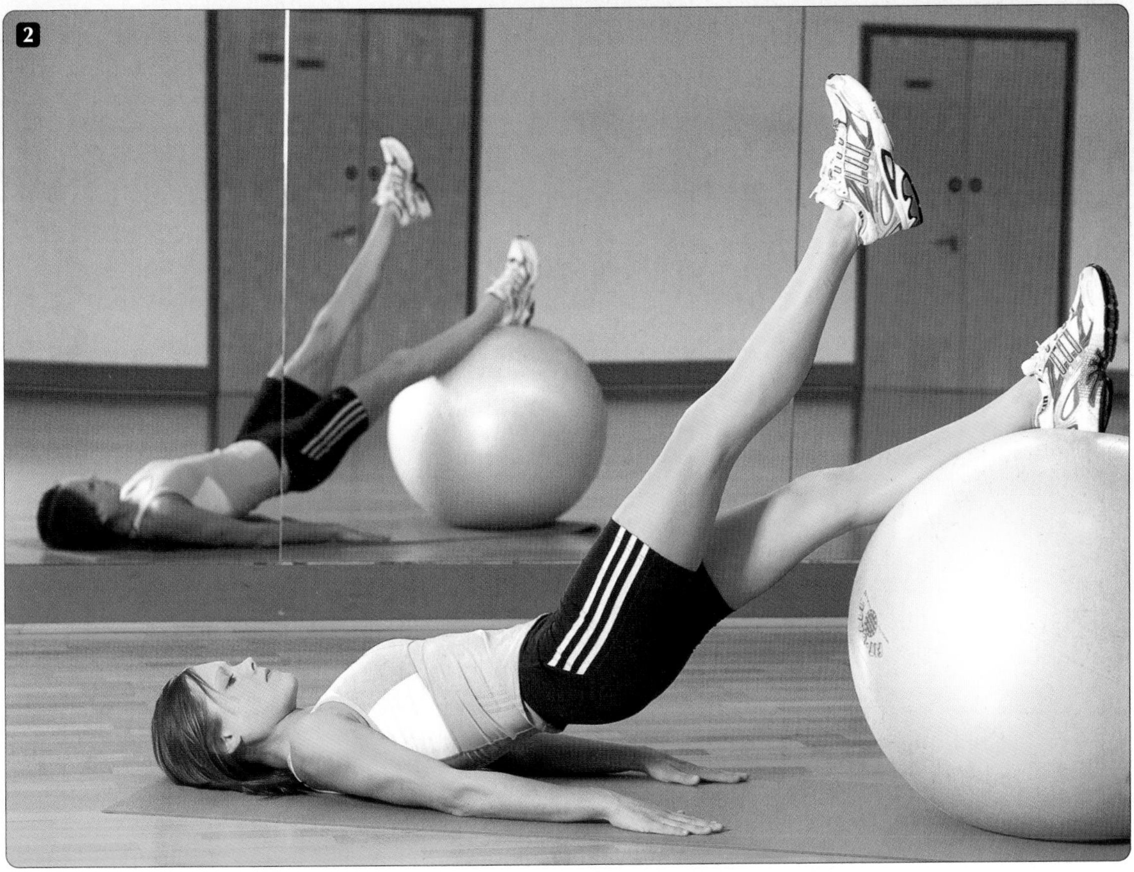

3 SIDE KNEEL

1 Kneel up on a mat and extend your left leg out to the side, keeping your big toe in line with your hip. Using your core muscles, lower your torso to the right and place your right hand on the floor beside you.

2 Now lift the left foot off the floor, keeping it in line with your body.

3 From this position, bend and straighten the knee. Swap sides.

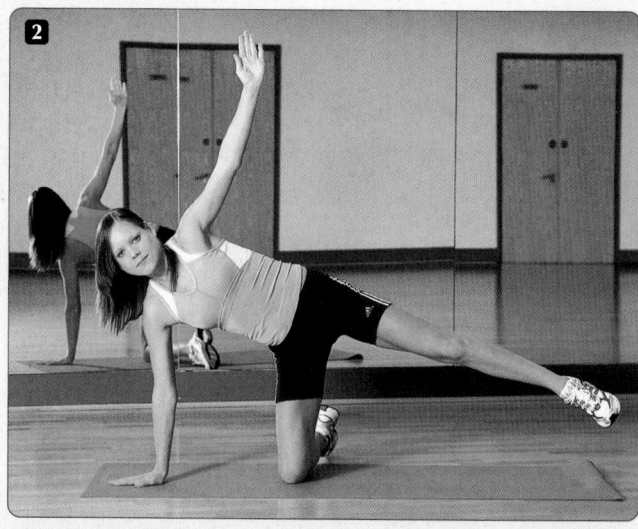

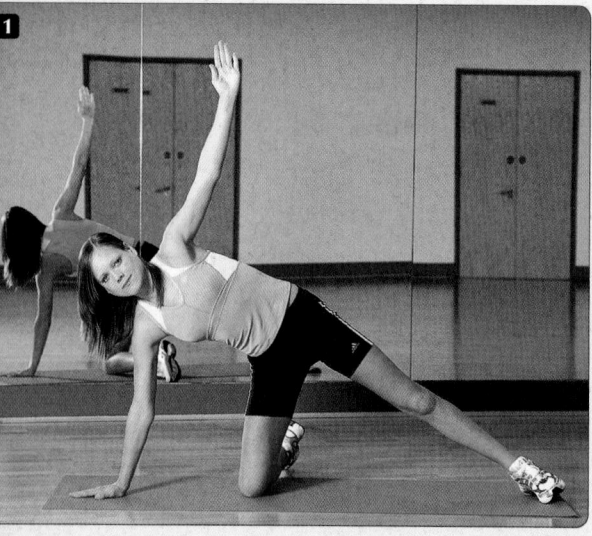

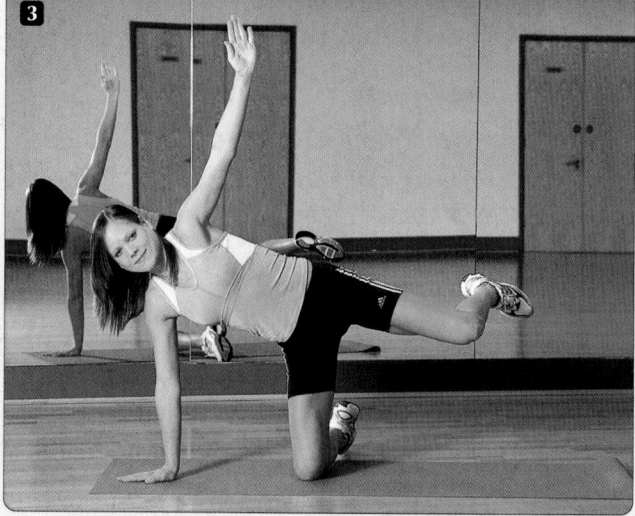

4 BALL DRIFT

1 Sit on an exercise ball and roll down and forwards until just your shoulders and head are on the ball. Place your feet hip distance apart. Adjust your position so that your body is in a straight line, using the glutes and abs to stabilise you.

2 Shift your weight over to the right foot, pause, then shift over to the left foot. Continue to alternate for the set.

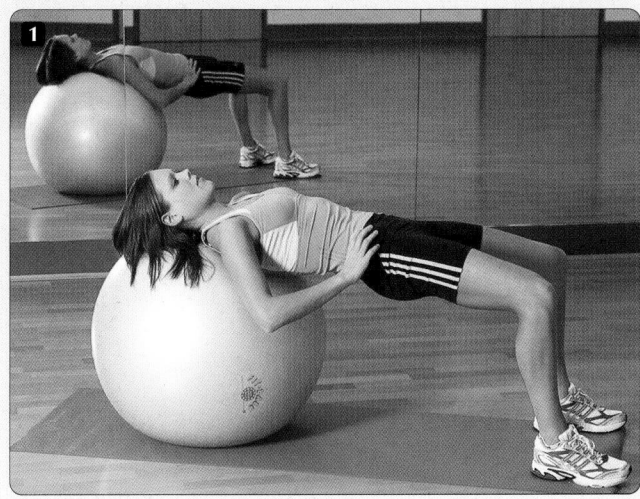

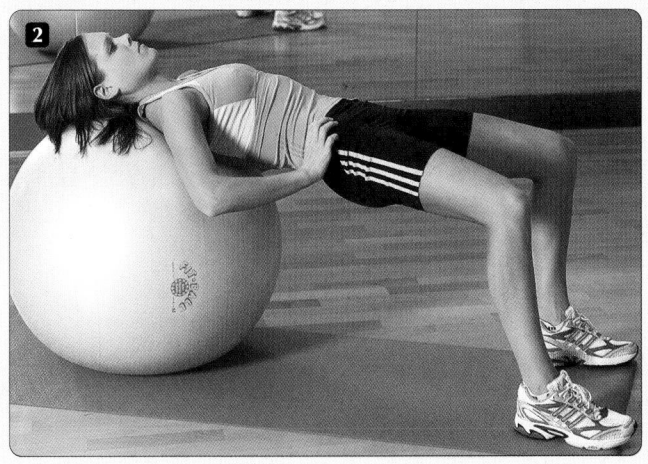

Making progress

The first six weeks

Focus on technique to establish neuromuscular patterns. Aim for the higher end of your chosen reps, the lower end of your sets ranges and use a slightly lower weight than you optimally can. You can work out the whole body at once or follow a split routine – training each body part two to three times per week.

The next six weeks

To consolidate and build on your gains, move to the lower end of your chosen reps, the higher end of your chosen sets range and up your weights. Continue to train the same number of times per week. Also feel free to play with different speeds of movement and training techniques (see page 141).

And after twelve weeks?

For maintenance, keep the overall intensity of your training the same (in other words, if you up the weight, decrease the reps) and take the frequency down to twice a week. If you want to continue developing strength, keep frequency as it is, or even increase it. This is the perfect time to add in some new exercises, from the targeted toning workouts, play with different training techniques and perhaps adopt a split routine. Variety is very important but make sure that it has some kind of logic to it. So if you decide to home in on your upper arms, do it with consistency and progressively build on your gains before moving on to something else.

FUELLING YOUR WORKOUTS,

How to get a balanced, healthy diet while you cut calories – and how to fuel up before, during and after your workouts.

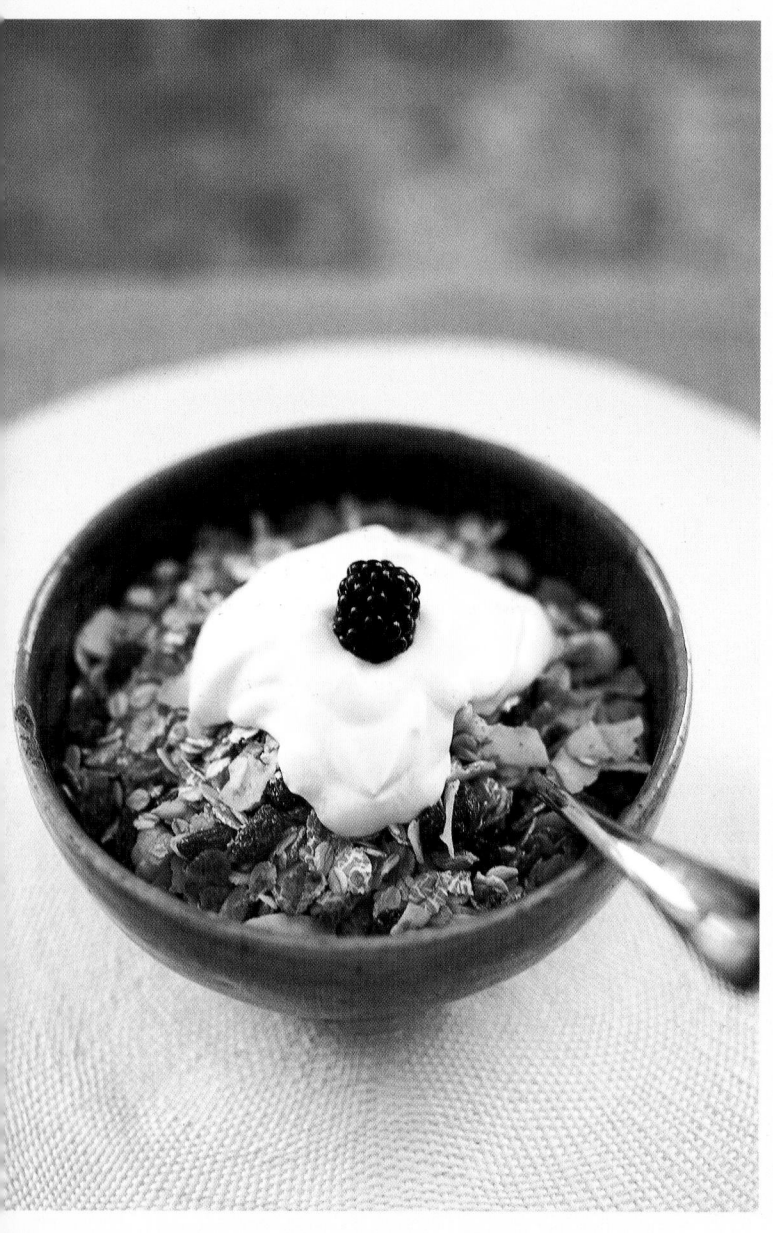

It's common knowledge these days that exercise and diet go hand in hand when it comes to losing weight. But, much as we know this, it can be tough to increase your activity levels *and* reduce your energy intake simultaneously. Often, the problem is simply that we try to reduce calorie intake too much – and to a level that cannot be sustained long term. So guess what? As soon as calorie intake goes back to 'normal' the weight creeps back on.

The advice contained in this chapter isn't a diet as such, the aim is simply to lay down the ground rules of healthy eating – showing you how to cut calorie intake sufficiently to shed body fat but not so much that you feel deprived or can't keep it up. I am a firm believer that food is one of the great joys in life – far from being just a necessary 'evil' to produce energy in the body. That's why 'soup' diets, meal replacements and other extreme regimes just don't cut it for me. Do you really want to eat like that for the rest of your life? If the answer is 'no' then you might as well stop right now because the results will last only as long as the diet does.

Losing fat, saving muscle

Research shows that when women diet 25–30% of the weight they shed isn't fat but water, muscle and even bone. Depressing, huh? And the quicker you lose the weight the

MAXIMISING WEIGHT LOSS

less of it is fat. But strength training changes all that. In a study at Tufts University dieting women were split into two groups – one group just dieted while the other group was put on a strength-training programme (twice a week) while they dieted. Both groups lost an average of 13lb (6kg) during the study but women in the diet-only group lost an average of 2.8lb (1.2kg) of lean body mass (muscle) while the women who strength trained actually gained 1.4lb (700g) of lean tissue – meaning that every ounce they lost was fat. So you see, once again – weights work for weight loss!

First, let's look at the principles of healthy eating in general. Then we'll explore the ways in which you might consider subtly altering your diet to ensure you get the best results from strength training.

Where should my calories come from?

With the amount of controversy in recent years regarding how much carbohydrate, fat and protein we should be eating, you could be forgiven for feeling bewildered. While some experts are sticking to their guns and advocating a high-carbohydrate, low-fat diet, others believe that there does seem to be some evidence for reducing carbohydrate intake a little and increasing protein percentage. Still others believe that the burgeoning obesity problem isn't due to too much fat per se, but the wrong *type* of fat. The US Institute of Medicine revised its dietary guidelines in 2002 to recommend a breakdown of between 45

and 65% carbohydrate, 10 and 35% protein and 20 and 35% fat (giving much wider margins for all nutrient groups, a lower minimum guideline for carbs and a *higher* maximum guideline for fats). They cite evidence that a high carb, low fat diet can reduce good HDL cholesterol, increase triglycerides and increase the glycaemic load. All undesirable effects. Then again, a high fat diet is linked to heart and cardiovascular disease, obesity and diabetes. So it would seem that it's a case of what *type* of carbs, fats and protein you should opt for.

Top class carbs

The majority of your daily energy should come from carbohydrate. It is the body's equivalent of four-star fuel. Since only a limited amount can be stored – and since carbohydrate is the only fuel that the brain can utilise without

STRONG WORDS

WEIGHING IN

When, say, 5g or 50g of carbohydrate is referred to note that it refers to the grams of pure carbohydrate in a food and *not* 50g of the food itself. So, for example, getting 50g of carbohydrate doesn't mean eating a banana or potato weighing that much it means eating something that contains 50g of carbohydrate along with its other nutrient constituents. If, however, it says 50g of chicken, it means 50g of chicken!

having to convert, supplies need to be constantly replenished. Besides, carbohydrate needs to be present in order for fat to be burned. Carbs also pack a micronutrient-fuelled punch – being rich in B vitamins, iron, magnesium and chromium, as well as fibre, and phytochemicals that can help prevent cancer and promote good health. Experts recommend 4–6g per kg of body weight per day for people weight training three to five times per week. For a 60kg woman that equals 240–360g per day of carbohydrate.

But carbs vary in their health-giving value. Carbohydrates used to be divided into 'simple' or 'complex' varieties. Simple referred to sugary carbohydrates like table sugar, honey and fruit sugars while complex meant starchy foods like bread, potatoes, rice and pasta. The premise was that starches were

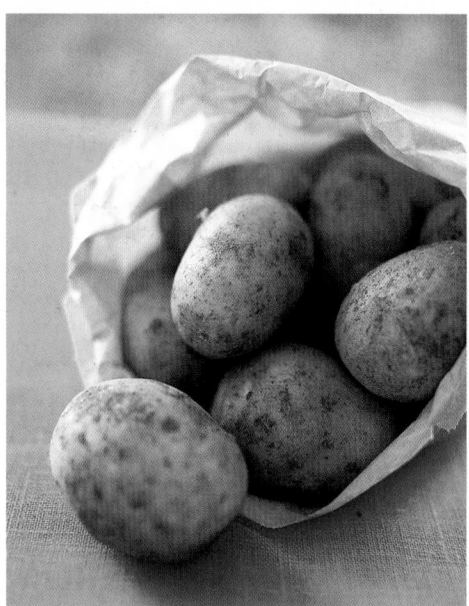

'good', sugars 'bad'. However, surprisingly, there is no evidence that high sugar intake is related to excess weight – it's only excess calories that can be linked scientifically to excess body fat.

But there is some evidence that the effect of some carbohydrates on the body's insulin levels is related to fat storage. Foods that are high on what is known as the glycaemic index (GI) cause a sharp rise in blood sugar, triggering the body to release insulin to get the sugar out of the bloodstream and restore levels to normal. The trouble is, insulin encourages the conversion and storage of the excess sugar as fat. What's more, this sudden surge and then plummeting of blood sugar can cause energy crashes. Low glycaemic index foods, in contrast, cause a more gentle insulin response, allowing blood sugar levels to remain more stable – a far preferable state of affairs.

The other point that is often overlooked is that we rarely eat foods on their own and that there are many factors that mitigate the carbohydrate's effect on blood sugar; such as the presence of fibre, fat, protein, acids such as vinegar and lemon juice and the way the food is cooked.

GI IQ

Unfortunately, whether a food is classified as a simple or complex carb doesn't tell you anything about its GI value. So it's a matter of looking foods up. But it isn't possible – or desirable – to base all your nutritional decisions on the GI chart. Otherwise you would be foregoing healthful foods like carrots, potatoes, watermelon and dried fruit, purely on the strength of their high GI.

In addition, research from the University of Sydney suggests that highly active, fit people have a less pronounced response to high glycaemic index foods and so don't have to worry so much about their effects on blood sugar. However, opting for mainly wholegrains, wholemeal bread, pasta and rice, pulses and beans and eating a wide range of fruits and vegetables should ensure a sustained energy supply as well as a nutritionally rich diet.

Fat facts

There has been a recent shift in expert opinion about dietary fat. While the message for years has been 'eat less fat!' it now appears to be 'eat healthier fats'. Although a gram of olive oil contains the same number of calories as a gram of butter or lard, evidence is increasingly showing that there are some important health benefits to be had from particular types of fat. At present, too much of the fat we eat comes from unhealthy saturated and trans fat sources (derived from meat and dairy products, pastry, fried food, refined and pre-packaged products, cakes and biscuits) and not enough comes from healthier monounsaturated fat (such as olive oil) and sources of the two essential fatty acids, Omega-3 and Omega-6. Aiming to get 12% of your total daily calories from monounsaturated fats, no more than 10% of total calories from saturated fat and a bare minimum of trans fats – will help you maintain a healthy body weight and improve your heart health significantly.

STRONG WORDS

QUALITY NOT QUANTITY

The American Journal of Epidemiology reports that overall carbohydrate intake is not associated with higher body weight, but that processed carb intake is. So steer away from those refined and packaged foodstuffs.

FIVE TOP LOW GI FOODS

• Sweet potato – far lower on the GI than normal potatoes and packed with betacarotene, vitamin C and E – and fibre too.

• Chickpeas – versatile and rich in a phytochemical called saponin which is thought to lower cholesterol

• Oats – the breakfast of Olympians – oats are high in fibre and energy and can help reduce cholesterol due to the type of soluble fibre they contain.

• Lentils – brown and green varieties are rich in potassium, iron, selenium and manganese – one study found a pre-workout lentil-based meal allowed study participants to keep going for longer than a high GI meal of the same calorific value.

• Grapes – a portable fruit fix that won't send blood sugar soaring. Opt for red ones which are rich in resveratrol, an antioxidant. Fibre-rich skins too.

FAT TYPES

A high intake of saturated fat is linked to heart disease. What's more, saturated fat appears to have no useful role to play in the body so the calories it provides are simply stored as body fat. Major sources include: meat, butter, dairy products, pastry, coconut and palm oil.

Polyunsaturated fats do have an important role in the body. The two most important types are Omega-6 (linoleic acid) and Omega-3 (linolenic acid). Omega 6 fatty acids may prevent blood clots, help to stabilise blood sugar and lower blood pressure. But most of us tend to have enough in our diets already. The main source of Omega 6 is any kind of vegetable oil.

Omega-3 fatty acids are the ones we don't tend to get enough of. Consuming Omega-3s is thought to be protective against atherosclerosis (the build-up of fat deposits on the artery walls causing them to narrow), helps to make the blood less sticky and can lower blood pressure. The major source is oily fish but you can also get significant amounts from some nuts, including walnuts, linseed and its oils and dark green leafy vegetables, such as kale and spinach.

Monounsaturated fats are found in the oils of the 'Mediterranean' diet. The best-known source is olive oil but rapeseed oil, nut oils, avocados, nuts and seeds are also good sources.

Trans fats

The effects of trans fats on health are so negative that no 'recommended limit' has been set. In other words, no amount at all is good for you. As well as lowering good HDL, they also raise unhealthy LDL and they have been purported to be linked with certain cancers. That said it can be challenging to avoid trans fats as they are added to so many foods and, in the UK, it isn't a legal requirement to list trans fat content on food labels. Anything in which vegetable oil has been hydrogenated, such as margarine, shortening, fried foods, breads, crackers, snack foods, spreads, processed foods and ready-meals, contains trans fats.

Reducing fat intake

Most of us eat a higher than necessary amount of fat in our diet regardless of its source (the average British diet contains 41% fat). In addition, many of us consume too many calories overall and so the surplus

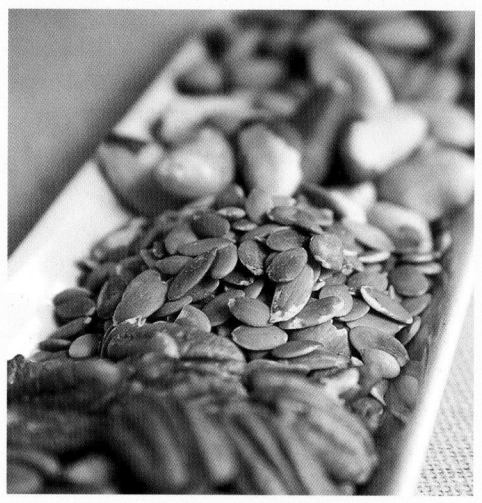

energy, regardless of where it came from, is converted to fat and stored. Fat, gram for gram, is significantly more fattening than either carbohydrate or protein (containing 9 calories per gram compared to 4 calories for carbs and protein) and just 2–3 calories out of every 100 are used in metabolising it. Whereas carbohydrate and protein need 6–8 and 25–30 respectively, out of every 100 consumed, to be processed and metabolised.

To lose weight, aim to cut down on fat overall so that around 25% of your total calories come from fat. And ensure that the majority of the fat you consume comes from the healthier sources (though I am not suggesting you should pile in the olive oil and avocado if you are aiming to lose body fat).

The power of protein

Protein is an essential part of a balanced diet. It helps build and repair all the body's cells, plays a part in the hormonal and immune systems, regulates fluid balance and is a component of every red blood cell. It also gives structure to our hair, skin and nails. But, most importantly, it forms the fabric of our muscles. Without sufficient protein you may as well forget about gaining strength or definition in your muscles.

Proteins are constructed from substances called amino acids, of which there are twenty, all with distinctive functions within the body. Of these twenty, eight are termed 'essential' because they must be supplied by the diet and cannot be made from other amino acids.

But what role does protein have in weight loss? Firstly, studies suggest that protein tends to be more satiating than carbohydrate as it spends longer in the stomach. So not skimping on protein means you are less likely to overeat. Secondly, around a quarter of the calories from protein are actually used up in its metabolism. Thirdly, due to its crucial role in repair and maintenance, it is less readily converted and stored as fat. And finally, as we know, one of the consequences of weight loss can be a loss in muscle mass and a subsequent decrease in metabolism and daily energy expenditure. Studies have shown that increasing protein intake to 1.6g per kg of body weight per day offsets lean tissue loss during dieting. So if you weigh 60kg, that would mean 96g of protein. This may take your protein intake slightly above the normal recommended guidelines but the reduction in

STRONG WORDS

A FAT LOT OF GOOD

Fat is an essential nutrient with an important role to play in a balanced diet. Certain vitamins, including A, D, E and K are fat-soluble, so can only be derived from fat sources and fat also helps the body absorb those all-important phytochemicals. Secondly, fat produces some important hormones, provides insulation and protection for our bodies and, for women, enables pregnancy and lactation to take place.

fat and carbohydrate intake will ensure that your overall calorie intake does not increase. This extra protein intake is also useful if you are training regularly as the increased breakdown of protein during training needs to be compensated for. This is the case particularly when you are new to exercise as the body has yet to become accustomed to conserving and recycling protein efficiently.

How many calories should I cut for weight loss?

Although many diets recommend cutting 500 calories per day – to create a 3500 calorie deficit in a week (equal to 450g of body fat) – that could equate to as much as a third or quarter of your total daily energy expenditure. Not only will this feel like a very significant drop in food intake it may also leave you devoid of energy so that your precious training gets pushed aside. A better solution is to cut your daily energy intake by 15%. This avoids the metabolic reactions that take place in response to greater calorie reductions – such as a lower metabolic rate, increased protein oxidation and depletion of stored carbohydrate in the muscles. Research shows that less than 1200 calories a day triggers hormonal reactions that enable the body to conserve, rather than burn, calories. Therefore the more modest 15% calorie reduction will help you shed fat (rather than water, lean body tissue and bone) and maintain the loss – without it feeling like starvation!

This begs the question, then, of how many calories you need on a daily basis. There are

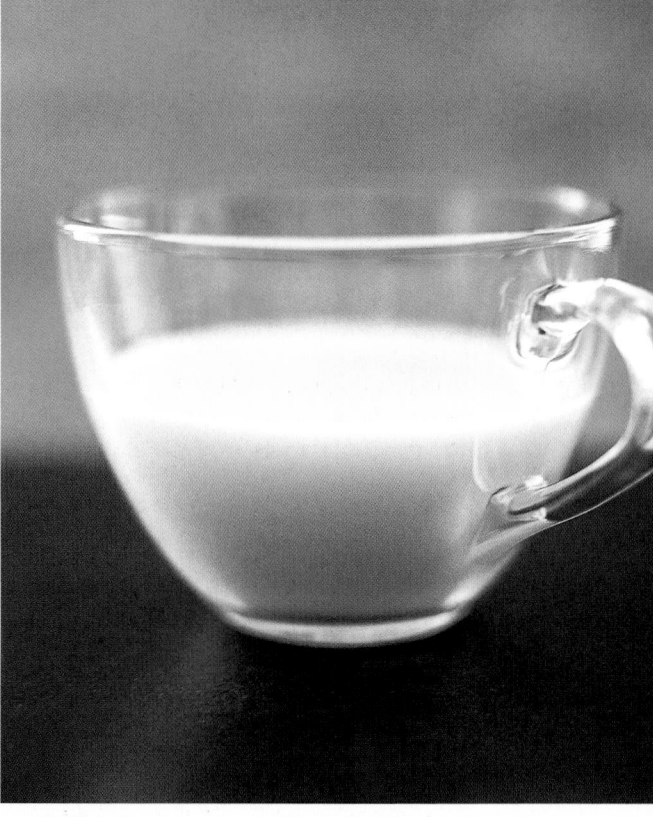

lots of ways of calculating this, based on your resting metabolic rate, weight, age and so on. The chart opposite will show you how to estimate your own daily energy needs. Once you have the figure, multiply it by 85% to get an idea of how much energy you will be aiming to take in when you cut your calories by 15%.

How much do you need?

How much energy you need is determined by your resting metabolic rate (RMR) plus the amount of extra energy you need to cater for your daily activity.

To get a rough idea of how many calories you need, fill in the following calculations:

1. My weight in kilograms (1 kilogram = 2.2 lb)

2. WOMEN
I am 18–30 years old: weight x 14.7.
Answer + 496 = RMR
OR
I am 31–60 years old: weight x 8.7.
Answer + 829 = RMR

MEN
I am 18–30 years old: weight x 15.3.
Answer + 679 = RMR
OR
I am 31–60 years old: weight x 11.6.
Answer + 879 = RMR

MY ESTIMATED RMR IS ....

3. Take this figure and multiply it by the number below most closely representing your typical daily activity level.

I am totally sedentary	1.2–1.3
I am mostly sedentary (no structured activity, office work)	1.5–1.6
I am moderately active (some walking each day, stair climbing and regular active leisure time activities)	1.6–1.7
I am very active (vigorously physically active each day)	1.8–2.1

MY RESULT IS ....

Making sense of the figures

Remember that you will be burning additional calories through strength training and any other activity that you do regularly. To factor this in, add up the calories expended on exercise during a typical week, divide by 7 and add this to your total. You can get a rough idea of the calorie expenditure of different activities using many website tools, such as www.caloriesperhour.com.

However, it isn't necessary to take in exactly the right number of calories every day. As long as, in general, your intake over the course of a week or so breaks down to your estimated daily requirement you will be fine.

STRONG WORDS

ALCOHOL – THE NON-NUTRITIOUS NUTRIENT

We've talked about the gram for gram content of fat, carbohydrate and protein – but there's a fourth source of calories in our diets that can add a substantial amount – alcohol. At seven calories per gram it isn't far behind fat in the calorie stakes and a single 'unit' of alcohol contains roughly 8g. The recommended daily allowance for women in the UK is up to three units per day (21 per week) and four units per day (28 units per week) for men. In its entirety this adds between 1100 and 1500 calories to your weekly energy intake. Anyone for a soda water?

More ways to weight loss

- Fidget! Research from the University of Minnesota found that people who couldn't sit still burned 100–500 calories more per day than more sedentary people!

- Eat mindfully. Eating on the move prevents you from noticing that you are eating. Try to sit down and pay attention to the taste, smell and texture of your food.

- Eat slowly. The hormone peptide YY, located in the intestines, is released when you are full – but it takes a while to kick in.

- Frontload your day. Pigging out at dinner after virtually starving all day results in a lower metabolism. The body is also more responsive to insulin in the morning so is better able to handle carbohydrate without causing a large glycaemic response.

- Reduce portions. Even healthy foods are fattening when eaten to excess.

- Boost fibre intake. Fibrous foods keep people feeling full longer and aid weight loss. Fibre also plays a healthy role in digestion by speeding the movement of waste through the intestines, inhibiting cholesterol absorption and attenuating the blood sugar response.

- Don't set yourself up for failure. Don't try to change everything about your diet at once. Focus on adding in some good stuff before you start subtracting the not-so-good stuff and you won't feel deprived.

Nutrition to maximise the benefits of weight training

There is no doubt at all that the quality and quantity of fuel that you put into your engine affects the performance you'll get. The American College of Sports Medicine's 2000 statement on nutrition and athletic performance confirms that nutrition can affect both performance and recovery in exercise.

What you might need more of...

Protein

The American College of Sports Medicine's statement asserts that protein requirements for active people are higher than average. They suggest that for strength training needs may be 1.6–1.7g per kg of body weight compared to 0.8g per kg in sedentary people. But even this amount doesn't necessitate downing loads of egg whites or protein shakes as it is quite possible to get enough protein from your normal diet. For example, if you were looking to take on board 1.4g per kg per day and you weighed 60kg that would mean 96g of protein, the equivalent of a 200ml glass of milk, a boiled egg, a chicken breast, a cup of baked beans, a small can of tuna and a handful of peanuts.

Iron

Iron is an essential mineral in the human body – it is involved in the formation of red blood cells and the carrying of oxygen to all the body's cells. Since iron is lost in sweat, and exercise increases sweat, it is more important than ever to get sufficient dietary iron when you are active. Studies suggest that regularly active women need an additional 0.3mg per day on top of the recommended daily amount of 14.8mg per day. Insufficient iron can allow haemoglobin to fall below optimal levels. This is not in itself classed as anaemia (which is an iron, rather than a haemoglobin deficiency) but it will hamper your training performance. It is estimated that up to 15% of women are iron deficient – if you think you may be one of them, ask your doctor for a haemoglobin and serum ferritin test. A value less than 12g.dl-1 on the latter is cause for concern.

Carbs

Despite the obvious role protein plays in building muscle carbohydrate is still the fuel of choice for muscles. Exercise physiologists have compared recovery time after exercising to exhaustion with a high protein or high carbohydrate diet. The high protein eaters took five days to replenish their glycogen stores following the intense workouts while the high carb dieters took just two days. What's more, other research found that multiple-set resistance exercise regime resulted in a 25–40% depletion of carbohydrate stores – the higher the volume of training the greater the level of depletion.

Water and fluids

Water, though calorie free and nutritionally empty, is a vital part of our diet. It is involved in every bodily process, from energy metabolism to digestion and muscle contraction, and makes up almost two thirds of our body composition.

Drinking water (and other fluids) regularly throughout the day is a healthy habit worth having. When you are exercising regularly you need to drink in order to replace fluid lost through sweating. Aim to drink 250–500ml of fluid 30 minutes before your workout, 100– 250ml every 15–20 minutes during it and 250–500ml afterwards depending on the length and intensity of the session.

Supplements

The advice on supplements always states that providing you have a healthy balanced diet you don't need them. The exceptions are in the case of:

- Diets low in energy for weight loss.

- Diets in which foods or food groups are omitted due to likes or dislikes.

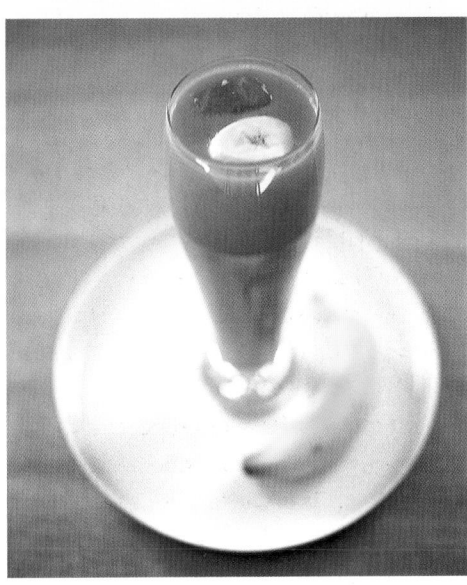

VEGGIES AND VEGANS

Protein, as we've learned, is the building block for muscle. So a true vegetarian diet presents more of a challenge in ensuring you get sufficient levels. While beans, lentils, nuts and seeds are high in protein, they are not what are known as 'complete' proteins because they lack some of the nine essential amino acids. Combine them with another wholegrain or vegetable, however, and you can get the full complement of amino acids. The soya bean is an exception in that it constitutes a complete protein all on its own – so eating the bean or its derivatives, like tofu or soya milk, is a smart veggie move.

As far as iron is concerned, providing you eat enough iron-fortified foods, you should get by. Cereals and bread tend to be fortified with iron but always have with orange juice rather than coffee as Vitamin C enhances iron absorption, while caffeine slows it. Also, don't rely entirely on that bag of spinach for, despite being quite abundant in iron, vegetable sources are absorbed at a lower rate than meat-derived sources.

Vitamin B12, part of the B complex, cannot be derived from a vegan diet as it is only present in meat, shellfish and dairy products. We don't need much – a glass of milk would give you sufficient B12 for the day – but if you don't eat any of the above food groups then you really must take a supplement, containing at least 2mcgs of B12, every day.

- Diets lacking in a particular type of food due to allergy or intolerance.

- Erratic and unbalanced diets.

In these cases a good multi vitamin-mineral supplement is recommended. But what about specific supplements for muscle-boosting, fat-loss enhancing or joint protection? Do you need them? Do they work? And above all, are they safe? Here are a few for which the evidence is promising…

Conjugated linoleic acid (CLA)

CLA is an essential fatty acid that has been lauded for increasing muscle gain, enhancing fat loss, improving immunity and even warding off cancer. The evidence in rodents has been utterly compelling but studies on humans have produced more mixed results. Those that have shown a beneficial effect have noted significant changes in body composition (a shift from fat to muscle) when subjects were exercising regularly. In other words, you can't sit on the couch and reap the benefits. No negative effects of CLA supplementation have yet been found.

Recommended dose: 2000–3000mg per day.

Creatine phosphate

Creatine is a protein that occurs naturally in the body and has a key role in the formation of ATP, the body's energy source, particularly to supply short bouts of high intensity activity such as lifting weights. The theory is that boosting creatine levels through taking a supplement enables you to work harder and recover faster, allowing you to do more total work in a session. In studies creatine supplementation has been shown to increase lean body weight but also to increase total body weight (mainly as a result of water retention).

Recommended dose: 3–7g per day over a 30-day period. Creatine supplements should be taken in cycles, so you might take it daily for a month and then have a break. Taking a low dose like this daily for a month causes less water retention than 'loading up' for shorter periods with as much as 20g per day.

Hydroxy beta-methyl butyrate (HMB)

HMB is the resultant product of the breakdown of leucine, one of the body's essential amino acids. Playing an important role in muscle growth and repair, some research suggests that HMB supplementation can help with muscle and strength gains in novice strength trainers but not in more experienced participants. It is believed that HMB assists the body in minimising protein breakdown following intense exercise.

Recommended dose: 1000mg per day.

Glucosamine sulphate

Glucosamine sulphate is a naturally occurring substance in the body which plays a role in keeping cartilage healthy and reducing 'wear and tear' on joints. Research has shown that supplementation may help with joint pain and osteoarthritis. For example, a study published in the *British Journal of Sports Medicine* found that 2000mg taken for twelve weeks

provided pain relief and improved function in 88% of subjects with knee pain. Other research suggests 1000–1500mg a day is sufficient and that the product works best when taken in conjunction with chondroitin (many supplements contain both so check the label).

Recommended dose: 1000–2000mg per day.

THE PERFECT PRE-AND POST-WORKOUT SNACKS

The goal of a pre-workout snack is to provide some carbohydrate and protein calories, ideally along with hydration. Aim to eat it 30 minutes to an hour before your workout, rather than ten minutes before, to reduce the likelihood of it repeating on you. Try…a pot of yoghurt, peanut butter on crisp breads, a banana or an isotonic sports drink.

In the hours following your workout, taking some protein and carbohydrate in enhances recovery and helps promote an increased secretion of growth hormone (which helps to control body fat). But don't overdo it, a sports bar, half a tuna sandwich or a pot of yoghurt is sufficient.

As for during your session, it's only necessary to take calories on board if you are planning to do a challenging aerobic workout after your resistance session. If this is the case the easiest way of getting some ready fuel in is to drink an isotonic sports drink.

MAKING IT PART OF YOUR ROUTINE

Knowing how to strength train effectively is one thing but fitting it into your life – and your existing fitness routine – is quite another. Here's how your weights regime fits into the bigger picture.

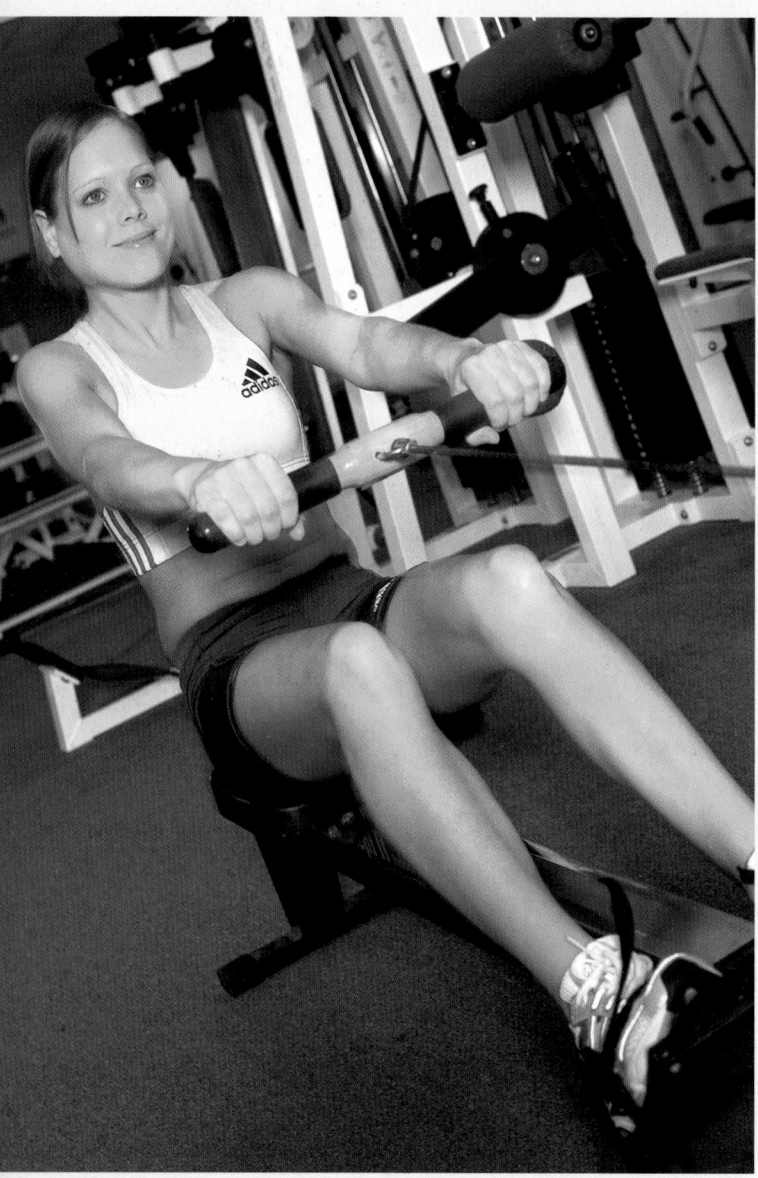

OK, I know this is a book about strength training – but the truth is that a balanced exercise programme – especially one with weight loss as its goal – needs to include both aerobic exercise and strength training (with flexibility work to keep muscles and joints healthy and supple). But how much is enough? And how hard do you have to work?

Creating a balanced programme

We've already looked at how often and how hard to strength train in Chapter 5. So what about aerobic activity? The American College of Sports Medicine recommends three to five sessions per week of moderate- to vigorous-intensity activity, lasting 20–60 minutes, to improve aerobic fitness, while general health guidelines suggest we get a dose of 30 minutes moderate activity on most days of the week. If you think that 30 minutes is a lot bear in mind that the human body was designed to be a lot more active than that! Clocking up 30 minutes is actually a bare minimum for health benefits and, quite honestly, won't go a long way towards aiding weight loss if done in isolation.

In fact, the American College of Sports Medicine's *Position Stand on Weight Loss*, published in 2001, recommends building up to 200–280 minutes of activity per week for sustained weight loss – that's 40–60 minutes a day, five days a week. Sounds like a lot, huh? But this can – and should – consist of both 'daily activity' and structured workouts. For example, if you clock up the 30-minute daily dose on five days and throw in three more effortful 20-minute sessions on your bike or on the treadmill, then you are there. The daily dose doesn't even have to be completed all at once. In fact, its role is to replicate the more active lifestyles our ancestors used to live and can be made up entirely of routine daily activities like walking, climbing stairs, carrying and lifting, gardening and doing household chores (see the box opposite for some ideas of where you could be more active).

You can easily get all the exercise you need – including your strength training – with three 50-minute sessions a week, coupled with general lifestyle activity on most days. In the gym you could follow your strength training session with a 30-minute swim or precede it with an aerobics class or treadmill run. That saves time while still allowing you to get the right balance of aerobic training and strength work. As we'll look at in a moment there is some feeling that concurrent strength and endurance work in the same session may reduce the benefits slightly, so if you have the motivation and time to train on separate days then you may gain slightly more – but in the greater scheme of things, the important thing is that you do it at all.

GETTING YOUR DAILY DOSE

Getting more active on a daily basis isn't about putting time aside for exercise, it's about using the time you have more effectively. It could be gardening, hosing down the wheelie bin, hand-washing the car, nipping to the shops on a bike, playing football with the kids or chasing sticks with the dog. Really think about your daily lifestyle. Ask yourself if you are guilty of any of the following:

- Do you use a shopping trolley when you could carry a basket?

- Do you park as close as you can to the supermarket/gym/station in the car park?

- Do you walk a dog and then stand still throwing a ball or stick?

- Do you walk to the closest sandwich shop at lunchtime?

- Do you sit up in the spectators' gallery while the kids are swimming instead of going for a swim or power walk yourself?

- Do you stand still on escalators or wait for lifts?

- Do you drive to the station when you could walk?

- Do you email colleagues in the same building?

- Do you use a remote control for the TV or stereo?

- Do you pile things at the bottom of the stairs rather than taking them up at the time?

The weekly regime

Where does strength training fit in if you are already an aerobics addict, yogi or runner? Not just in terms of finding the time to do both but also with respect to how to schedule both types of sessions to best effect. If you are already doing, or planning to do, aerobic exercise alongside strength training, you may be worried that you might reduce the effectiveness of what you are doing.

The general consensus about order of aerobic exercise and strength training is that concurrent strength and endurance training doesn't compromise endurance gains but *can* reduce strength gains. Since our focus is strength training this is an important consideration. One of the main factors seems to be the proximity of the two types of training. For example, following a tough treadmill run with resistance training may mean you aren't maximising the benefits to be gained from the latter. Research shows that it is more effective to do the two types of exercise on different days. But if that doesn't fit into your real life, then in what order should you perform the two types of activity?

Results are conflicting. Some research found that strength development was not hindered when strength training immediately *preceded* endurance training, or when resistance training took place at least half an hour after endurance training. However, a recent study at Brigham Young University in Utah found that performing aerobic exercise *before* resistance work was more beneficial than the other way round – for two reasons. First, the resistance training made the treadmill run feel harder and, secondly, EPOC (the 'afterburn' calories that the body uses to restore systems to normal after exercise) was greatest when resistance work followed a treadmill run, thereby maximising calorie expenditure. Keep the intensity of the preceding endurance activity moderate rather than high, too, if you don't want to compromise your strength training – a study from the University of Queensland found that high-intensity endurance exercise could inhibit performance in a subsequent resistance training session.

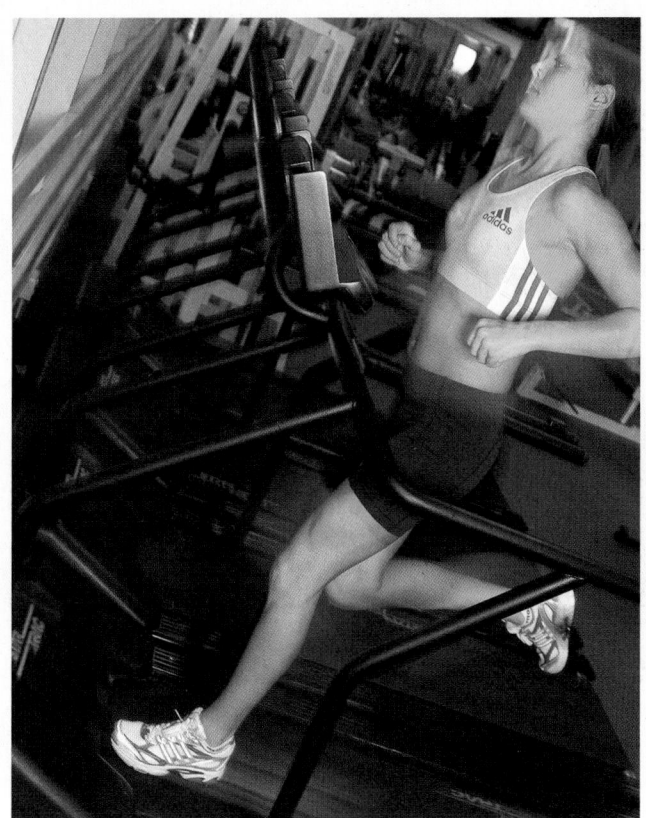

But knowing what we know about the different adaptations caused by aerobic training and strength training, we have to ask, are circuits really an effective method of building strength, or less of a 'Jack of All Trades' and more 'Master of None'? This question was addressed by the Australian-based Fitness Network, who came up with the following recommendations for making circuits effective:

- Bear in mind that if you are doing 20–30 repetitions of an exercise, you are working not on strength but on muscular endurance. If you want to build strength, then intersperse sets of 6–12 challenging repetitions with 1 to 3-minute 'aerobic' recovery periods.

- If you are already familiar with strength training the overload provided by circuit training is unlikely to be sufficient to trigger further strength increases. In one study, it was shown that strength gains from circuit training for ten to twelve weeks were 5–25%, while the same period of time spent resistance training created improvements of 50–200%.

- The aerobic pay-off of circuit training isn't as great as standard aerobic training as the time spent at each station is short and the resistance work causes a build-up of lactic acid in the muscles therefore reducing the intensity at which you can work at the next station. Circuit training can improve aerobic capacity (VO_2 max) by 5–8% according to

On the circuit

Then there's another solution. Perform the two in the very same session. That, of course, is the premise behind circuit training. You do a strength training exercise, followed by a period of aerobic activity – each one being a 'station' on the circuit. The circuit might be completed two or three times in all. Some circuit training uses weight training machines, like the international franchise-based Curves gyms, while others use free weights and body weight for resistance.

one study but conventional aerobic training is likely to elicit far greater gains in the range of 10–35%.

- Ensure the circuit doesn't 'pre-fatigue' muscles with isolation exercises, such as triceps extensions or biceps curls, as this will limit the effectiveness of subsequent compound moves like squats, push-ups and step-ups.

- The bottom line? If you enjoy circuit training and want a general workout – then go ahead. Additionally, if you are very mesomorphic and don't want to build muscle, this may be a good activity to utilise. But if your aim is to build strength, tone and maximise weight loss, you are better off doing your aerobic exercise and strength work separately.

Fitting in other activities

It's all very well talking about strength and endurance exercise when the distinction between them is so clear. But what about, say, rock climbing or yoga? Where do these fit in?

Activities that are highly strength-dependent, like rock climbing, in which you are pulling and pushing your own body weight, are effectively a form of resistance training – so don't expect to do your weights workout on Saturday and not suffer on your wall climbing session on Sunday. However, activities that may leave your muscles a bit sore, like Spinning or kickboxing, aren't overloading the muscles in the same way as strength training (they are improving muscular endurance, not strength) so you could do them back to back without a problem.

Finally, activities like Pilates and yoga are good for building strength from within rather like the Foundation Workout. For inexperienced exercisers they are effectively like strength training but there will come a time when the challenge placed on your body, in terms of overload, won't be great enough to instigate further muscle development.

Keeping it balanced

When deciding whether you are ready for a strength training session there are two good rules of thumb to follow: firstly, if your muscles are still substantially sore from an activity it is best to delay your next strength training session. A bit of residual soreness is fine but if every move you make has you groaning in pain, forget it! Delayed onset muscle soreness (DOMS) is usually worst two days after the activity that caused it.

The second rule is the hard-easy rule. If you have worked really hard in one session (be it aerobic exercise or another type of activity) make your next workout a little more forgiving or take a rest day.

YOU KNOW WHAT?

A study showed that calorie expenditure and heart rate were significantly higher during exercises using the lower body or lower and upper body together, compared to just the upper body. So think below the belt, if making a tighter notch in it is your goal!

Staying on track

A lack of visible results is the prime cause of dropping out of exercise programmes. Hopefully, that won't be your experience if you follow the advice in this book but that doesn't mean your resolve won't wobble occasionally. Here are some ways to stay on course…

Get practical

Do you keep missing your workout because the gym shuts so early? Or doesn't open early enough? If that's the case, swap gyms. Find somewhere that is more suited to your lifestyle. Maybe somewhere near to work rather than to home, for example. Or consider whether you could switch to home workouts, at least while you ride out a particularly busy period. Do you grab your kitbag and find it full of last week's smelly clothing and towel? Be organised by putting clean kit in your gym bag as soon as you get home from your last visit. Keep some spare kit at work or in the car as a back-up.

Beat boredom

If you are finding your workouts dull maybe it's time to find a new environment. Perhaps join a gym, so that you have the stimulation of other people around you, enlist a workout buddy (it always brings out your competitive streak!) or put some invigorating music on. New research from Brunel University saw up to an 18% improvement in adherence to exercise regimes with the help of the right music. You can also shake things up by adding new exercises to your repertoire, changing the structure of your workout or

setting yourself a few goals. For example, pledge to deadlift 40kg in six weeks' time or hold a ball kneeling balance for a minute.

Re-focus

If you feel as if you are just going through the motions of your workout, you may have lost sight of what you are really doing it for. Think back to when you started strength training, and write down the reasons you started. Have you got closer to any of those goals? Is picking up your toddler easier? Can you lift heavy boxes that you previously had to ask your partner to shift? Do you walk to work now when you wouldn't have dreamed of doing so before? Give yourself some recognition for what you have achieved and make sure you know where you are heading next.

Make time

It's not so much that we don't have time to exercise, more that we don't schedule it in, simply hoping that we'll squeeze it in at some point. Realise that while exercise will take up minutes or hours of your week, the time spent doing it will enable you to use the rest of your day more productively. Not convinced? Well, studies show that exercise can improve mental function (such as decision making and problem solving skills), it can alleviate mild depression and dissipate tension. What's more, when you exercise regularly, you actually become more stress-resilient so the day's problems will bounce off you rather than knock you down.

Find a role model

You might not want to look like one of those cover models on *Muscle & Fitness* magazine, but do you covet Nicole Kidman's shapely arms or Kelly Holmes' fantastic abs? Think of somebody who has a physique – or part of a physique – that you like and stick a picture of them on the fridge, or by your desk, to remind you that you need to keep on track if you want to reap visible results.

Pushing off a plateau

People often say that getting started with exercise is the most difficult bit, but I beg to differ! In the first few weeks the improvements come thick and fast, there's the novelty factor and you can't imagine why you didn't do it before. But a few weeks or months down the line perhaps you begin to feel as if you aren't making progress any more, the novelty has worn off and it all feels a bit of a drag.

This is a very common experience and is probably the reason why more than half of those who take up exercise have given it up within six months. So what can you do to stay on course? Well, for starters, it's worth knowing that it is easier to make progress at the outset. This is because you are further away from your natural potential so you have more room for improvement. As you get fitter it is tougher to overload the body in order to instigate further changes. So it's not your imagination! But don't be disheartened by this truth. With what you have learned about manipulating your programme, it shouldn't be too difficult to ring the changes

and find a new way of challenging your body and making further progress.

Shake up your routine

Playing with different reps and sets isn't the only way to shake up your strength training regime. Here are a few other ideas…

Use unilateral movements

In other words, do exercises that you would normally do with both sides of the body or both limbs, with just one. For example, do a unilateral bench press, using alternate dumbbells, or use the leg press or leg curl machines with one leg at a time. Research shows that in free weight exercises unilateral work demands more core stability, so there's an added benefit, too.

Try metabolic circuits

This is a term used to describe a form of strength circuit-training. It is best performed with dumbbells or medicine balls – or just your body weight – and is most effective when lower and upper body exercises are alternated. (For example, a bench press is followed by a lunge.) The idea is to work swiftly – without compromising form – performing each exercise in the circuit for fifteen seconds, taking a 30-second rest afterwards. (Or, if you performed the exercise for 30 seconds, you'd take a one-minute rest – creating the same 1:2 work to rest ratio.) You then move on to the next exercise immediately. Once the circuit is complete, you repeat it – as many times as is appropriate for you.

Cut the rest

Shorter rest periods (less than a minute) won't maximise strength gains but they will stimulate the release of more growth hormone, contributing to fat loss.

Add instability

Instead of exercising on a weights bench, use an exercise ball to make your body work harder in order to stabilise itself. Or perform standing exercises on an unstable surface such as a core board or a balance pad.

Jump to it

Add power to your moves. Plyometrics is a system of exercise that makes use of the body's 'stretch-shortening' system. The notion is that the energy stored in the muscle allows for greater force to be produced rapidly. For example, instead of performing a squat with both feet on the ground you'd leap up off the floor, land back into a squat and go straight into the next one. However, this isn't a strategy to try until you are fairly experienced. I also recommend doing the moves initially without weight to get your body accustomed to it. If you want to give it a try do it at the start of your workout, when muscles are freshest, and aim for only a few repetitions.

Change the speed

A study published in the *Journal of Strength and Conditioning Research* from Appalachian State University in North Carolina found that varying the speed of the exercise played a part in increasing strength and power in an eight-week programme. Slow, controlled movements on some days were interspersed with fast, power-based moves on others.

Try a new technique

Yes! There is more than one way to lift a weight. Read on to find out about some of the popular methods...

Superslow training

In 'superslow' training, the weights are lifted and lowered very slowly (up to fifteen seconds per repetition) – the theory is that this forces more motor units to get a piece of the action. Some research has found much bigger strength gains from the superslow technique, compared to regular-speed training, but brand new research, published in *Medicine & Science in Sport & Exercise* found that faster training resulted in an 11% greater increase in strength than slow training did. The discrepancy in these findings once again goes to show that there is no single way to work that beats all the others. Throwing in the odd superslow session will do no harm and adds variety to your regime. But bear in mind that you will almost certainly have to drop the weight you use by 10–20% and perform fewer repetitions to reach fatigue.

Breakdown training

Aptly named, as this is no walk in the park. But breakdown training can be an effective way of blasting off a plateau, when you don't seem to be able to make further gains. The general idea is that you do your set as usual, with your standard weight, until you reach momentary muscle failure, then immediately decrease the resistance by 10–20% and continue to eke out as many reps as you can with this slightly lower weight. The premise behind this is that it forces the muscle to recruit more fibres to complete the work. Research at the South Shore YMCA in Massachusetts found that breakdown training worked well both for beginners and more experienced trainers. In eight weeks, beginners increased their weight load by an average of 25lb (11.3kg), compared to 18lb (8kg) in a control group doing regular strength training. Experienced weight trainers saw significant improvements after just six weeks – performing a greater number of chin-ups and dips and lifting considerably more weight.

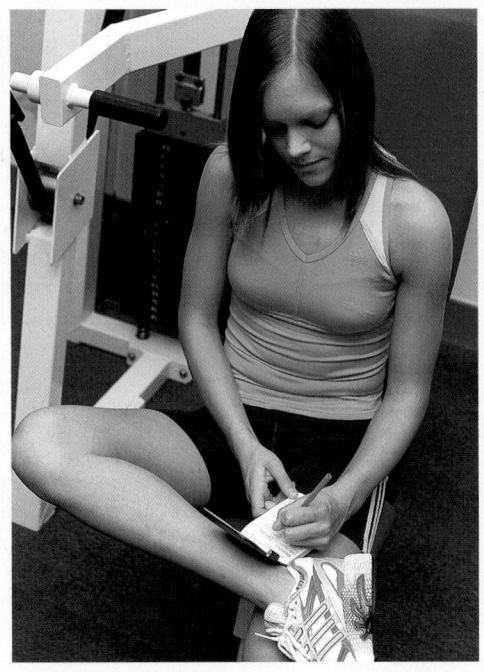

Eccentric training

Also called negative resistance training, this technique focuses only on the part of the muscle action in which the muscle is lengthening to control the movement initiated (for example, the lowering of the dumbbells in a bench press). Why would you do this? The theory is that muscles are stronger during the eccentric phase so working through this part of the movement can result in greater strength gains. As an example, you might get a partner to assist you in placing a barbell in your hands once you are in the top of a biceps curl position and then lower it with control. You can also do it sans partner. For example, you could lift a weight with both hands but lower it with just one. Research shows that the post-

BACK AND BICEPS WORKOUT

	1/3/06	5/3/06	8/3/06	10/3/06
Aerobic training	15 mins x-trainer	30 mins run	15 mins x-trainer	15 mins rower
Deadlift	4 x 4 30kg	4 x 5 30kg	4 x 5 30kg	4 x 6 30kg
Lat pulldown			3 x 8 40kg	
Assisted pull-ups	3 x 8 70kg	3 x 8 70kg		3 x 8 70kg
Seated row	3 x 10 30kg		3 x 10 30kg	
Single arm-row		3 x 8 15kg		3 x 8 15kg
Prone flye	2 x 8 4kg superslow	2 x 8 4kg superslow	2 x 8 4kg superslow	2 x 8 4kg superslow
Barbell curl				
Biceps curls	3 x 10 8kg	3 x 10 8kg	3 x 10 8kg	3 x 10 8kg

(3 x 8 70kg means 3 sets of 8 reps with a 70kg weight)

workout muscular aches (delayed onset muscle soreness or DOMS) you get from eccentric training is greater than from standard training, so be warned.

Supersetting

This is a time-efficient but challenging technique in which you pair up two exercises, usually those that work opposing muscle groups (such as the biceps and triceps), and perform an exercise for each with no rest in between. You only rest when you have finished the whole set. A variation on supersetting is 'compound' supersetting in which you alternate two exercises for the *same* muscle group with no rest between each one. So, you might team up bench presses with chest flys, for example. This is a very intensive way to train – but a great way to shake things up now and again, and has been shown to elicit size gains as well as strength.

Whatever technique or method you follow, don't do it forever. Variety is the secret to continued improvement – and interest.

The write way to keep on track

It is vital to keep a record of your strength training. It's impossible to remember how many reps and sets you did and what weight you used for every single exercise. A training log doesn't have to focus solely on your strength training either. It can include all your physical activity notes about what you ate and drank, your mood, your menstrual cycle… The only difference between a training journal for, say, running and a strength training log is that

STRONG WORDS

PUT YOUR MIND WHERE YOUR MUSCLE IS

Take off that iPOD and transport your mind inside your muscles. Imagine the fibres shortening and lengthening and the blood flowing through them. Really focus on perfect posture and as you inhale, visualise the energy flowing to the muscle. Only close your eyes while you do this if you are securely situated on a fixed machine – otherwise, focus on your 'third' eye, a spot slightly above your eyes and in the middle.

you need a lot more space for the latter. Most people use a simple notebook to keep track of their strength workouts or create blank sheets on the computer that they fill in. Don't forget to include information such as if you used a particular technique, such as superslow or supersetting, and, where relevant, comment on whether things worked well or otherwise. You may find it a bit tedious at first, to fill in the blanks after every workout, but once you see your weights climbing you won't be able to wait to fill in the next column!

AGES AND STAGES

Safe, effective strength training throughout life's ages and stages

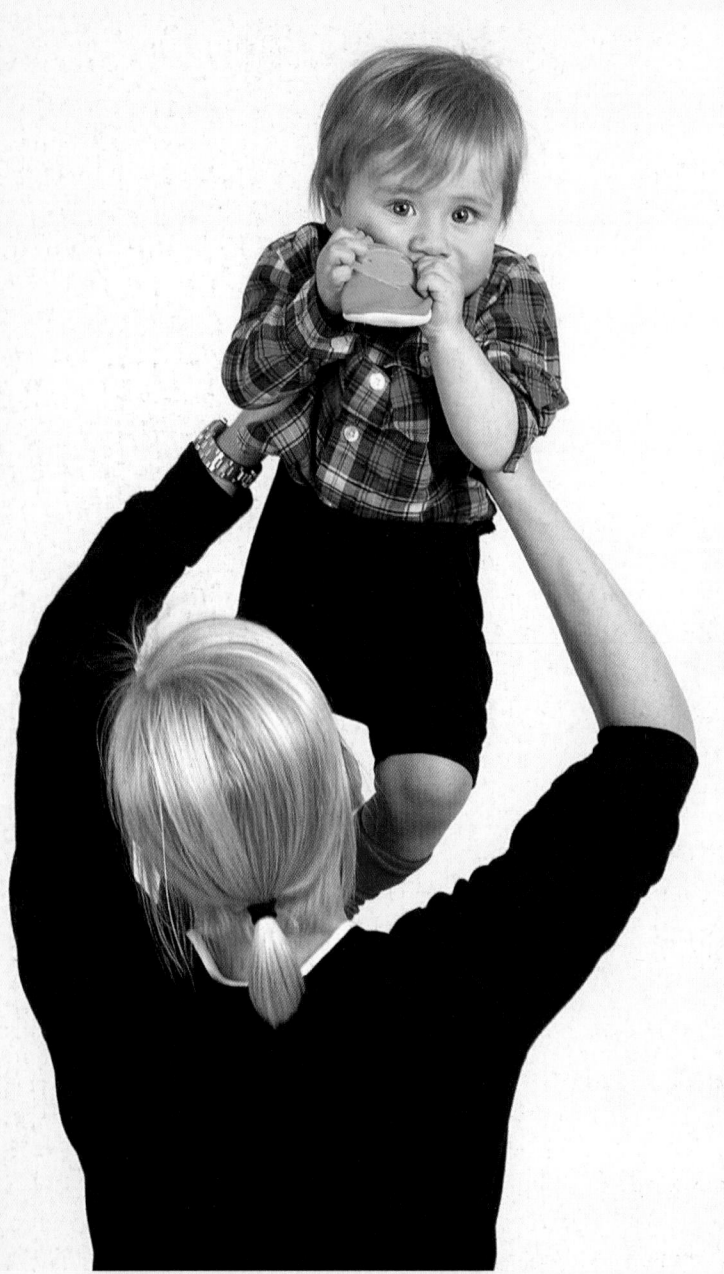

Is strength training an activity you can benefit from at any age? You bet! But there are some precautions to take and some factors to be aware of when training during pregnancy, after giving birth and during or post-menopause. This section gives you a little more information, but always consult your doctor if you are in doubt about whether strength training is appropriate.

Pregnancy – lifting for two

Internationally recognised guidelines from the American College of Obstetricians and Gynaecologists (ACOG) state that exercise during pregnancy is not just safe but desirable. But does that include strength training? It does, but there are a couple of considerations to bear in mind. As with all types of training, pregnancy is a time to maintain what you already have rather than aim to achieve more. So put your goals aside for a few months and focus on holding on to the strength you have achieved thus far.

Here are a few other safety points to consider:

- Use slow, controlled movements because the effects of the hormone relaxin make your joints 'looser' and more liable to be injured.

- Stick to lighter weights to reduce the risk of injury.

- Don't hold your breath during exercises, which can increase blood pressure. Avoid the Valsalva manoeuvre (forcefully exhaling without actually releasing air which causes lower abdominal pressure similar to that of a bowel movement).

- Don't exercise in overheated environments and ensure you stay well hydrated.

- Avoid exercises that put you in a position where you could be at risk of dropping a weight on to your belly. So, for example, you would be safer to use the chest press machine rather than doing a dumbbell or barbell bench press.

- Beginning in the second trimester avoid lifting weights while standing as the increased blood volume you have can cause blood to pool in your legs and cause dizziness or lightheadedness. Some experts believe that lying flat on your back decreases blood flow to the uterus too, so you may want to consider sticking with seated exercise.

- Be aware that some pregnant women are more prone to losing their balance as their centre of gravity shifts forwards and upwards.

Don't exercise without medical advice if

- You are pregnant with multiple babies.

- You have had previous miscarriages or premature births.

- You have hypertension.

- You have experienced bleeding.

- You feel any pain or discomfort from doing so
.

- You don't feel confident about doing so.

STRONG WORDS

REASONS TO STAY STRONG

Half of all pregnant women experience back pain – probably due to the increased lordotic curve that results from pregnancy – but exercise to strengthen the abdominals prior to pregnancy will reduce the risk of being one of the unlucky 50%.

Exercise that strengthens the upper body – particularly in terms of keeping the upper and mid-back muscles strong – will also help avert the slumped posture many women adopt in pregnancy due to the increasing weight of their breasts and the changing centre of gravity.

Recent research shows that physical activity may reduce the occurrence of gestational diabetes and pre-eclampsia by as much as 50% and 40% respectively.

Post-pregnancy

There are no hard and fast rules about when it is appropriate to resume exercise after pregnancy. ACOG recommends no physical stress for two weeks after delivery and not to return to full daily activities for a further four weeks. Additionally, if you have had a Caesarean delivery, you should avoid exercise for eight to ten weeks, to allow for full healing. Joint laxity, as a result of the relaxin, takes about twelve weeks to dissipate after pregnancy but that doesn't mean you can't begin some very gentle controlled exercises.

Take the floor

First on the list should be Kegel exercises. You will *not* regain strength or tone in the pelvic floor muscle without them. The easiest way to identify these muscles is to stop the flow of urine while you are on the loo, without clenching your buttocks. Once you've got a hold on that, you basically need to do this movement every day for the rest of your life. Recent research suggests that you don't need to contract to your maximum; a slightly less than maximal contraction is more effective. Try 'the elevator' in which you contract upwards progressively over five levels – then release progressively over another five. Another good exercise to try is to imagine 'knitting' the walls of the vagina together – so you are squeezing together rather than pulling upwards.

Mummy's tummy

Over two thirds of women experience an opening in the abdominal wall by the third trimester of pregnancy (known as diastis recti). It is vital not to do standard abdominal exercises post-pregnancy if this is the case, as it can prevent the gap from closing up. Even without diastis recti the rectus abdominis can stretch by as much as 20cm during pregnancy while the transversus abdominis, which is responsible for providing core stability and protecting the lower back, will need to be strengthened and its function restored. All women should wait until their post-birth check up before resuming standard abdominal exercises. Exercises for the abdominals that are safe to do before then are shown below.

On the pull

Finally, as you get to grips with being a new mum, try to focus your strength training efforts on the back of the body and pulling – rather than pushing – movements. Everything about motherhood – from nursing to changing nappies to putting baby in a car seat – involves forward movements and, without balancing work in the gym or with resistance, you may end up with a very 'forward' posture with hunched, rounded shoulders, tight chest muscles, a weak back and flabby buttocks.

NAVEL TO SPINE CONTRACTIONS:

Inhale and, as you exhale, draw the navel gently into the spine. Hold for a few seconds without holding your breath. Build up to 20 second holds.

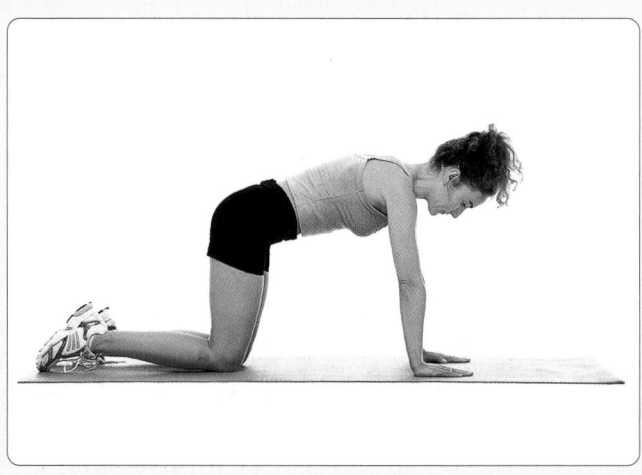

FRONT LYING ABDOMINAL RAISE:

Lie face down with your hands under your fore-head, head in line with the body. Keeping the rest of the body relaxed, inhale and, as you exhale, peel the navel off the floor, lifting the abdominals. Hold for 6 seconds, breathing freely, then relax. Do not lift the hipbones off the floor or contract the back.

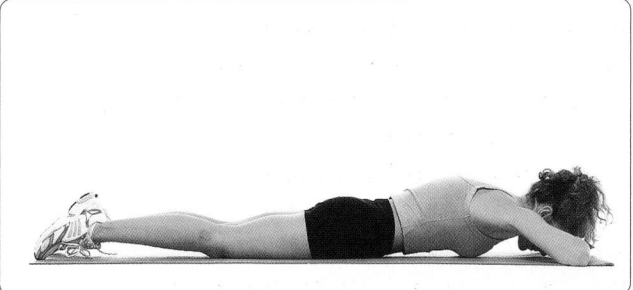

PELVIC TILTS:

Lie on the floor with the knees bent, feet flat and spine in neutral. Inhale and, as you exhale, draw the navel to spine and tilt the pelvis so the pubic bone curls towards you. Feel your back pressing lightly into the floor.

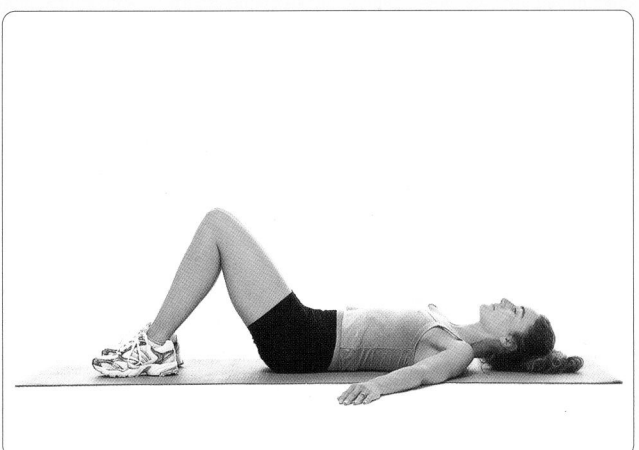

Menopause and strength training

Despite the huge emotive significance that menopause has in our society – the turning of the corner, the slippery slope towards old age, the passing of femininity – the menopause, put simply, is the signal of the end of reproductive potential. There is no longer enough of the hormones oestrogen and progesterone to facilitate or sustain pregnancy. The average woman reaches menopause at 52 years old but the changes associated with the menopause can begin as much as a decade earlier. During this 'peri-menopause' stage, levels of the female hormones are depleting, influencing everything from mood to fat distribution and bone density and causing unwelcome effects like hot flushes and vaginal dryness.

For many women menopause goes hand in hand with weight gain and loss of lean muscle tissue. But research has not found any proof that weight gain is a direct result of menopause. In fact, one study found that women aged 42 to 50 gained the same amount of weight over that period whether or not they had been through the menopause, suggesting that lifestyle factors are more to blame. Peri-menopausal symptoms vary widely from woman to woman but there is a lot of evidence to suggest that regular exercise can soften the experience of the menopause. The Melpomene Institute found that physically active women rated their health through menopause much better than non-active women did. They were also less likely to suffer – or suffered less severely – with mental and physical symptoms of the menopause. Research shows that exercise is associated with a 55% decline in the frequency and intensity of hot flushes, for example.

So what about strength training? Well, the evidence suggests that resistance training can attenuate the loss of lean tissue, along with the accompanying decline in metabolic rate and the drop in levels of the muscle-building hormone testosterone. And a high lean body mass doesn't just look good – it is also associated with a high level of the type of oestrogen known as oestrone which is thought to protect against reproductive tissue cancers. A study from the University of Vienna put early post-menopausal women on an intense strength-training programme for fourteen months. At the end of the study measures of strength, endurance, quality of life and even bone mineral density had improved in women during the critical early post-menopausal years. Talking of which…

Aging bones and osteoporosis

The old 'use it or lose it' adage is often applied to muscle, but the same goes for bone density (the thickness and strength of the bone). The more you do sooner, the better. Peak bone mass – the maximum amount of bone you ever attain – occurs around the age of 20 and, from 30 or so, a slow decline begins. In the decades prior to menopause we lose 0.75–1% per year – but in the years following it bone density can plummet by as much as 5% per year which is why the bone-thinning condition osteoporosis – that causes

frailty, a high risk of fracture and loss of height – affects one in three women over the age of 50 in the UK.

According to the UK Health Development Agency, regular weight-bearing exercise can reduce the accelerated rate of bone loss in post-menopausal women, even in the absence of hormone replacement therapy (HRT). Regular physical activity can reduce the risk of hip fractures by around 50%.

The best recipe for preventing osteoporosis is combining weight-bearing aerobic exercise with strength training. If you want proof, then consider that swimmers and cyclists, whose activity *isn't* weight bearing, have been found to have similar bone density as normally active people, while bodybuilders and gymnasts have bone density 30% higher than average.

A stronger skeleton

Why is strength training so good? Partly because, unlike running or jumping it can work the entire skeleton not just the lower half. You can actually target any muscle you like with specific exercises. The most common vulnerable sites for osteoporotic fractures are the spine, hip and wrist. Also, because when muscles contract and pull on bone the force that the bone experiences causes it to increase its mass to better tolerate the contractions next time. The evidence suggests that resistance training successfully maintains or slightly improves hip and spine bone mass.

As I've said before, lifting light weights numerous times is not of much benefit – and this holds true in terms of bone health,

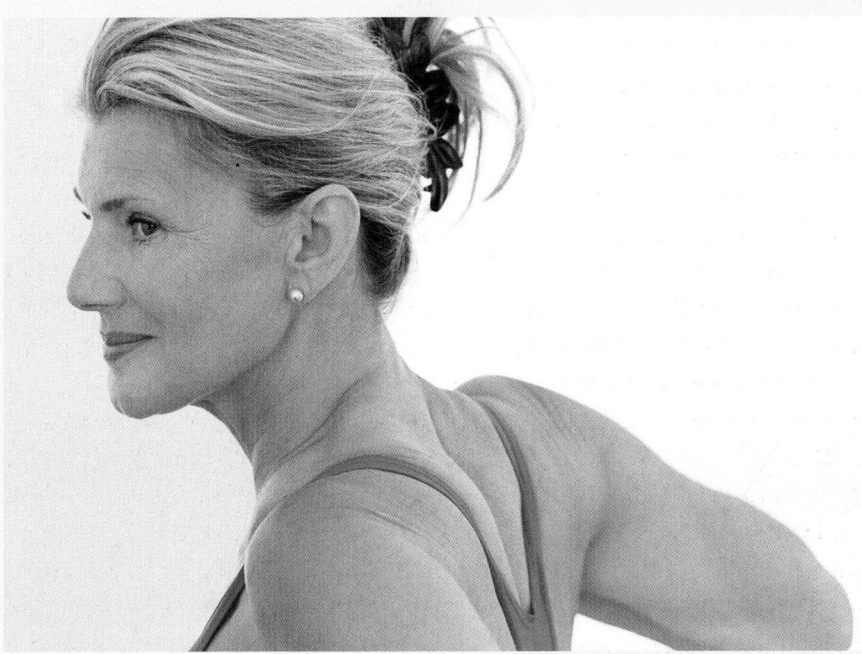

according to expert Kerry Winters-Stone. It seems that high intensity is the name of the game – research shows that women who benefit as far as bone is concerned are working three sets with heavier weights.

If you already have osteoporosis you can still work with weights but you should do so under the guidance of your doctor. Start slowly, with lighter weights, in order to master the technique and movements involved. A weighted vest can be a good alternative to free weights for some exercises (for example, squats and lunges), as it keeps the weight close to the body and leaves the hands free. Alternatively, use resistance tubing so that you don't over-stress your joints or risk weight-related injuries.

Training and aging

Like it or not, with advancing age comes a natural decline in muscle mass and range of motion. The average adult loses 5–10% of muscle mass between the ages of 20 and 50. The strength of the back, leg and arm muscles plummets by as much as 60% between the ages of 30 and 80, spinal extension range decreases rapidly and ankle joints can lose half their range of motion between the ages of 55 and 85. With strength and muscle-mass loss comes a knock-on effect on metabolic rate and on our ability to do tasks that were once a cinch. Results from a large-scale epidemiological study found that 40% of the female population aged 55–64, 45% of women aged 65–74 and 65% of women aged 75–84 were unable to lift 4.5kg. It's a worrying prospect – but over and over again research shows that most of this decline occurs because we don't do anything to stop it. If we maintained muscle mass in the first place we'd offset the drop in metabolic rate, not gain excess body fat and continue to be active on a daily basis. A Scandinavian study published in the *International Journal of Sports Medicine* demonstrated that 70-year-olds who had lifted weights regularly for more than ten years had as much muscle as 28-year-olds.

Never too late

But what if the rot has already set in? Happily it isn't to late too do something to reverse the situation. Some classic research in a report in the *Journal of the American Geriatrics Society* showed that women aged 60–77 who strength trained for sixteen weeks could walk 20% faster, had gained a 50% increase in muscle strength and were able to sit or stand more comfortably for longer. Low bone mass, poor daily function, reduced muscle strength and postural instability are predictors of the risk of fracture in an elderly person, so any activity that can preserve strength and attenuate these risk factors is well worth doing. Once again, strength training takes centre stage.

What's more, a study published in the *Journal of Applied Physiology* in 2005 found that, in older women, six months of resistance training resulted in a 4% increase in resting metabolic rate as well as a 9% increase in total daily energy expenditure (amounting, on average, to 177 calories per day). And the average age of the women was 72 years old!

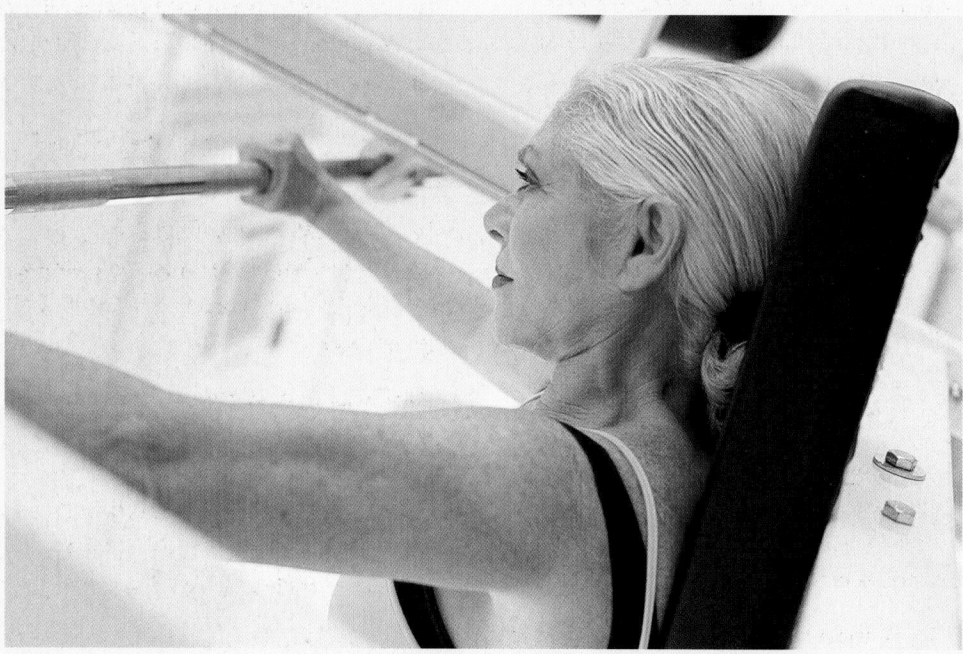

Another important consideration is that, often, studies in which older adults are put on exercise programmes don't result in them increasing their energy expenditure because they spontaneously decrease the amount of energy they burn the rest of the day. This has led some experts to suggest that gentler forms of activity like tai chi and walking are more suitable. But it is likely that this compensatory response is because the level of intensity of exercise in the study is too high, so the subjects are exhausted for the rest of the day. However, it appears from research that resistance training is less likely to have this effect than aerobic exercise. In fact, if the level of intensity is appropriate to begin with, and increased slowly but surely, it is possible that subjects could become *more* spontaneously active, as they have a better ability to cope with daily demands due to enhanced strength and aerobic capacity.

Exercise also reduces the risk of falls and accidents among older people through developing bone health and maintaining normal muscle strength and joint structure and function. Regular workouts can give older people a level of functional capacity associated with people ten to fifteen years younger.

Exercising safely in later life

- Warm up thoroughly. Levels of elastin (the stretchy component in connective tissue) deteriorate with age making muscles and tendons more injury-prone.

- Think about functional exercises rather than

STRONG WORDS

IS STRENGTH TRAINING SAFE AFTER BREAST CANCER?

According to a study from the University of Pennsylvania in 2005 the answer is yes. A randomised controlled trial assessed the safety and effects of twice-weekly weight training among recent breast cancer survivors. Those who strength trained showed significant increases in lean mass as well as significant decreases in body fat and a self-perceived better quality of life.

about honing in on single muscle groups. For example, a squat is much more akin to daily activities than is a leg extension. A shoulder press overhead is more useful than a triceps kickback…

- Allow yourself longer to recover between sessions.

- Heed the ACSM guidelines for strength training for older adults. These recommend 10–15 repetitions for adults 50–60 years of age or older.

- Watch your protein intake. Studies show that many older adults are not eating enough protein and, if you are strength training this is even more important. The ACSM guidelines suggest 1.0–1.25g of high-quality protein per kg of body weight per day.

Directory

You've got the book, you've done the workout – now you want the t-shirt, and the shoes, and the exercise ball! You should find everything you need to help you get stronger on these pages…

Equipment

Bowflex
A home gym machine on which you can perform over 60 exercises, based on rods and pulleys.
0800 013 1606 or www.bowflex.co.uk

ICON Health & Fitness
Home aerobic machinery such as treadmills and elliptical trainers.
0113 387 7122 or www.nordictrack.com/uk

Life Fitness
A comprehensive and reliable range of weight-training equipment and aerobic machines.
www.lifefitness.com

4My Way of Life
Exercise mats and balls, resistance tubing, balance pads and other core stability items.
0870 241 5471 or www.4mywayoflife.com

Nautilus
An extensive range of strength-training products, from weight stations, racks, benches and bars to dumbbell sets,
01908 267 345 or www.nautilus.com

The Physical Company
A huge range of exercise mats and balls, medicine balls, resistance tubing, core stability equipment and a wide range of free weights, including dumbbells and barbells.
01494 769 222 or www.physicalcompany.co.uk

ProActive Health
A massive range of products from weights benches to yoga mats, treadmills to core boards, mini trampolines to body bars.
0870 848 4842 or www.proactive-health.co.uk

I don't know what dumbbells to buy – any advice?
Why not start off with a set of dumbbells in different weights? You can get a set of three different weights quite cheaply and these will give you more scope than just having one set. Alternatively, you could invest in dumbbells on which you attach weight plates so that the amount you lift can be varied quite significantly. The best thing to do, if you don't have the opportunity to try a few different weights at the gym, is to go to a sports store where you can actually see and pick up what is on offer.

I like…
One of the best bargains around is the V-Fit trio of dumbbells from Argos, available for home delivery (www.argos.co.uk). Two at 1.5kg, two at 3kg and two at 5kg give a beginner plenty of scope.

What essentials should I have in my gym bag?

What gets you through a workout varies from person to person. But everyone should have a drinks bottle to hand, to ensure that you stay hydrated while you train. You will almost certainly need a gym towel, too – not only to wipe off your sweat but also to protect your skin from other people's. The Marsupialtowel is a great version that has a Velcro pocket on it for locker keys and iPODs (www.marsupialtowel.com). The other essential, in my opinion, is a training log and pen so you can jot down your reps, sets and weight lifted at the time of training. And finally, a pair of weight-training gloves, if you are precious about your hands! Lifting weights will eventually cause hard skin to build up below your fingers if you don't wear gloves.

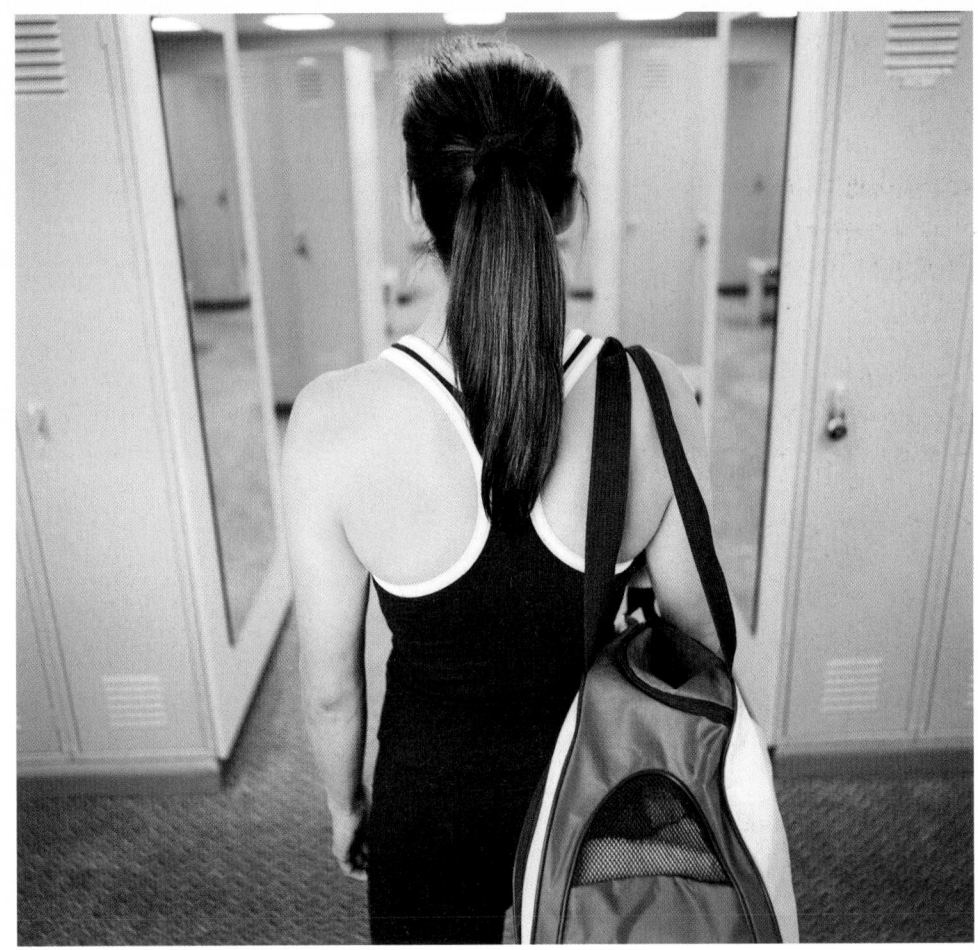

I like…

A new take on elastic resistance, called the Digiband. Thanks to the Digiband's 'powermarks', little oval-shaped icons with a kg weight printed in them, you can keep tabs on how much weight you're pushing or pulling. When you stretch the band enough to make the oval turn into a circle you are working at the resistance stated. Cheap, lightweight and available in three strengths, it is available from www.proactive-health.co.uk.

Clothing

What should I wear to workout in?

You can wear anything that is loose and comfortable (especially if you are exercising at home!). Avoid clothes that are too baggy or flowing as they may get caught in machinery – and besides, they don't allow you to keep tabs on your body position and technique. Breathable fabrics are best for wicking away sweat from the body and allowing it to evaporate – look for brand names Coolmax, Climacool and Dri-fit.

Adidas

Performance-orientated clothing, accessories and footwear.
0161 419 2500 or www.adidas.co.uk

Casall

Stylish activewear, underwear and accessories for fitness.
www.casall.co.uk

Gaiam

Good for products relating to health, wellness, fitness and yoga.
0870 241 5471 or www.gaiamdirect.co.uk

Less Bounce

A sports bra specialist.
0800 036.3840 or www.lessbounce.com

New Balance

Clothing, footwear and accessories.
01925 423000 or www.newbalance.co.uk

Nike

Clothing, footwear and accessories including weight-training gloves.
0800 056 1640 or www.nike.com

Pretty Sporty

A women-only clothing and accessories store for active women.
01494 872 277 or www.prettysporty.co.uk

Sweaty Betty

Own-brand and other high-end brands of sportswear, footwear, equipment and accessories for women.
www.sweatyBetty.com

What sort of shoes should I wear?

A pair of cross-trainers, with adequate support, stability and cushioning is fine for strength training. If you are going to be combining resistance training with high-impact aerobic exercise at the gym, however (such as running or aerobics), then you are better off investing in shoes designed for your particular activity and wearing them for your gym workout. Running shoes are not ideal for aerobics or kickboxing type classes as they don't have any lateral support and lack forefoot cushioning.

Supplements

With supplements, you tend to get what you pay for – cheap brands are often less effective and don't contain sufficient doses of the active ingredients. Buy supplements from a reputable source and check the dosage and concentration of the relevant ingredient. Here are some good places to start…

www.highfive.co.uk (for own brand energy, protein and creatine supplements).

www.thenutricentre.com (for a variety of brands and a useful search facility).

www.seeknatural.co.uk or 0870 321 0079 (for a variety of brands and products).

www.solgar.co.uk (for own-brand vitamin and mineral supplements).

Useful organisations

National Register of Personal Trainers
By searching this national database of qualified, experienced personal trainers you should be able to find the right person to help you get the basic techniques of strength training correct and keep you motivated.
0870 200 6010 or www.nrpt.org.uk

National Strength and Conditioning Association
A US-based body that conducts extensive research into the effects of strength training, maintains a comprehensive website, publishes journals and offers courses for becoming a qualified strength coach.
www.nsca-lift.org

www.strongwomen.com
Run by Dr Miriam Nelson, a leading researcher in women's health and the role of strength training, this US-based site has some useful tips and articles.

Recommended reading

An Action Plan for Osteoporosis
(Kerri Winters-Stone, Human Kinetics)

The Complete Guide to Post-natal Fitness
(Judy deFiore, A&C Black)

The Weight Loss Bible
(Joanna Hall, Kyle Cathie)

Strength Training Anatomy
(Frederic Delavier, Human Kinetics)

Glossary

Aerobic Literally means 'with oxygen', but usually refers to exercise that relies on aerobic metabolism

Atherosclerosis Accumulation of fat on the artery walls resulting in a narrowing of the vessels and risk of heart attack or stroke.

Anaerobic In the absence of oxygen (although this is never entirely the case). But usually refers to short, sharp efforts in exercise, in which energy cannot be supplied fast enough through aerobic metabolism. Strength training is an example.

Basal metabolic rate The rate at which your body ticks over at rest, usually measured following a 12 hour fast and a night's sleep.

Body composition The ratio of body fat to lean tissue

Body mass index A method of estimating and classifying body composition based on weight and height

Bone mineral density A measure of the amount of bone mineral content

Cardiac output The amount of blood pumped from the heart in one minute

Cardiorespiratory Relating to the heart and lungs

Cardiovascular Relating to the heart and blood vessels

Cartilage A tough connective tissue found throughout the body

Concentric A muscular contraction that takes place while the muscle is shortening

Compound An exercise that uses multiple muscle groups

Contraction Muscle pulling to create force

Core stability Control and appropriate strength and function of the stabilising muscles throughout the body. Often refers specifically to those of the abdominals and back

Diastolic The lower part of a blood pressure reading, representing the phase during which the heart muscle relaxes

Eccentric A muscular contraction that takes place while the muscle is lengthening

Engage To consciously recruit a muscle

Extensor A muscle that straightens a joint

Fast-twitch fibre A type of muscle fibre that reaches maximum tension very fast but also fatigues quickly

Flexor A muscle that bends a joint

Glycaemic Index A classification of the effect of a carbohydrate food on blood sugar levels

Glycogen The body's storage form of carbohydrate, stored in the liver and in muscles

Heart rate The number of times the heart beats per minute

Hypertrophy A growth in physical size of a muscle

Isometric A muscular contraction in which the muscle stays the same length

Lean body mass The proportion of the body made up of non-fat tissue (including muscle, connective tissue and bone)

Ligament Connective tissue that joins bone to bone

Lumbar spine Lower spine

Maximal oxygen uptake (VO2 max) The maximum amount of oxygen a person can extract from the air and utilise in the working tissues

Metabolic rate The amount of energy expended by a person in a given amount of time

Metabolism The process of energy production and usage in the body

Motor Unit A nerve and the muscle fibres it enervates

Muscle fibre A single muscle cell (a muscle may contain as many as 450000 fibres)

Myofibril A bundle of muscle fibres

Myoglobin A form of oxygen stored in the muscles

Neuromuscular Relating to nerves and muscles

Osteoporosis A condition marked by a substation decrease in bone density that leaves the bones brittle and liable to fracture

Peri-menopause The years preceding the menopause when hormonal changes are already taking place

Periodization A planned training programme consisting of different phases or cycles with a specific purpose and progression towards a specific goal

Progressive overload The principle that states that in order for the body to continue getting fitter, the workload needs to be gradually but consistently increased

Prone Face down

Resting heart rate The number of times the heart beats per minute at rest

Sarcomere The functioning unit within a muscle fibre

Slow twitch fibre A type of muscle fibre that is fatigue resistant but slow to reach maximal power. Best suited to low power, long duration activities.

Somatotyping A system of classification of body types by shape and proportions

Submaximal Below maximum effort or intensity

Supine Face up

Synovial fluid The sticky substance found in joints which adds cushioning and lubricates joint structures.

Systolic The top part of a blood pressure reading, which represents the phase during which the heart muscle contracts

Total Energy Expenditure The amount of energy used in a day, including resting metabolic rate

Tendon Connective tissue that joins bone to muscle

Valsalva Manoeuvre A technique in which one increases the pressure within the abdominal and chest cavity by forcibly breathing out while keeping the throat closed to trap and pressurise air in the lungs

Index

Acknowledgements

My greatest appreciation goes to Pat Fox, strength and conditioning specialist at the Human Performance Centre, South Bank University – not just for his valuable feedback and contributions to the text but also for showing me how to kneel on a balance ball and perfect my deadlift! Sincere thanks also to Sarah Connors, from the Back on Track Sports Injury Clinic in London, for her time and input in developing the Foundation Workout – true strength comes from within…

Adidas and Casall provided the fantastic clothing for the photo shoots, while the Physical Company and Gaiam kindly loaned us a wealth of fitness equipment and gadgets. Rachel Fradgley, Jill Christie, Juliet Murrell and Lulu Valentine did a sterling job being supermodels and Guy Hearn took the fantastic photographs. Thanks to you all.

Good Housekeeping

easy to make!
Family Meals
in Minutes

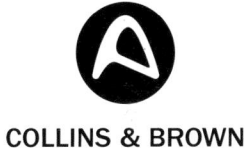

COLLINS & BROWN

First published in Great Britain in 2009
by Collins & Brown
10 Southcombe Street
London W14 0RA

An imprint of Anova Books Company Ltd

The Good Housekeeping website is
www.allaboutyou.com/goodhousekeeping

1 2 3 4 5 6 7 8 9

ISBN 978-1-84340-495-8

A catalogue record for this book is available from the British
Library.

Reproduction by Dot Gradations Ltd
Printed and bound by Times Offset, Malaysia

This book can be ordered direct from the publisher. Contact the
marketing department, but try your bookshop first.

www.anovabooks.com

NOTES

- Both metric and imperial measures are given for the recipes. Follow either set of measures, not a mixture of both, as they are not interchangeable.
- All spoon measures are level.
  1 tsp = 5ml spoon; 1 tbsp = 15ml spoon.
- Ovens and grills must be preheated to the specified temperature.
- Use sea salt and freshly ground black pepper unless otherwise suggested.
- Fresh herbs should be used unless dried herbs are specified in a recipe.
- Medium eggs should be used except where otherwise specified. Free-range eggs are recommended.
- Note that certain recipes, including mayonnaise and some cold desserts, contain raw or lightly cooked eggs. The young, elderly, pregnant women and anyone with an immune-deficiency disease should avoid these, because of the slight risk of salmonella.
- Calorie, fat, salt and carbohydrate counts per serving are provided for the recipes.
- If you are following a gluten- or dairy-free diet, check the labels on all pre-packaged food goods.
- Recipe serving suggestions do not take gluten- or dairy-free diets into account.

Picture credits
Photographers: Craig Robertson (Basics photography and pages
32, 38, 39, 40, 45, 51, 54, 59, 60, 68, 69, 71, 74, 75, 79, 81, 86,
96, 100, 110, 111, 113, 115, 118, 119, 120); Nicki Dowey (pages
34, 35, 47, 52, 53, 64, 72, 73, 78, 114, 121, 126); Neil Barclay
(pages 36, 41, 42, 44, 46, 55, 58, 61, 63, 65, 76, 84, 87, 91, 94,
97, 99, 101, 102, 104, 107, 116, 123, 124, 125); Lucinda Symons
(pages 14, 16, 33, 56, 92, 93, 105)

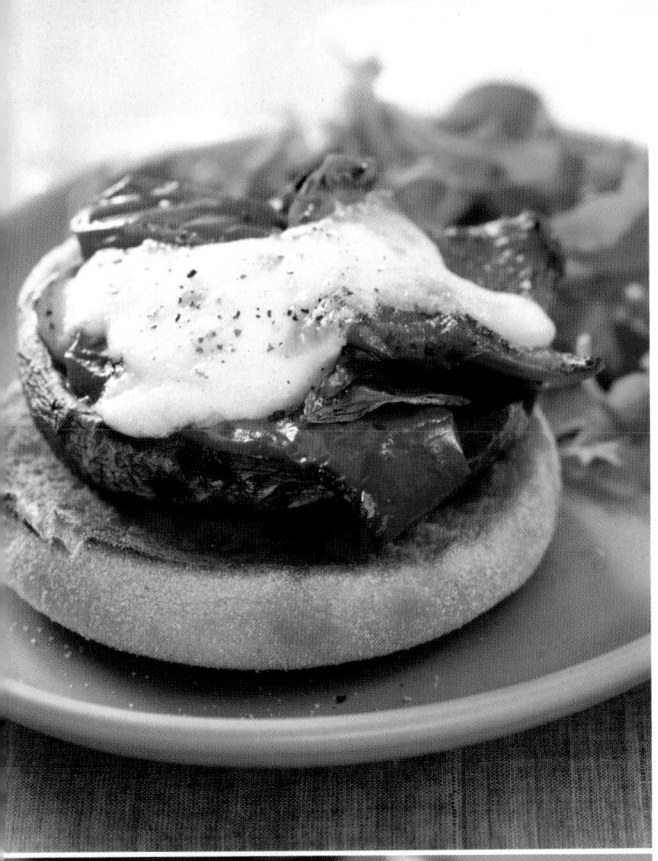

Contents

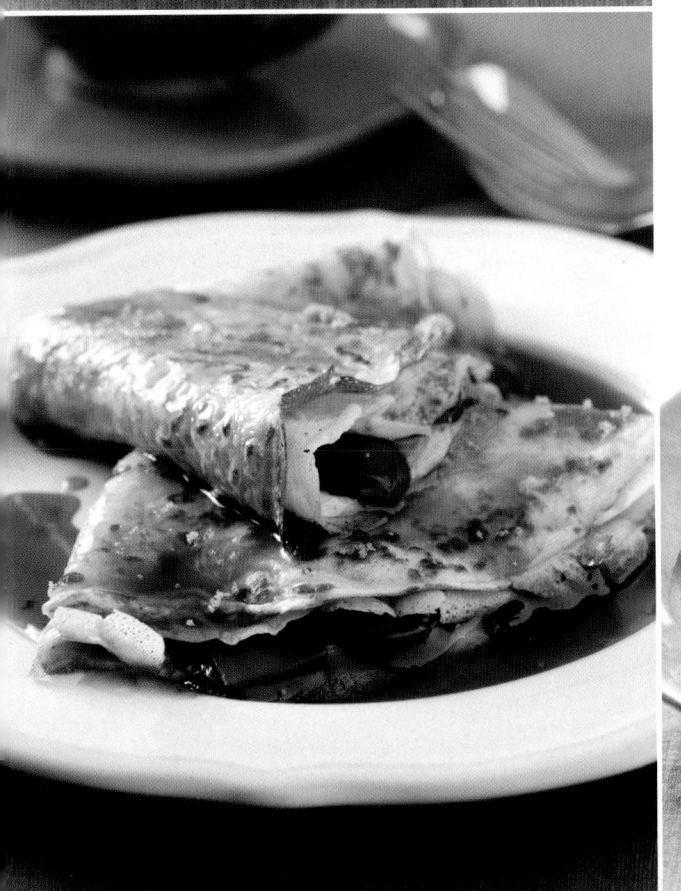

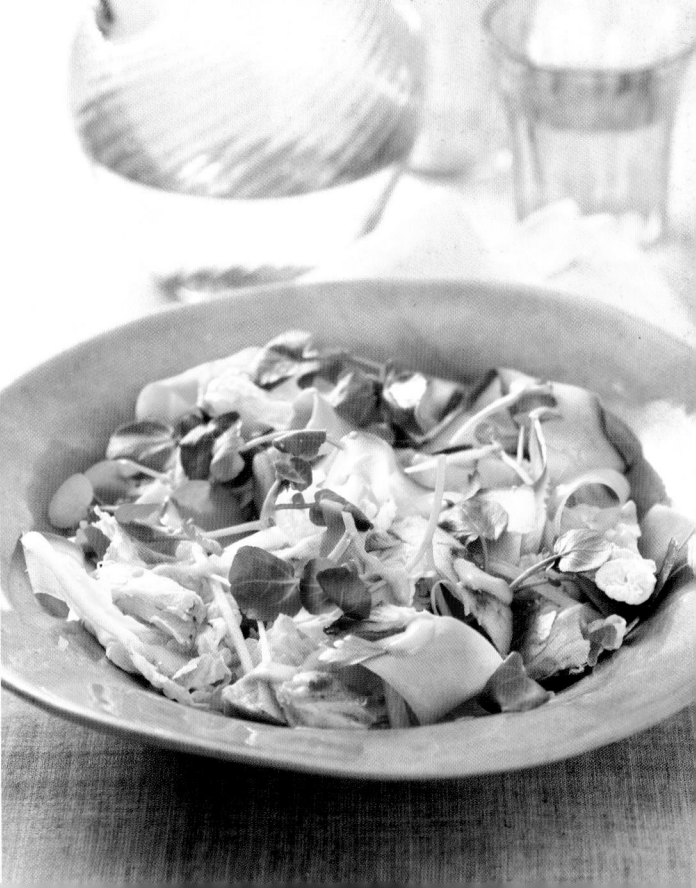

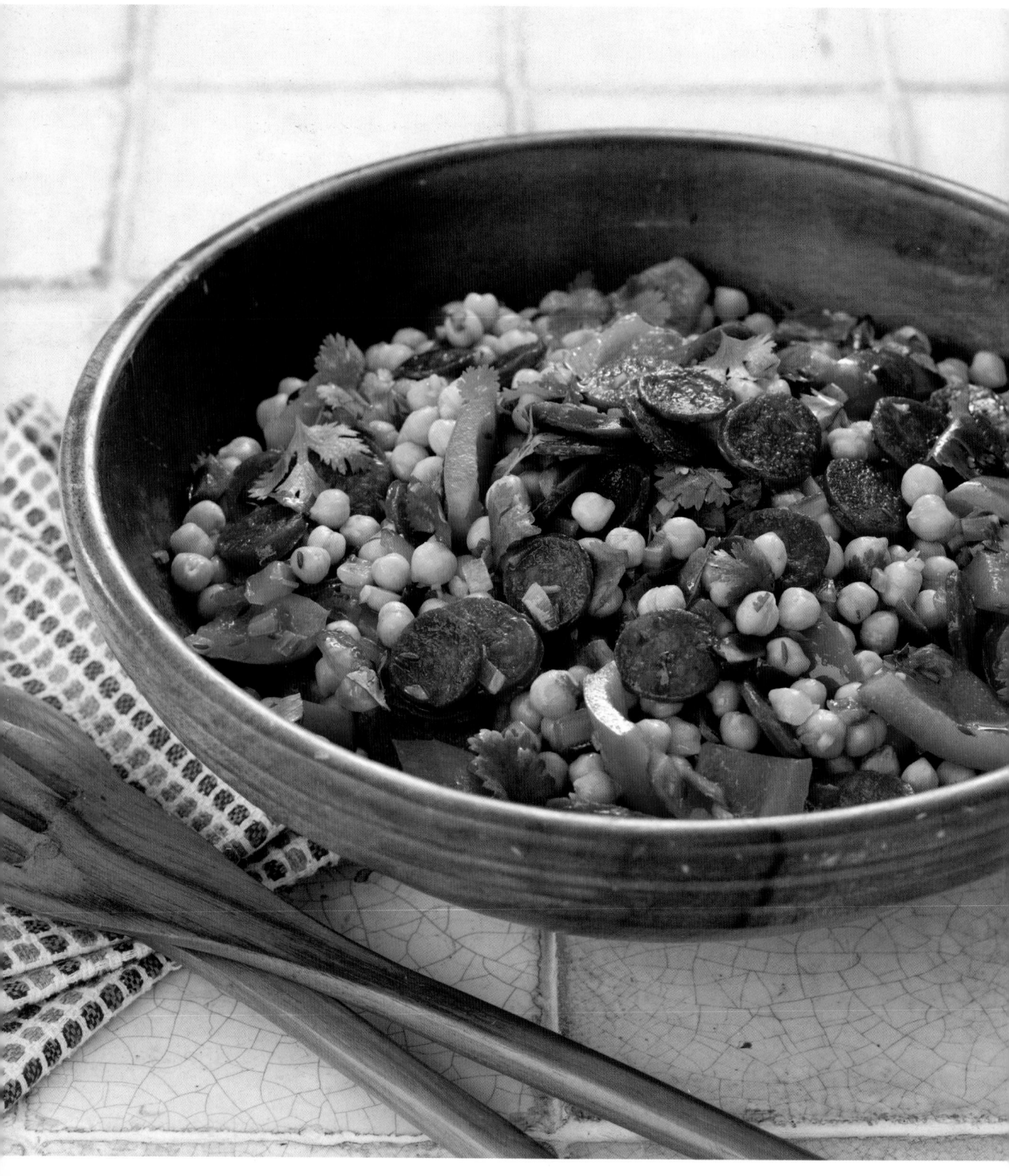

Foreword

Cooking for the family should be just as fun as baking cakes, but we know from readers queries that it's one of the most difficult meals to decide what to make. When you're pressed for time and ravenous, it is still just as easy to whip up something quick and delicious as when you have lots of hours to spare.

One way of simplifying it is to make a plan of meals for the week before you go shopping. I cook from scratch every night, and most of those meals are on the table in half an hour. By cooking a roast on a Sunday, I have what I call one free meal the next night. The other nights I use a handful of basic recipes – stir-fries with rice, noodle soups, sauces with pasta varying the ingredients as to what's available. That way it feels like you're having something different, even if the base is pretty much the same.

For inspiration I'll flick through this book. It has a tantalising array of recipes – from light bites, such as fast fish soup, when you're feeling just a little bit peckish to more substantial suppers, such as pasta with pesto and beans. We've also included a section with longer recipes – Cook Once, Eat Twice – those ones that take a bit more time, such as lasagne and Bolognese, that can also be frozen for another time. All the recipes are triple tested so they're guaranteed to work for you the very first time you make them.

Emma

Emma Marsden
Cookery Editor
Good Housekeeping

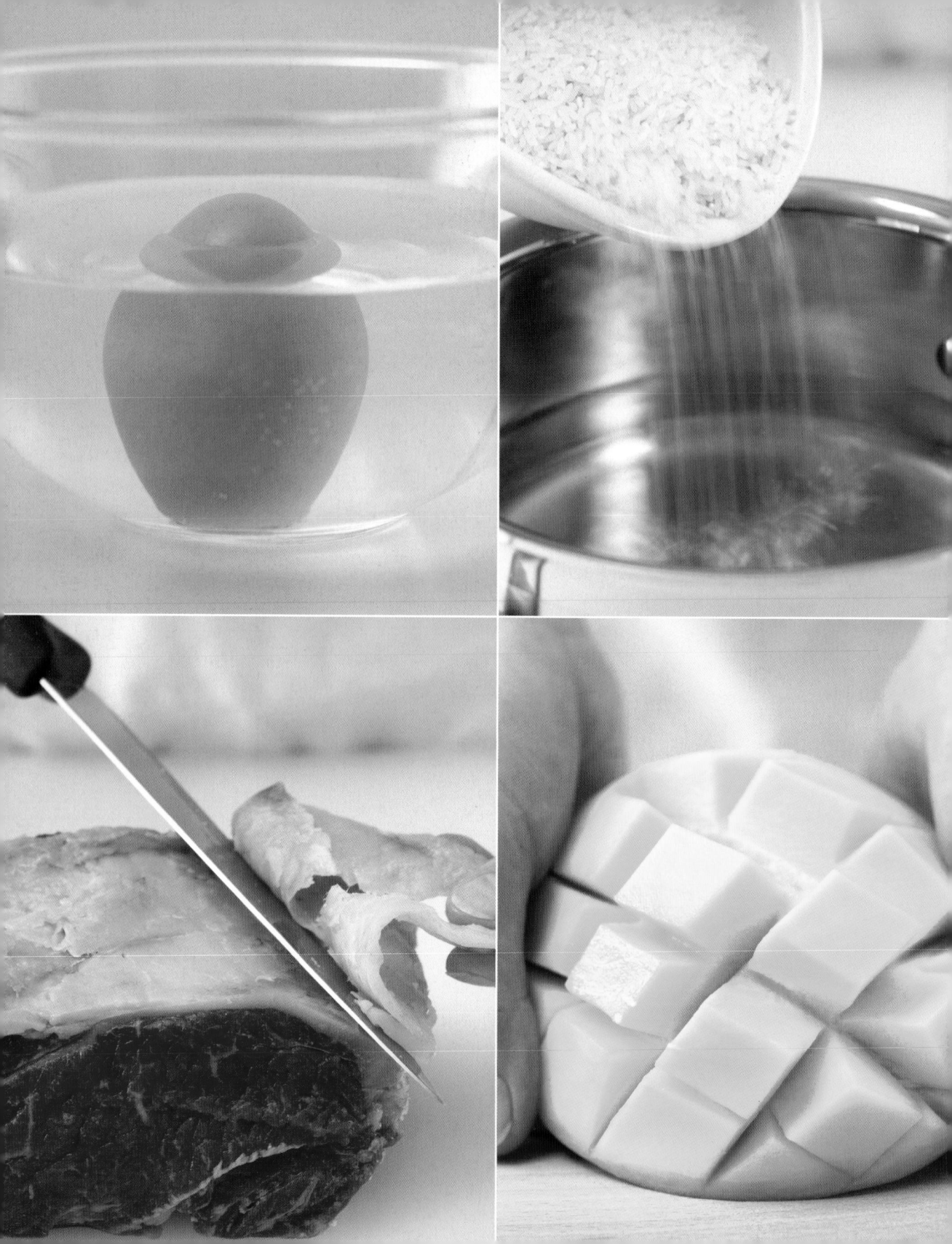

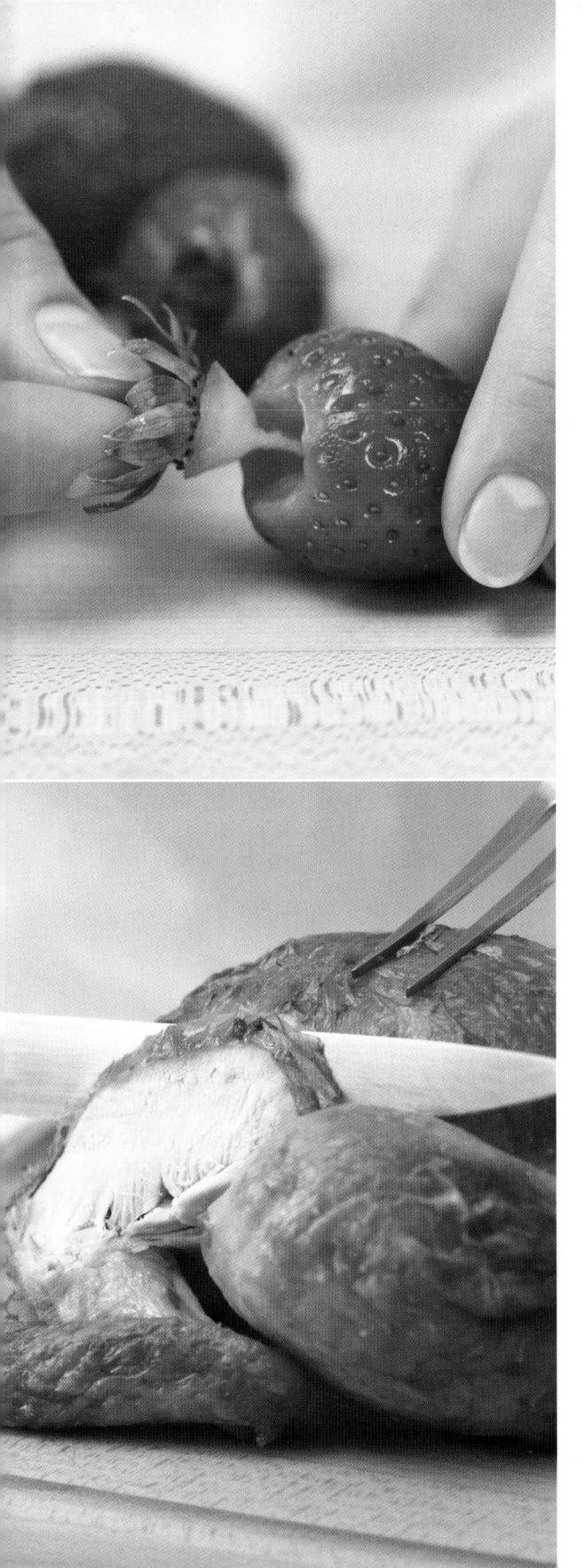

O

The Basics

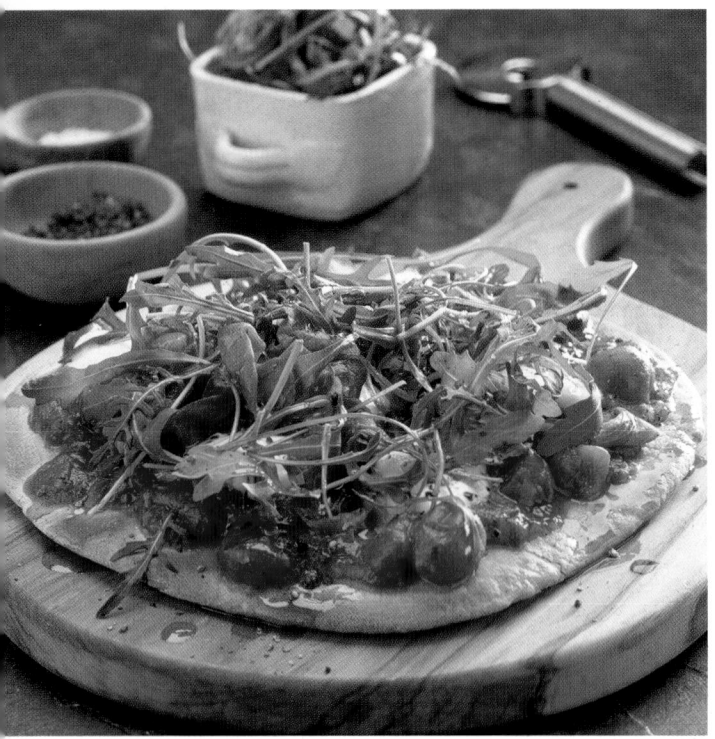

Different types of midweek meals

Midweek meals are not always about speed. It's nice to have a varied repertoire of meals that include filling lasagnes, pies and casseroles, as well as the more obvious quick suppers such as pasta dishes, stir-fries and main-course salads.

Light Bites and Midweek Suppers – nutritious snacks and slightly more substantial dishes that are quick to make; serve with a green salad or follow with fruit.

Meals in Minutes – simple recipes that can be prepared, cooked and on the table within approximately 30 minutes. These are ideal for those nights when you don't have any leftovers to reuse but have time to pop into the supermarket for one or two key ingredients.

Cook Once, Eat Twice – these recipes take time and are usually cooked from scratch. You can make double the quantity and freeze half for an easy meal another day, or divide into portions and keep in the fridge for one or two family members to reheat later in the week.

Waste Not – we include tips on how to make the most of the bits & bobs that end up tucked away at the back of your fridge. Why waste leftovers when they can be transformed into another meal?

Planning Midweek Meals

It can be quite a challenge to make sure that every member of the family eats healthy and balanced meals, especially if they come home at different times after various activities. If you plan each week's menu in advance, it will take the stress out of deciding what to cook each day and you can turn leftovers into meals in their own right.

Before shopping

Before doing your weekly shop, have a good look at the ingredients in your fridge and vegetable rack and think of ways to use them up. You can then go out and buy the ingredients you need to make the most of your fridge items. For example:
- A half used pack of olives – add to a pasta dish, or to the Mozzarella, Parma Ham and Rocket Pizza on page 57
- A couple of rashers of bacon – perfect for making the Quick and Easy Carbonara on page 64
- A small piece of Camembert – perfect for making the Camembert and Tomato Tarts on page 34
- A couple of potatoes – perfect for topping the Lamb and Leek Hotpot on page 96

The weekly menu

This needn't be a hefty document – simply jot down an idea for every day of the week, including some dishes that you've already made and stored in the fridge or freezer, some recipes that make creative use of leftovers and some quick meals that need a trip to the shops for one or two fresh ingredients. Include vegetables or other accompaniments in your plan, but remember that you can always change your mind if you find a bargain in the supermarket.

Time savers

Use pre-prepared ingredients every now and again to save time in the kitchen. These can be bought fresh or be frozen and then thawed on the day of use:

Packs of chopped root vegetables
Perfect for casseroles
Prepared cauliflower and broccoli florets
Perfect for vegetable bakes such as the Cheese and Vegetable Bake (page 55)
Packs of chopped stir-fry vegetables
Perfect for stir-fries
Bags of washed and prepared salad
Perfect accompaniments, or use in the Throw-it-all-together Salad (page 39)
Frozen broad beans and peas
Perfect for making the Easy Pea Soup (page 45) and Spiced Egg Pilau (page 52)
Frozen fresh chopped herbs
Perfect for the Falafel, Rocket and Soured Cream Wraps (page 36) and the Chilli Bean Cake (page 54)
Ready-made garlic paste
Perfect for many recipes
Roasted vegetables in oil, such as red peppers, artichokes and sunblush or sun-dried tomatoes
Perfect for Mozzarella Mushrooms (page 32)
Jars of tomato sauce
Perfect for Aubergine Parmigiana (page 60) and Mozzarella, Parma Ham and Rocket Pizza (page 57)
Ready-rolled puff pastry
Perfect for Camembert and Tomato Tarts (page 34) and Express Apple Tart (page 117)

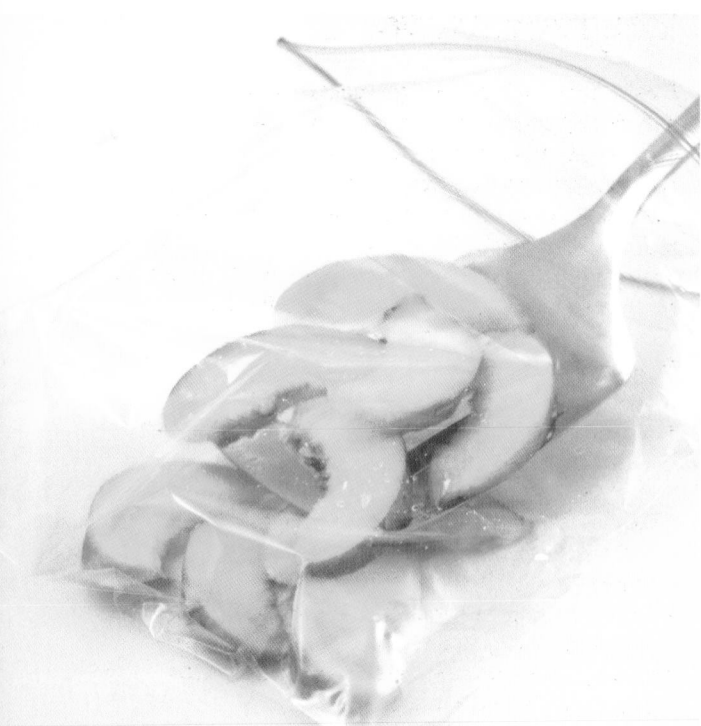

Making the most of your fridge, freezer and microwave

Having the right equipment can make life so much easier in the kitchen. Consider the space you have available: do you have room for a separate fridge and freezer? The microwave is energy-efficient, quick and easy to use – the busy cook's perfect kitchen companion.

The fridge

The fridge is a vital piece of equipment and keeps food fresh for longer. However, it is the main culprit for waste. The bigger it is, the more it becomes a repository for out-of-date condiments and bags of wilted salad leaves that lurk in its depths.

Safe storage
- Cool cooked food to room temperature before putting in the fridge
- Wrap or cover all food except fruit and vegetables
- Practise fridge discipline. The coldest shelves are at the bottom so store raw meat, fish and poultry there
- Separate cooked foods from raw foods

To make sure the fridge works properly:
- Don't overfill it
- Don't put hot foods in it
- Don't open the door more than necessary
- Clean it regularly

Vegetables and Fruit

Green vegetables	3–4 days
Salad leaves	2–3 days
Hard and stone fruit	3–7 days
Soft fruit	1–2 days

Dairy Food

Cheese, hard	1 week
Cheese, soft	2–3 days
Eggs	1 week
Milk	4–5 days

Fish

Fish	1 day
Shellfish	1 day

Raw Meat

Bacon	7 days
Game	2 days
Joints	3 days
Minced meat	1 day
Offal	1 day
Poultry	2 days
Raw sliced meat	2 days
Sausages	3 days

Cooked Meat

Joints	3 days
Casseroles/stews	2 days
Pies	2 days
Sliced meat	2 days
Ham	2 days
Ham, vacuum-packed (or according to the instructions on the pack)	1–2 weeks

The freezer

This is an invaluable storage tool and if you use it properly – particularly with batch cooking (see Cook Once, Eat Twice chapter) – you can save time and avoid wastage. Make sure you allow food time to thaw: if you leave it overnight in the fridge, your meal will be ready to pop into the oven when you get home from work. You can have all sorts of stand-bys waiting for you: breads, cakes, pastry, frozen vegetables and fruit such as raspberries and blackberries, cream, stocks, soups, herbs and bacon.

How to store food:
- Freeze food as soon as possible after purchase
- Label cooked food with the date and name of the dish
- Freeze food in portions
- Never put warm foods into the freezer, wait until they have cooled
- Check the manufacturer's instructions for freezing times
- Do not refreeze food once it has thawed

What not to store in the freezer:
- Whole eggs – freeze whites and yolks separately
- Fried foods – they lose their crispness and can go soggy
- Vegetables – cucumber, lettuce and celery have too high a water content
- Some sauces – mayonnaise and similar sauces will separate when thawed

To make sure the freezer works properly:
- Defrost it regularly
- Keep the freezer as full as possible

Thawing and reheating food:
Each recipe will give you instructions on how to reheat the particular dish, but generally:
- Some foods, such as vegetables, soups and sauces, can be cooked from frozen – dropped into boiling water, or heated gently in a pan until thawed
- Ensure other foods are thoroughly thawed before cooking
- Cook food as soon as possible after thawing
- Ensure the food is piping hot all the way through after cooking

The microwave

A conventional microwave oven cooks by microwaves that pass through glass, paper, china and plastic and are absorbed by moisture molecules in the food. They penetrate the food to a depth of about 5cm (2in), where they cause the molecules to vibrate and create heat within the food, which cooks it. The manufacturer's instruction booklet will tell you all you need to know to get the best out of the microwave oven, but here are a few handy tips:

Microwave safety:
- The oven will work only if the door is closed
- The door has a special seal to prevent microwaves from escaping
- Never switch on the microwave when there is nothing inside – the waves will bounce off the walls of the oven and could damage the magnetron (the device that converts electricity into microwaves)
- Allow sufficient space around the microwave for ventilation through the air vents
- If using plastic containers, use only microwave-proof plastic – ordinary plastic buckles

What to use a microwave for:
- Cooking ready-prepared meals
- Cooking vegetables and fish
- Reheating foods and drinks
- Softening butter and melting chocolate
- Drying herbs
- Scrambling eggs

What not to use a microwave for:
- Browning meat (unless the oven comes with a browning unit)
- Soufflés
- Puff pastry
- Breaded or battered foods

Microwave tips:
- Consult the manufacturer's handbook before you use the microwave for the first time
- Use a plastic trivet so that the microwaves can penetrate the underside of the food
- Cover fatty foods such as bacon and sausages with kitchen paper to soak up any fat
- Stir liquids at intervals during microwaving
- Turn large items of food over during microwaving
- Clean the interior regularly

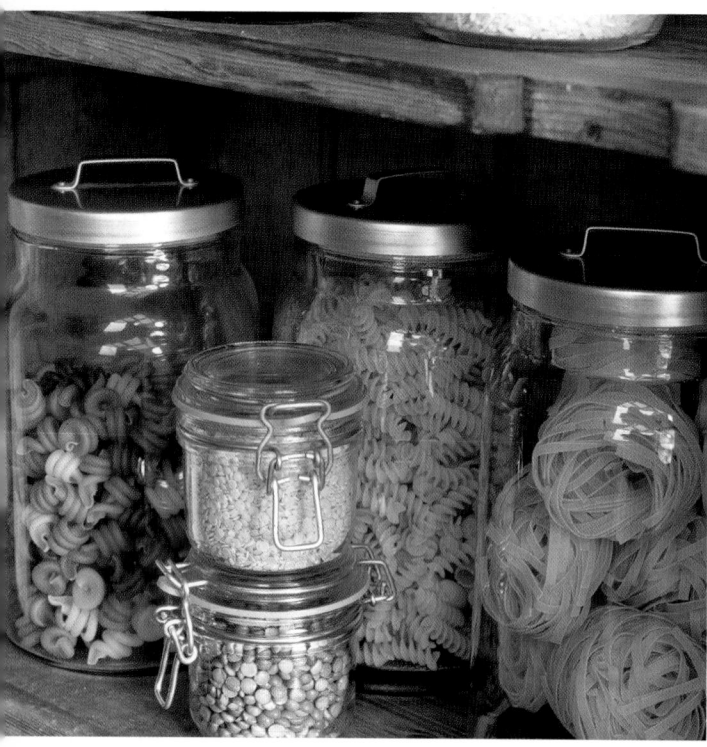

The storecupboard

A well-stocked storecupboard can help you rustle up a quick meal at short notice. However, resist the urge to fill the cupboard with interesting bottles that you 'might use one day'.

A few rules on storage

- Keep food cupboards cool and dry
- Line shelves for easy cleaning and clean regularly
- Organize shelves – put new goods to the back and use up those in front
- Canned food, once opened, should be transferred to a bowl and kept in the fridge
- Store dried pulses, herbs, beans and spices in sealed containers. Light can affect these
- Check use-by dates regularly

Stocking your storecupboard

Dried

- ✓ Pasta and noodles
- ✓ Rice (long-grain, Arborio and other risotto rice, pudding rice)
- ✓ Pulses
- ✓ Pizza bases
- ✓ Nuts (pinenuts, walnuts, almonds)
- ✓ Dried fruits
- ✓ Stock cubes
- ✓ Spices and herbs
- ✓ Salt and pepper
- ✓ Flour (plain, self-raising, wholemeal and cornflour)
- ✓ Dried yeast
- ✓ Gelatine
- ✓ Baking powder, cream of tartar, bicarbonate of soda
- ✓ Sugar
- ✓ Tea
- ✓ Coffee
- ✓ Cocoa powder

Bottles and jars

- ✓ Mayonnaise
- ✓ Tomato ketchup and purée
- ✓ Tabasco sauce
- ✓ Worcestershire sauce
- ✓ Sweet chilli sauce
- ✓ Pasta sauces
- ✓ Thai fish sauce
- ✓ Curry paste
- ✓ Chutneys
- ✓ Pickles
- ✓ Olives
- ✓ Capers
- ✓ Mustards
- ✓ Oils
- ✓ Vinegar
- ✓ Jam
- ✓ Marmalade
- ✓ Honey

Cans

- ✓ Chopped and whole tomatoes
- ✓ Fish (salmon, tuna, anchovies)
- ✓ Beans, chickpeas and lentils
- ✓ Coconut milk/cream
- ✓ Fruits

Storecupboard Recipes

Storecupboard Omelette

a drizzle of olive oil or knob of butter, 1 large onion, finely chopped, 225g (8oz) cooked new potatoes, sliced, 125g (4oz) frozen petit pois, thawed, 6 eggs, beaten, 150g pack soft goat's cheese, sliced, salt and ground black pepper.

1 Heat the oil or butter in a 25.5cm (10in) non-stick, ovenproof frying pan. Add the onion and fry for 6–8 minutes until golden. Add the potatoes and petit pois and cook, stirring, for 2–3 minutes. Preheat the grill.

2 Spread the mixture over the base of the pan and pour in the eggs. Tilt the pan to coat the base with egg. Leave the omelette to cook undisturbed for 2–3 minutes, then top with the cheese.

3 Put the pan under the hot grill for 1–2 minutes until the egg is just set (no longer, or it will turn rubbery) and the cheese starts to turn golden. Season with salt and pepper and serve immediately.

Variations

- Use 100g (3½oz) sun-dried tomatoes instead of the new potatoes.
- Throw in a handful of halved pitted black olives as you pour the egg into the pan.

Storecupboard saviours

Here are some more ideas for recipes you can produce from a well-stocked storecupboard and just one or two fresh ingredients:

- Sticky Chicken Thighs (page 35)
- Spiced Egg Pilau (page 52)
- Warm Spicy Chorizo and Chickpea Salad (page 61)
- Moroccan Chicken with Chickpeas (page 95)

Mixed Beans with Lemon Vinaigrette

400g can mixed beans, drained and rinsed, 400g can chickpeas, drained and rinsed, 2 shallots, finely sliced, fresh mint sprigs and lemon zest to garnish
For the lemon vinaigrette
juice of 1 lemon, 2 tsp runny honey, 8 tbsp extra virgin olive oil, 3 tbsp freshly chopped mint, 4 tbsp roughly chopped flat-leafed parsley, salt and ground black pepper.

1 Put the beans, chickpeas and shallots in a large bowl.

2 To make the lemon vinaigrette, whisk together the lemon juice, seasoning and honey. Gradually whisk in the olive oil and stir in the chopped herbs.

3 Pour the vinaigrette over the bean mixture, toss well, then garnish with the mint sprigs and lemon zest and serve.

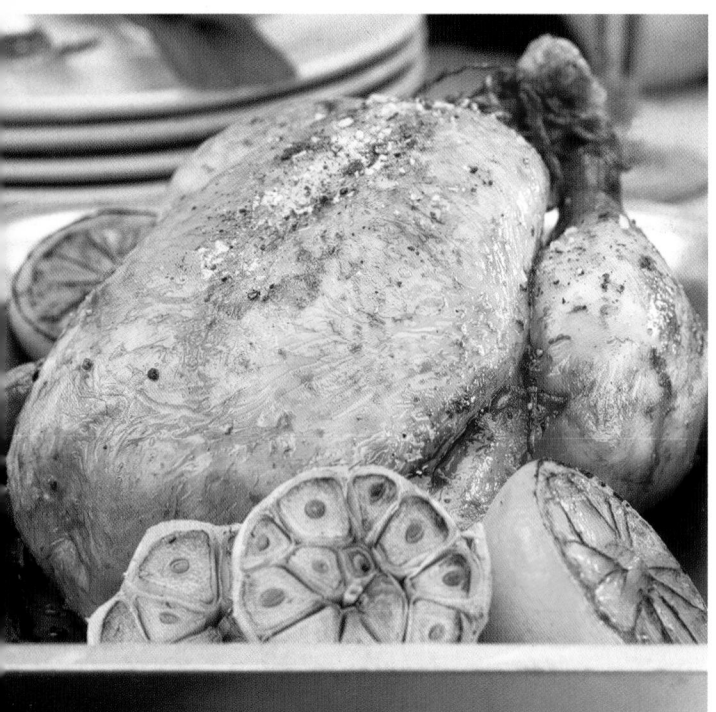

Ways of using leftovers

There are many ways of using leftover food and slightly over-ripe fruit and vegetables that are starting to wilt. You can:

- Simply add the ingredients to a stir-fry, pasta bake, soup, risotto ... the list is endless
- 'Stretch' the ingredients – sometimes the amount left over is so small it won't go very far in a family setting. Try adding to it. You can cook a little more of it (for example rice), or try adding lentils and tomatoes to leftover mince to create a whole new take on Bolognese sauce
- Make the most of fruit and vegetables that are starting to wilt – use fruit in a crumble, use vegetables in soups and bakes

The chart opposite gives some examples of typical fridge leftovers you could use in recipes in this book.

Expiry dates

These are a major area of debate. Supermarkets are extremely strict on expiry dates and will throw any food out the moment it is 'out of date'. Once you have purchased a product, you are asked to use it within the 'use by' date. After this, you are encouraged to throw it out and start again. However, with the odd exception – and using your judgement on certain danger foods like fish and eggs – you can simply check if it's okay to use by smell, look and feel. Follow your instincts, if it smells bad, bin it.

Using leftovers

We all struggle with portion sizing and often have some extra rice, potatoes or other ingredients left at the end of each meal. There is a difference between leftovers and waste food. Leftovers are the bits and pieces that sit in a clingfilm-covered bowl in your fridge, challenging you to use them creatively. If you ignore them for four or five days they become waste. Why not try making the most of your leftover bits & bobs?

How can I tell if my eggs are fresh?

A fresh egg should feel heavy in your hand and will sink to the bottom of the bowl or float on its side when put into water (1).
Older eggs, over two weeks old, will float vertically (2).

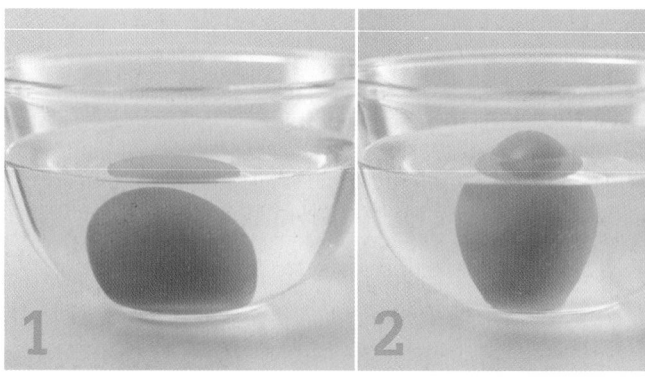

Planned leftovers

	First Use	Second Use	Third Use
Chicken	Perfect Roast Chicken (page 105)	Leftover Chicken Soup (below right) OR Throw-it-all-together Salad (page 39)	Chicken Stock (page 23)
Simple Bolognese Sauce	Spaghetti Bolognese (page 26)	Lasagne (page 26)	Cottage Pie (page 26)

Versatile leftovers

Leftover	Recipe
Bowl of cooked pasta	Pasta with Pesto and Beans (page 53) Simple Salmon Pasta (page 65)
Bacon rashers	Quick and Easy Carbonara (page 64)
Mixed vegetables	Cheese and Vegetable Bake (page 55)
Savoy cabbage	Spanish-style Pork (page 87)
Salad	Throw-it-all together Salad (page 39)
Tomato sauce	Aubergine Parmigiana (page 60)
Over-ripe bananas	Instant Banana Ice Cream (page 115) Sticky Banoffee Pies (page 121)
Turning apples	Express Apple Tart (page 116)
Turning pears	Pear and Blackberry Crumble (page 112)
Fromage frais	Chicken with Spicy Couscous (page 75)
Custard	Cheat's Chocolate Pots (page 125)
Pancake batter	Chocolate Crêpes (page 111)

Alternative suggestions

You may not always feel like transforming your leftovers into meals – or there may not be enough to do so. Another option is to freeze the odd ingredient for later use.

Small amounts of herbs – freeze in ice cube trays

One or two chillies – these freeze well and are easy to chop from frozen

Double cream – lightly whip the cream and then freeze

Cheese – hard cheeses will become crumbly once thawed, but can be used for grating or in cooking

Bread – whiz in a food processor to make breadcrumbs: these freeze well in a sealed plastic bag. Use to sprinkle over bakes for a crisp topping, or to coat fish or chicken before frying, grilling or baking – or use for bread sauce to serve with game or turkey

Leftover Roast Chicken Soup

3 tbsp olive oil, 1 onion, chopped, 1 carrot, chopped, 2 celery sticks, chopped, 2 fresh thyme sprigs, chopped, 1 bay leaf, a stripped roast chicken carcass, 900ml (1½ pints) boiling water, 150–200g (5–7oz) chopped roast chicken, 200g (7oz) mashed or roast potato, 1 tbsp double cream.

1 Heat the oil in a large pan. Add the onion, carrot, celery and thyme and fry gently for 20–30 minutes until soft but not brown. Add the bay leaf, chicken carcass and the boiling water to the pan. Bring to the boil, then simmer for 5 minutes.

2 Remove the bay leaf and carcass and add the chopped roast chicken and cooked potato. Simmer for 5 minutes.

3 Whiz the soup in a food processor, pour back into the pan and bring to the boil. Stir in the cream and serve immediately.

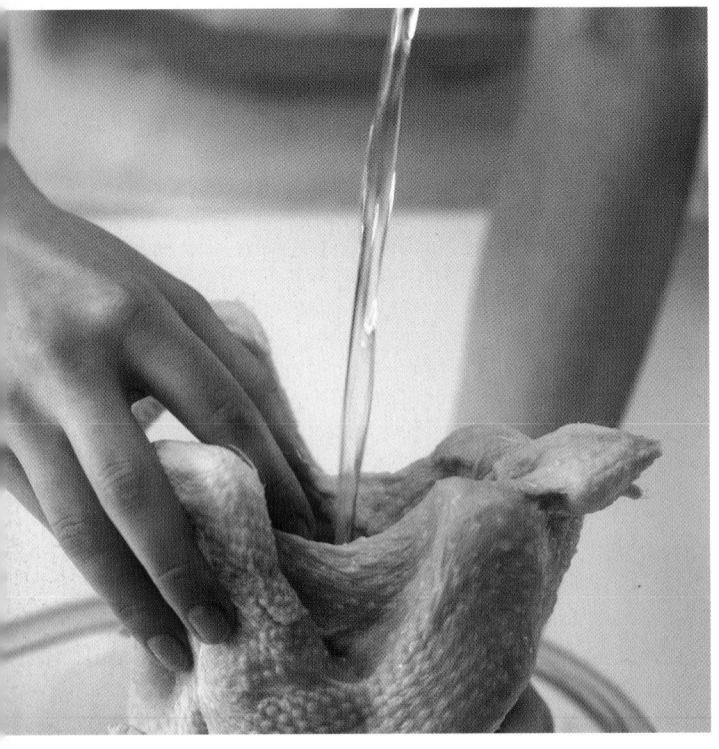

Preparing meat and poultry

Ready-prepared chicken pieces are perfect for midweek suppers, but a small bird doesn't take long to roast and is simple to prepare. Steaks and other cuts of meat can easily be made more tender and succulent for quick and tasty meals.

Hygiene

Raw poultry and meat contain harmful bacteria that can spread easily to anything they touch.
Always wash your hands, kitchen surfaces, chopping boards, knives and equipment before and after handling raw poultry or meat.
Don't let raw poultry or meat touch other foods.
Always cover raw poultry and meat, and store in the bottom of the fridge, where it can't touch or drip on to other foods.

Cleaning

Before stuffing a chicken or other bird for roasting, clean it thoroughly. Put the bird in the sink and pull out any loose fat with your fingers. Run cold water through the cavity and dry the bird well using kitchen paper.

Roasting and carving chicken

A roast chicken has a luxurious aroma and flavour; it makes an excellent Sunday lunch or special meal with very little preparation. These simple guidelines make carving easy, giving neat slices to serve.

Roasting times

Roast for 20 minutes per 450g (1lb) plus 20 minutes at 180°C (160°C fan oven) mark 4.

How to check your chicken is cooked

Test by piercing the thickest part of the leg: the juices should run clear.

Carving

1 Starting at the neck end, cut slices about 5mm (¼in) thick.

2 To cut off the legs, cut the skin between the thigh and breast. Pull the leg down to expose the joint with the ribcage. Cut through that joint. (For small birds, cut through the joint between thigh and drumstick.)

3 To carve meat from the leg of large chickens, remove the leg from the carcass as above. Joint the two parts of the leg. Holding the drumstick by the thin end, stand it up on your carving board and carve slices parallel with the bone. Carve the thigh flat on the board or upright.

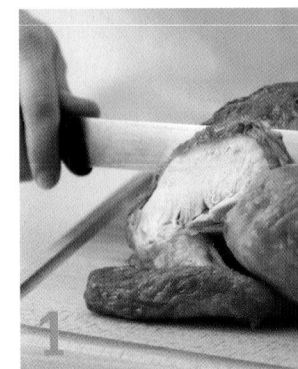

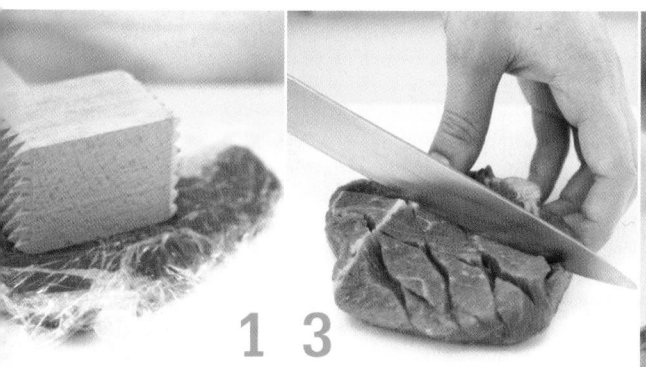

Tenderising steak

Some cuts of steak benefit from tenderising. There are two ways to do it: by pounding or scoring.

1 To pound, lay the steaks in a single layer on a large piece of clingfilm or waxed paper. Lay another sheet on top of the slices and pound gently with a rolling pin, small frying pan or the flat side of a meat mallet.

2 Scoring is useful for cuts that have long, tough fibres, such as flank. It allows a marinade to penetrate more deeply into the meat. Lay the steak on the chopping board and, using a long, very sharp knife, make shallow cuts in one direction over the whole surface.

3 Make another set of cuts at a 45 degree angle to the first. Turn the meat over and repeat on the other side.

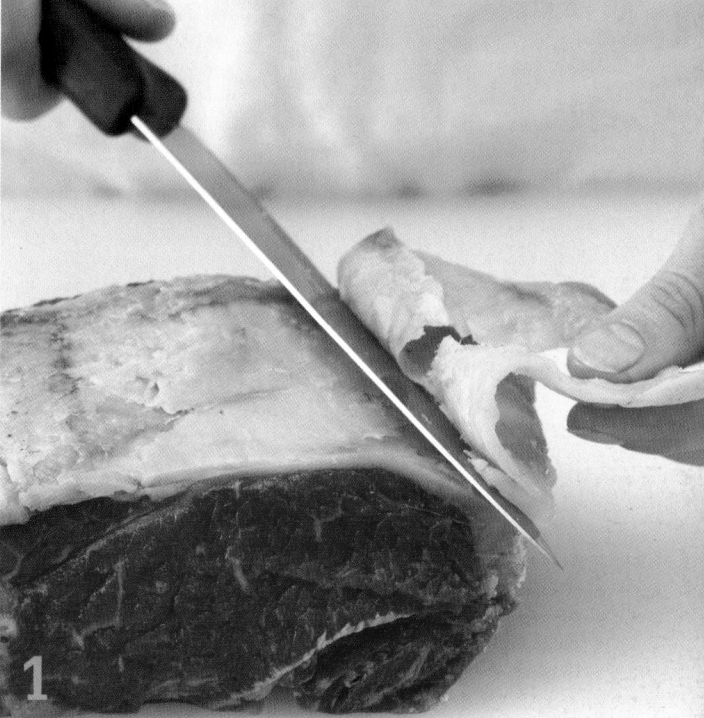

Trimming meat

When preparing meat for cutting into chunks, try to separate the individual muscles, which can be identified by the sinews running between each muscle.

Trimming a joint

1 Cut off the excess fat to leave a thickness of about 5mm (¼in) – a little fat will contribute juiciness and flavour. This isn't necessary for very lean cuts.

2 Trim away any stray pieces of meat or sinew left by the butcher.

3 If the joint has a covering of fat, you can lightly score it – taking care not to cut into the meat – to help the fat drain away during cooking.

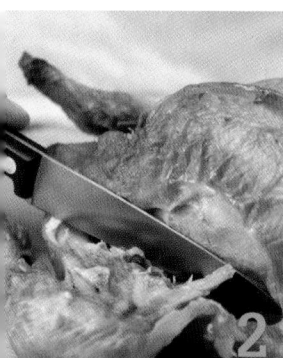
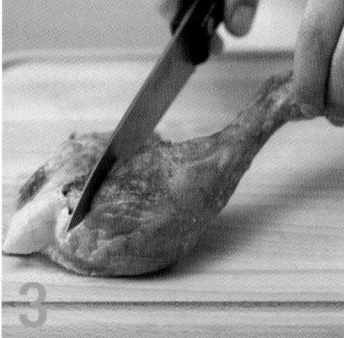

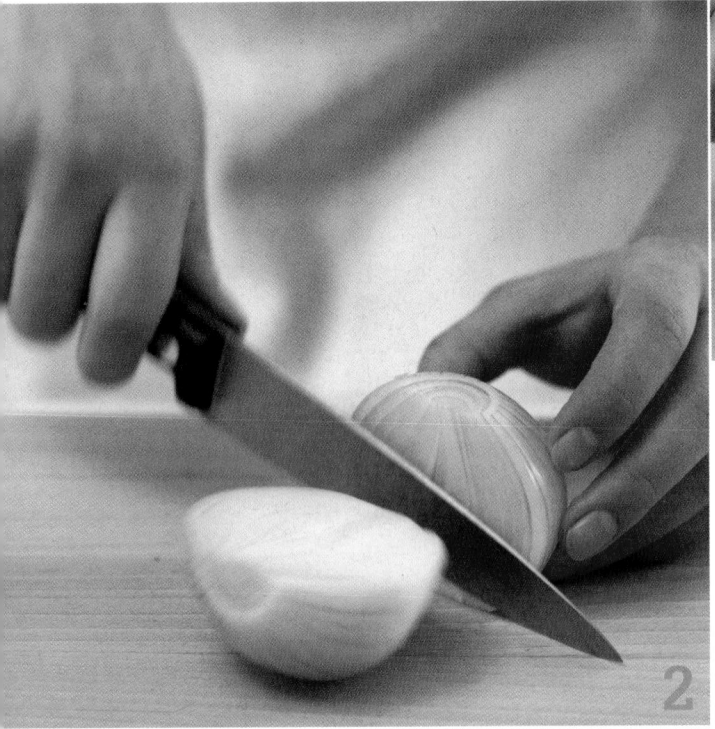
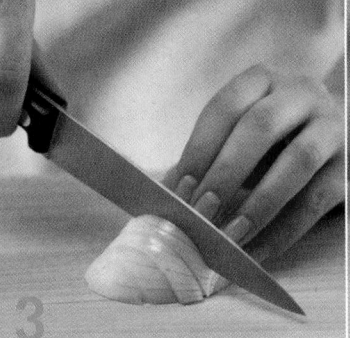
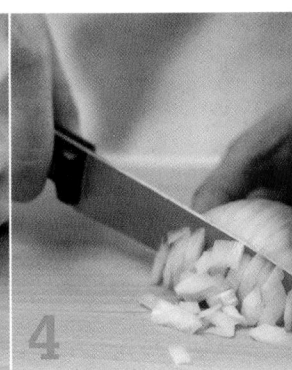

Preparing vegetables

Nutritious, mouthwatering and essential to a healthy diet – vegetables are a must in every kitchen. Some vegetables turn brown after peeling, and need to be placed in acidulated water (water and lemon juice) to slow the discolouration down – the recipe will tell you when this is necessary.

Onions

1 Cut off the tip and base of the onion. Peel away all the layers of papery skin and any discoloured layers underneath.

2 Put the onion root end down on the chopping board, then, using a sharp knife, cut the onion in half from tip to base.

3 **Slicing** Put one half on the board with the cut surface facing down and slice across the onion.

4 **Chopping** Slice the halved onions from the root end to the top at regular intervals. Next, make 2–3 horizontal slices through the onion, then slice vertically across the width.

Shallots

1 Cut off the tip and trim off the ends of the root. Peel off the skin and any discoloured layers underneath.

2 Holding the shallot with the root end down, use a small sharp knife to make deep parallel slices almost down to the base while keeping the slices attached to it.

3 **Slicing** Turn the shallot on its side and cut off slices from the base.

4 **Dicing** Make deep parallel slices at right angles to the first slices. Turn it on its side and cut off the slices from the base. You should now have fine dice, but chop any larger pieces individually.

Peeling tomatoes

1 Fill a bowl or pan with boiling water. Using a slotted spoon, add the tomato for 15–30 seconds, then remove to a chopping board.

2 Use a small sharp knife to cut out the core in a single cone-shaped piece. Discard the core.

3 Peel off the skin; it should come away easily depending on ripeness.

Seeding unpeeled tomatoes

1 Halve the tomato through the core. Use a small sharp knife or a spoon to remove the seeds and juice. Shake off the excess liquid.

2 Chop the tomato as required for your recipe and place in a colander for a minute or two, to drain off any excess liquid.

Peppers

Red, green and yellow peppers all contain seeds and white pith which taste bitter and should be removed. **Cut the pepper in half vertically**, discard the seeds and core, then trim away the rest of the white membrane with a small sharp knife. Alternatively, slice the top off the pepper, then cut away and discard the seeds and pith. Cut the pepper into strips or slices.

Leeks

As some leeks harbour a lot of grit and earth between their leaves, they need careful cleaning.

1 Cut off the root and any tough parts of the leek. Make a cut into the leaf end of the leek, about 7.5cm (3in) deep.

2 Hold under the cold tap while separating the cut halves to expose any grit. Wash well, then shake dry. Slice, cut into matchsticks or slice diagonally.

Celery

To remove the strings in the outer green stalks, trim the ends and cut into the base of the stalk with a small knife; catch the strings between the blade and your thumb. Pull up towards the top of the stalk to remove the string.

Mushrooms

Button, white, chestnut and flat mushrooms are all prepared in a similar way.
Shiitake mushrooms have a hard stalk; cut it off and use for making stock if you like.

1 Wipe with a damp cloth or pastry brush to remove any dirt.

2 With button mushrooms, cut off the stalk flush with the base of the cap. For other mushrooms, cut a thin disc off the end of the stalk and discard. Quarter or slice as needed.

Fennel

1 Trim off the top stems and the base of the bulbs. Remove the core with a small sharp knife if it is tough.

2 The outer leaves may be discoloured and can be scrubbed gently in cold water, or you can peel away the discoloured parts with a knife or a vegetable peeler. Slice or chop the fennel.

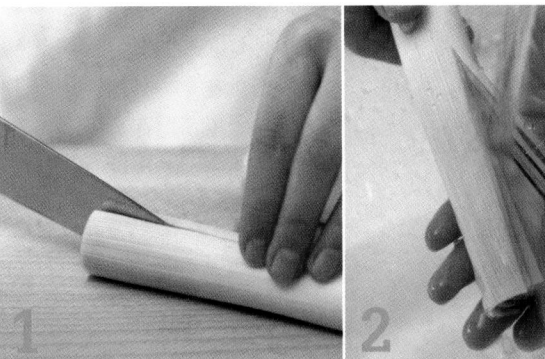

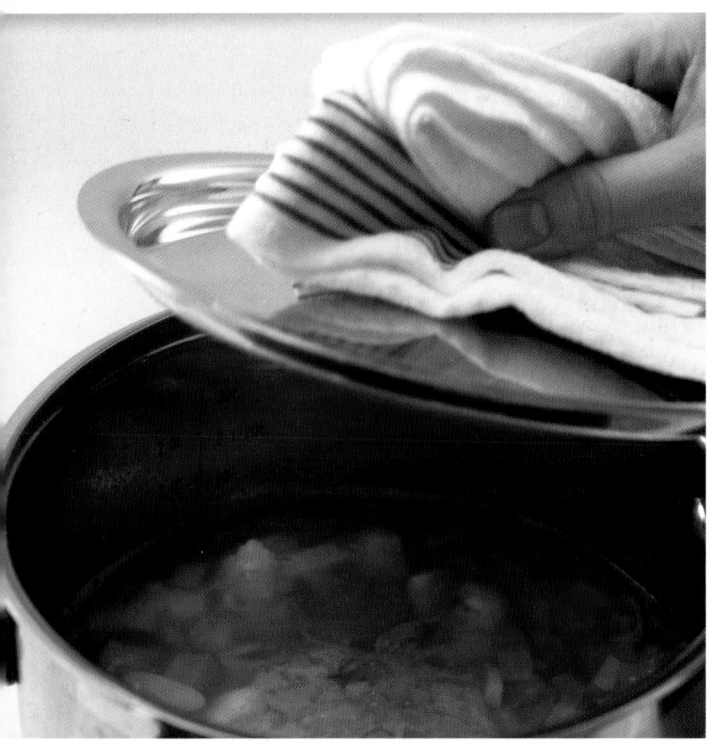

Making stock

Good stock can make the difference between a good dish and a great one. It gives depth of flavour to many dishes. There are four main types of stock: vegetable, meat, chicken and fish.

Stocks

Vegetable stock

For 1.1 litres (2 pints), you will need:
225g (8oz) each onions, celery, leeks and carrots, chopped, 2 bay leaves, a few thyme sprigs, 1 small bunch parsley, 10 black peppercorns, ½ tsp salt.

1 Put all the ingredients in a pan and pour in 1.7 litres (3 pints) cold water. Bring slowly to the boil and skim the surface. Partially cover and simmer for 30 minutes. Adjust the seasoning. Strain the stock through a fine sieve and leave to cool.

Meat stock

For 1.1 litres (2 pints), you will need:
450g (1lb) each meat bones and stewing meat, 1 onion, 2 celery sticks and 1 large carrot, sliced, 1 bouquet garni (2 bay leaves, a few thyme sprigs and a small bunch parsley), 1 tsp black peppercorns, ½ tsp salt.

1 Preheat the oven to 220°C (200°C fan oven) mark 7. Put the meat and bones in a roasting tin and roast for 30–40 minutes, turning now and again, until they are well browned.

2 Put the bones in a large pan with the remaining ingredients and add 2 litres (3½ pints) cold water. Bring slowly to the boil and skim the surface. Partially cover and simmer for 4–5 hours. Adjust the seasoning.

3 Strain the stock through a muslin-lined sieve into a bowl and cool quickly. Degrease (see opposite) before using.

Chicken stock

For 1.1 litres (2 pints), you will need:
1.6kg (3¹/₂lb) chicken bones or a stripped roast chicken carcass, 225g (8oz) each onions and celery, sliced, 150g (5oz) chopped leeks, 1 bouquet garni (2 bay leaves, a few thyme sprigs and a small bunch parsley), 1 tsp black peppercorns, ¹/₂ tsp salt.

1 Put all the ingredients in a large pan with 3 litres (5¹/₄ pints) cold water.

2 Bring slowly to the boil and skim the surface. Partially cover the pan and simmer gently for 2 hours. Adjust the seasoning if necessary.

3 Strain the stock through a muslin-lined sieve into a bowl and cool quickly. Degrease (see right) before using.

Fish stock

For 900ml (1¹/₂ pints), you will need:
900g (2lb) fish bones and trimmings, washed, 2 carrots, 1 onion and 2 celery sticks, sliced, 1 bouquet garni (2 bay leaves, a few thyme sprigs and a small bunch parsley), 6 white peppercorns, ¹/₂ tsp salt.

1 Put all the ingredients in a large pan with 900ml (1¹/₂ pints) cold water. Bring slowly to the boil and skim the surface.

2 Partially cover the pan and simmer gently for 30 minutes. Adjust the seasoning if necessary.

3 Strain through a muslin-lined sieve into a bowl and cool quickly. Fish stock tends not to have much fat in it and so does not usually need to be degreased. However, if it does seem to be fatty, you will need to remove this by degreasing it (see right).

Degreasing stock

Meat and poultry stock needs to be degreased. (Vegetable stock does not.) You can mop the fat from the surface using kitchen paper, but the following methods are easier and more effective. There are three main methods that you can use: ladling, pouring and chilling.

1 **Ladling** While the stock is warm, place a ladle on the surface. Press down to allow the fat floating on the surface to trickle over the edge until the ladle is full. Discard the fat, then repeat until all the fat has been removed.

2 **Pouring** For this you need a degreasing jug or a double-pouring gravy boat, which has the spout at the base of the vessel. When you fill the jug or gravy boat with a fatty liquid, the fat rises. When you pour, the stock comes out while the fat stays behind in the jug.

3 **Chilling** This technique works best with stock made from meat, whose fat solidifies when cold. Put the stock in the fridge until the fat becomes solid, then remove the pieces of fat using a slotted spoon.

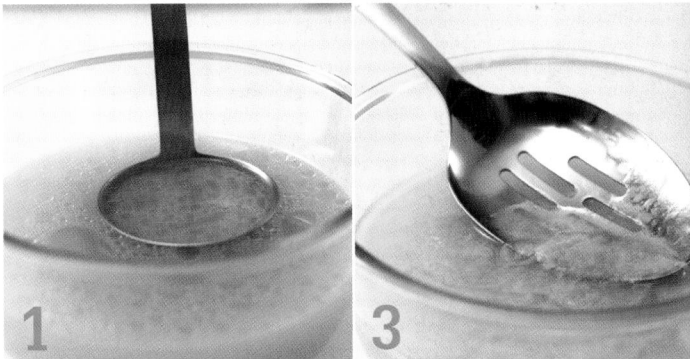

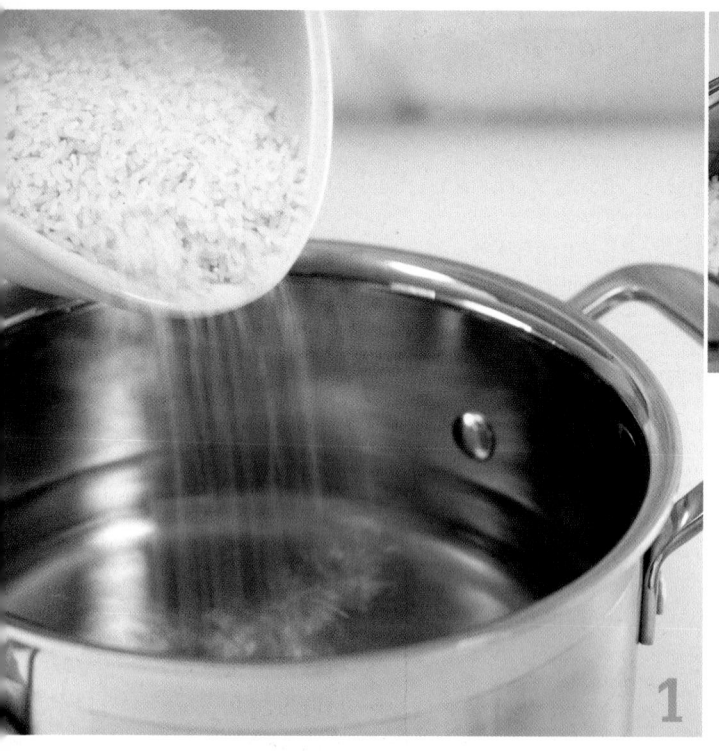

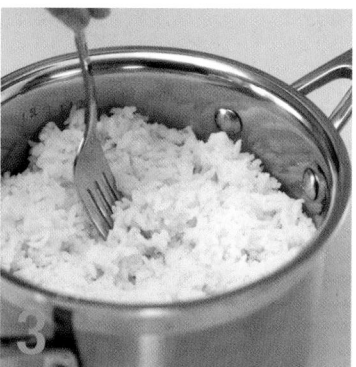

Cooking rice, pasta, grains and potatoes

Wholesome and healthy, rice, grains and potatoes are everyday staples. Easy to prepare and cook, they are also very economical and they store well.

Cooking rice

There are two main types of rice: long-grain and short-grain. Long-grain rice is generally served as an accompaniment; the most commonly used type of long-grain rice in South-east Asian cooking is jasmine rice, also known as Thai fragrant rice. It has a distinctive taste and slightly sticky texture. Long-grain rice needs no special preparation, although it should be washed to remove excess starch. Put the rice in a bowl and cover with cold water. Stir until this becomes cloudy, then drain and repeat until the water is clear.

Long-grain rice

1 Use 50–75g (2–3oz) raw rice per person; measured by volume 50–75ml (2–2½fl oz). Measure the rice by volume and put it in a pan with a pinch of salt and twice the volume of boiling water (or stock).

2 Bring to the boil. Turn the heat down to low and set the timer for the time stated on the pack. The rice should be al dente: tender with a bite at the centre.

3 When the rice is cooked, fluff up the grains with a fork.

Perfect rice

If you cook rice often, you may want to invest in a special rice steamer. They are available in Asian supermarkets and some kitchen shops and give good, consistent results.

Cooking pasta

Use about 1 litre (1³/₄ pints) of water per 100g (3¹/₂oz) of pasta. Filled pasta is the only type of pasta that needs oil in the cooking water – the oil reduces friction, which could tear the wrappers and allow the filling to come out. If the recipe calls for cooking the pasta with a sauce after it has boiled, undercook the pasta slightly when boiling it. Rinse pasta after cooking only if you are going to cool it to use in a salad, then drain well and toss with oil.

Dried pasta

1   Heat the water with about 1 tsp salt per 100g (3¹/₂oz) of pasta. Bring to a rolling boil, then add all the pasta and stir well for 30 seconds, to keep the pasta from sticking.

2   Once the water is boiling again, set the timer for 2 minutes less than the cooking time on the pack and cook uncovered.

3   Check the pasta when the timer goes off, then every 60 seconds until it is cooked al dente: tender, but with a bite at the centre. Drain in a colander.

Fresh pasta

Fresh pasta is cooked in the same way as dried, but for a shorter time. Bring the water to the boil. Add the pasta to the boiling water all at once and stir well. Set the timer for 2 minutes and keep testing every 30 seconds until the pasta is cooked al dente: tender, but with a bite at the centre. Drain in a colander.

Couscous

Often mistaken for a grain, couscous is actually a type of pasta that originated in North Africa. It is perfect for making into salads or serving with stews and casseroles. The tiny pellets do not require cooking and can simply be soaked.

1   Measure the couscous in a jug and add 1¹/₂ times the volume of just-boiled water or stock.

2   Cover the bowl and leave to soak for 5 minutes. Fluff up with a fork before serving.

3   If using for a salad, leave the couscous to cool completely before adding the other salad ingredients.

Boiling potatoes

1   Peel or scrub old potatoes, scrape or scrub new potatoes. Cut large potatoes into even-sized chunks and put them in a pan with plenty of salted cold water.

2   Cover, bring to the boil, then reduce the heat and simmer until cooked – about 10 minutes for new potatoes, 15–20 minutes for old.

Mashed Potatoes

For four people, you will need:
900g (2lb) floury potatoes such as Maris Piper, 125ml (4fl oz) full-fat milk, 25g (1oz) butter, salt and ground black pepper.

1   Peel the potatoes and cut into even-sized chunks. Boil as above until just tender, 15–20 minutes. Test with a small knife. Drain well.

2   Put the potatoes back in the pan and cover with a clean teatowel for 5 minutes, or warm them over a very low heat until the moisture has evaporated.

3   Pour the milk into a small pan and bring to the boil. Pour on to the potatoes with the butter and season.

4   Mash the potatoes until smooth.

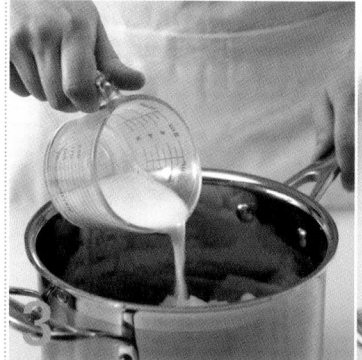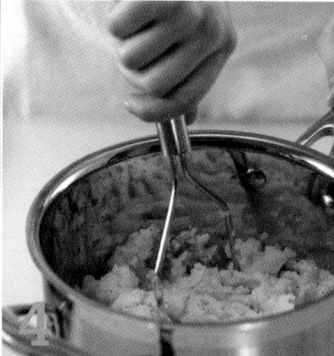

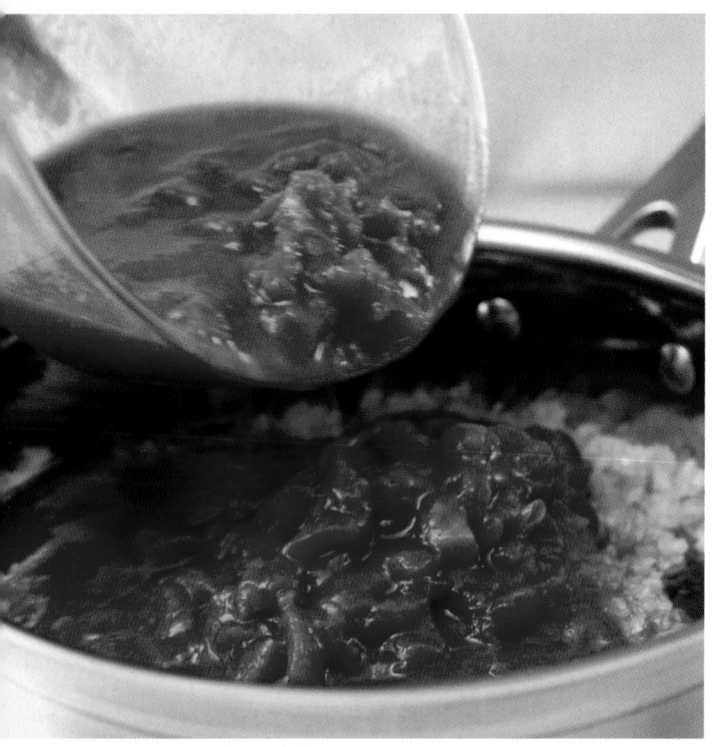

Making sauces

If you're cooking a sauce for a meal, it makes sense to cook double the quantity and freeze half. Once you've made a big batch, you can create speedy midweek meals that are all different! A simple tomato or Bolognese sauce can be the basis for many a warming treat. Pasta is always a great standby for a quick supper – here's a handful of ideas for when you're short of time or inspiration.

Simple Bolognese Sauce

This sauce tastes even better the day after it's been made.
1 tbsp olive oil, 1 large onion, finely chopped, 1 carrot, finely chopped, 1 celery stick, finely chopped, 1 garlic clove, crushed, 125g (4oz) button mushrooms, chopped, 450g (1lb) minced meat, 300ml ($\frac{1}{2}$ pint) stock, 300ml ($\frac{1}{2}$ pint) red or dry white wine, 400g can chopped tomatoes, 1 tbsp tomato purée, 2 tsp dried oregano, 2 tbsp freshly chopped parsley, salt and ground black pepper.
To serve freshly cooked pasta, freshly grated Parmesan.

1   Heat the oil in a frying pan. Add the onion, carrot, celery and garlic and fry gently for 5 minutes or until soft. Add the mushrooms and fry for a further minute.

2   Stir in the meat and cook, stirring, over a high heat until browned. Stir in the stock, wine, tomatoes, tomato purée, oregano and seasoning. Bring to the boil, cover and simmer for 1 hour or until the meat is tender and the sauce is well reduced.

3   Adjust the seasoning and stir in the parsley before serving with pasta and Parmesan.

Variations

Cottage Pie Preheat the oven to 200°C (180°C fan oven) mark 6. Add 1 tbsp plain flour once the meat has browned. Omit the tomatoes and add 450ml ($\frac{3}{4}$ pint) beef stock. Add 1 medium carrot, diced, with the mushrooms. Spoon the sauce into a 1.7 litre (3 pint) ovenproof dish and top with 1kg (2$\frac{1}{4}$lb) mashed potato. Cook for 20–25 minutes.
Lasagne Preheat the oven to 200°C (180°C fan oven) mark 6. When the bolognese sauce is nearly finished, make a double quantity of cheese sauce (page 55). Spoon half the bolognese sauce into a shallow 1.7 litre (3 pint) ovenproof dish. Top with 2 sheets of lasagne (the 'no precooking required' type) and half the cheese sauce. Repeat with the rest of the bolognese, lasagne and cheese sauce. Sprinkle with 1 tbsp grated cheese. Cook for 35 minutes.
Chilli con Carne After cooking the vegetables for 5 minutes, add 1 seeded, chopped red pepper and cook for a further 5 minutes. Add 2 tsp mild chilli powder with the mince. Drain a 400g can of red kidney beans and add to the pan for the final 5 minutes of cooking time. Serve with rice, jacket potatoes or in a flour tortilla. Grate some Cheddar cheese over, if you like.
'Stretch' the mince Replace half the mince with 200g (7oz) red lentils and add them after browning the mince. There's no need to soak them, just stir them in.

Eight quick pasta sauces

Tomato and Basil

Heat 1 tbsp olive oil in a pan, add 3 crushed garlic cloves and cook for 30 seconds only. Add a 500g carton creamed tomatoes or passata, 1 bay leaf and 1 thyme sprig. Season with salt and ground black pepper and add a large pinch of sugar. Bring to the boil, then reduce the heat and simmer, uncovered, for 5–10 minutes. Remove the bay leaf and thyme and add 3 tbsp freshly chopped basil.

Tomato, Prawn and Garlic

Put 350g (12oz) cooked peeled prawns in a bowl with 4 tbsp sun-dried tomato paste and stir well. Heat 1 tbsp olive oil and 15g ($\frac{1}{2}$ oz) butter in a frying pan and gently cook 3 sliced garlic cloves until golden. Add 4 large chopped tomatoes and 125ml (4fl oz) dry white wine. Leave the sauce to bubble for about 5 minutes, then stir in the prawns and 20g ($\frac{3}{4}$oz) freshly chopped parsley.

Creamy Pesto

Put 5 tbsp freshly grated Parmesan, 25g (1oz) toasted pinenuts, 200g carton low-fat fromage frais and 2 garlic cloves into a food processor. Whiz to a thick paste. Season generously with salt and ground black pepper. Add 40g (1$\frac{1}{2}$oz) each torn fresh basil leaves and roughly chopped fresh parsley and whiz for 2–3 seconds.

Lemon and Parmesan

Cook pasta shells in a large pan of boiling salted water for the time stated on the pack. Add 125g (4oz) frozen petit pois to the pasta water for the last 5 minutes of the cooking time. Drain the pasta and peas, put back in the pan and add the grated zest and juice of $\frac{1}{2}$ lemon and 75g (3oz) freshly grated Parmesan. Season with ground black pepper, toss and serve immediately.

Mushroom and Cream

Heat 1 tbsp olive oil in a large pan and fry 1 finely chopped onion for 7–10 minutes until soft. Add 300g (11oz) sliced mushrooms and cook for 3–4 minutes. Pour in 125ml (4fl oz) dry white wine and bubble for 1 minute, then stir in 500ml (18fl oz) low-fat crème fraîche. Heat until bubbling, then stir in 2 tbsp freshly chopped tarragon. Season with salt and ground black pepper.

Courgette and Anchovy

Heat the oil from a 50g can anchovies in a frying pan. Add 1 crushed garlic clove and a pinch of dried chilli and cook for 1 minute. Add 400ml (14fl oz) passata, 2 diced courgettes and the anchovies. Bring to the boil, then reduce the heat and simmer for about 10 minutes, stirring well, until the anchovies have melted.

Walnut and Creamy Blue Cheese

Heat 1 tsp olive oil in a small pan, add 1 crushed garlic clove and 25g (1oz) toasted walnut pieces and cook for 1 minute – the garlic should just be golden. Add 100g (3$\frac{1}{2}$oz) cubed Gorgonzola and 150ml ($\frac{1}{4}$ pint) single cream. Season with ground black pepper.

Broccoli and Thyme

Put 900g (2lb) trimmed tenderstem broccoli in a pan with 150ml ($\frac{1}{4}$ pint) hot vegetable stock. Bring to the boil, then cover and simmer for 3–4 minutes until tender – the stock should have evaporated. Add 2 crushed garlic cloves and 2 tbsp olive oil and cook for 1–2 minutes to soften the garlic. Add 250g carton mascarpone, 2 tbsp freshly chopped thyme and 100g (3$\frac{1}{2}$oz) freshly grated pecorino cheese and mix together. Season with salt and ground black pepper.

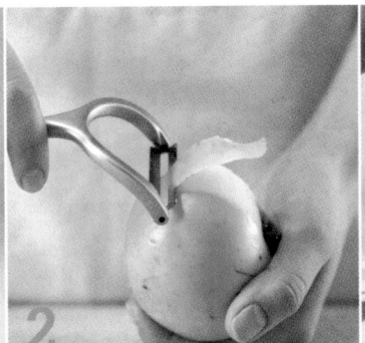
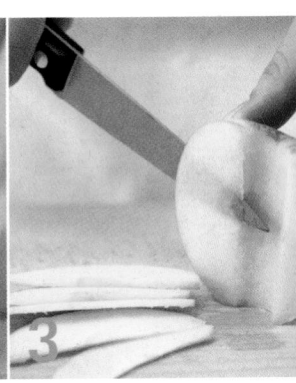

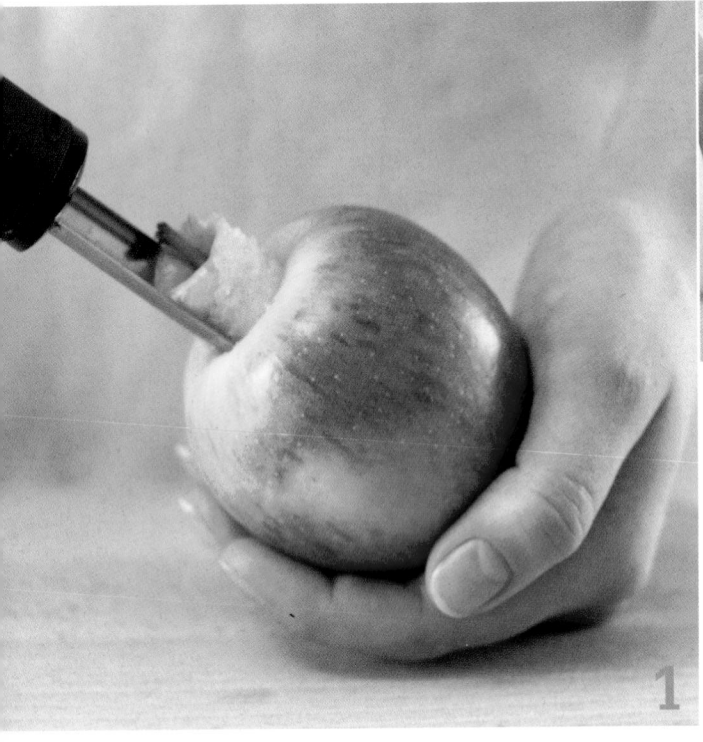

Apples

1 **To core** an apple, push an apple corer straight through the apple from the stem the base. Remove the core and use a small sharp knife to pick out any stray seeds or seed casings.

2 **To peel**, hold the fruit in one hand and run a swivel peeler under the skin, starting from the stem end and moving around the fruit, taking off the skin until you reach the base.

3 **To slice**, halve the cored apple. For flat slices, hold the apple cut side down and slice with the knife blade at right angles to the hollow left by the core. For crescent-shaped slices, stand the fruit on its end and cut slices into the hollow as if you were slicing a pie.

Preparing fruit

Soft fruits – strawberries, blackberries, raspberries and currants – are generally quick to prepare. Always handle ripe fruits gently as they can be delicate.

Pears

1 **To core**, use a teaspoon to scoop out the seeds and core through the base of the pear. Trim away any remaining fragments with a small knife. If you halve or quarter the pear, remove any remaining seeds.

2 **To peel**, cut off the stem. Peel off the skin in even strips from tip to base. If not using immediately, toss the pears in lemon juice.

3 **To slice**, halve the cored, peeled pear lengthways. Check for any remaining fragments of core, then slice with the pear halves lying cut side down on the board.

4 **To make pear fans**, slice at closely spaced intervals from the base to about 2.5cm (1in) from the tip, making sure you don't cut all the way through.

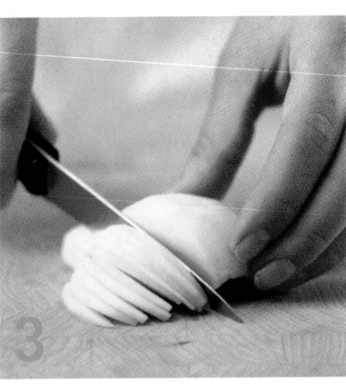

Berries

Most soft fruits can be washed very gently in cold water. Shop-bought blackberries will usually have the hull removed. If you have picked blackberries yourself the hulls and stalks may still be attached, so pick over the berries carefully and remove any that remain. Raspberries are very delicate so handle very carefully; remove any stalks and hulls. Leave strawberries whole.

1 Place the berries in a bowl of cold water and allow any small pieces of grit, dust or insects to float out.

2 Transfer the fruit to a colander and rinse gently under fresh running water. Drain well, then leave to drain on kitchen paper.

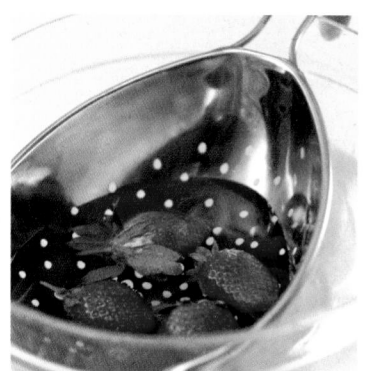

Hulling strawberries

1 Wash the strawberries gently and dry on kitchen paper. Remove the hull (the centre part that was attached to the plant) from the strawberry using a strawberry huller or a small sharp knife.

2 Put the knife into the small, hard area beneath the green stalk and gently rotate to remove a small, cone-shaped piece.

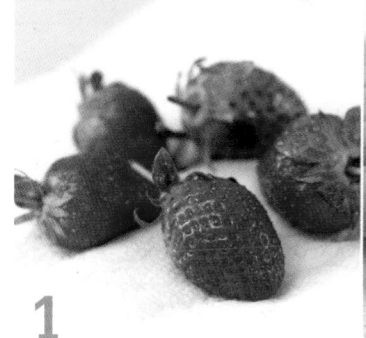

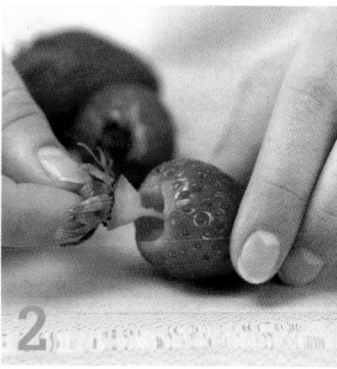

Stripping currants

Blackcurrants, redcurrants and whitecurrants can all be stripped quickly and simply from the stem in the same way.

1 Using a fork, strip all the currants off the stalks by running the fork down the length of the stalk.

2 Put the currants into a colander and wash them gently.

Mangoes

1 Cut a slice to one side of the stone in the centre. Repeat on the other side.

2 Cut parallel lines into the flesh of one slice, almost to the skin. Cut another set of lines to cut the flesh into squares.

3 Press on the skin side to turn the fruit inside out, so that the flesh is thrust outwards. Cut off the chunks as close as possible to the skin. Repeat with the other half.

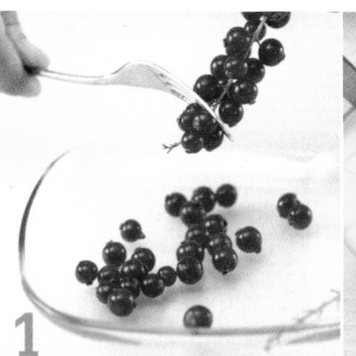

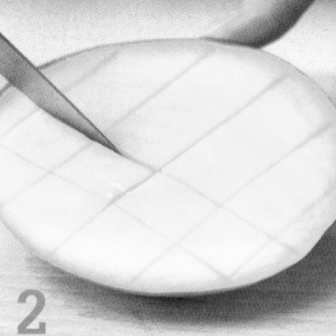

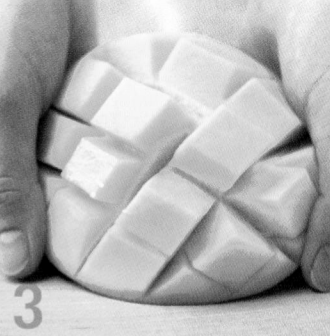

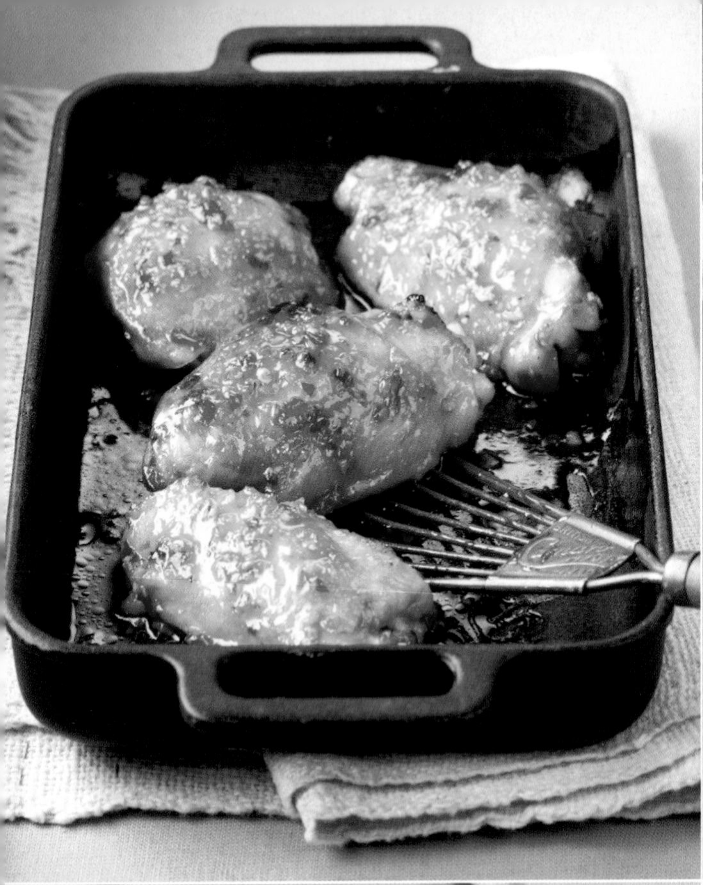

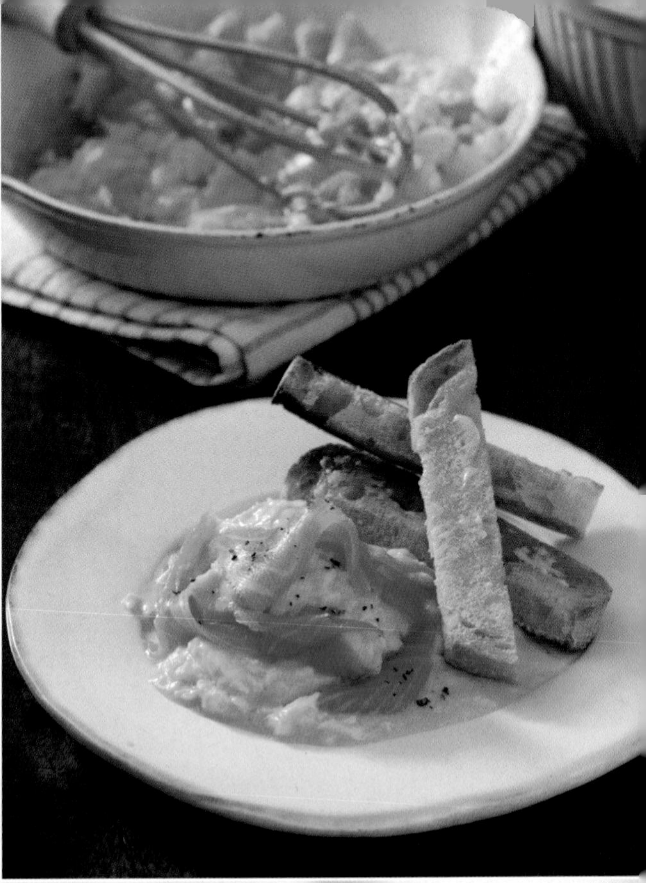

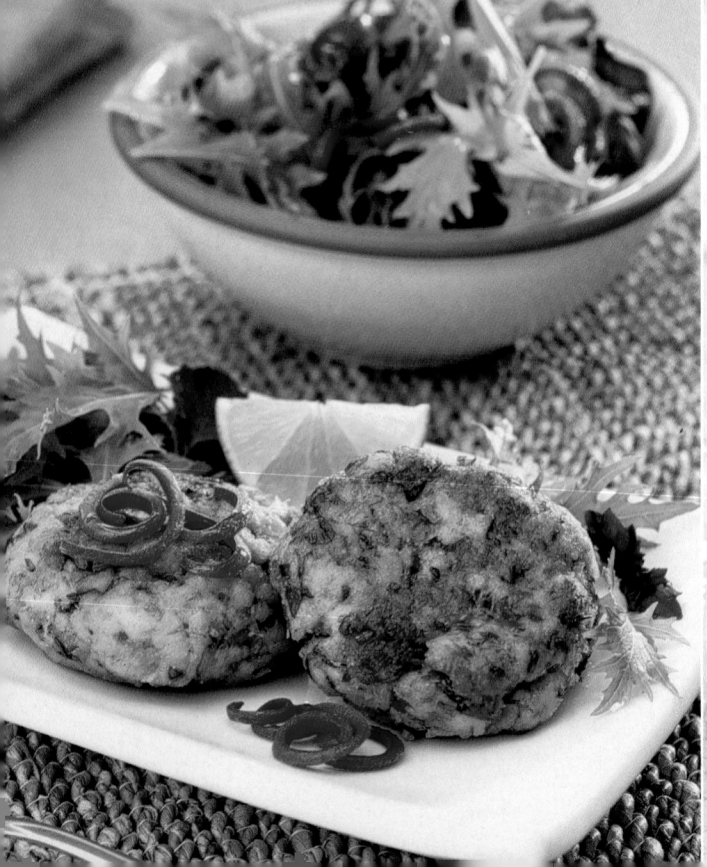
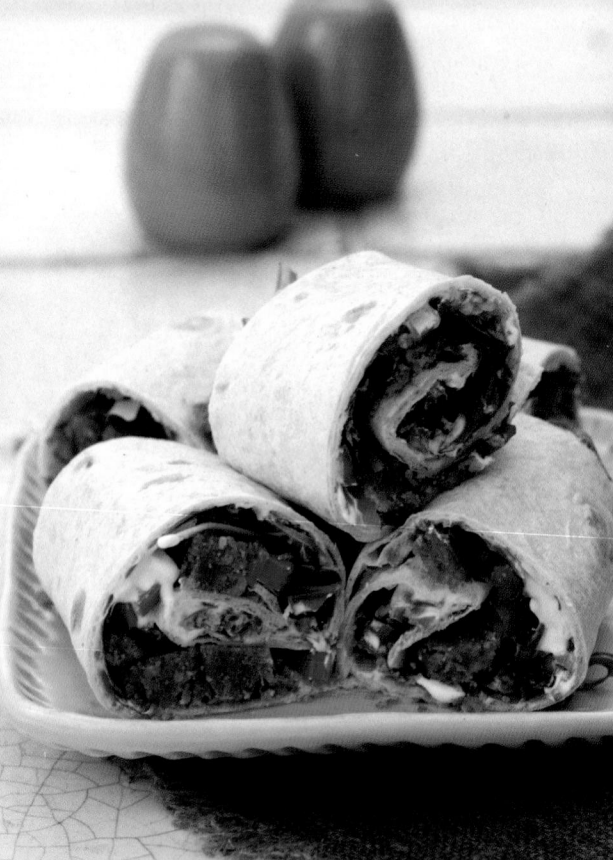

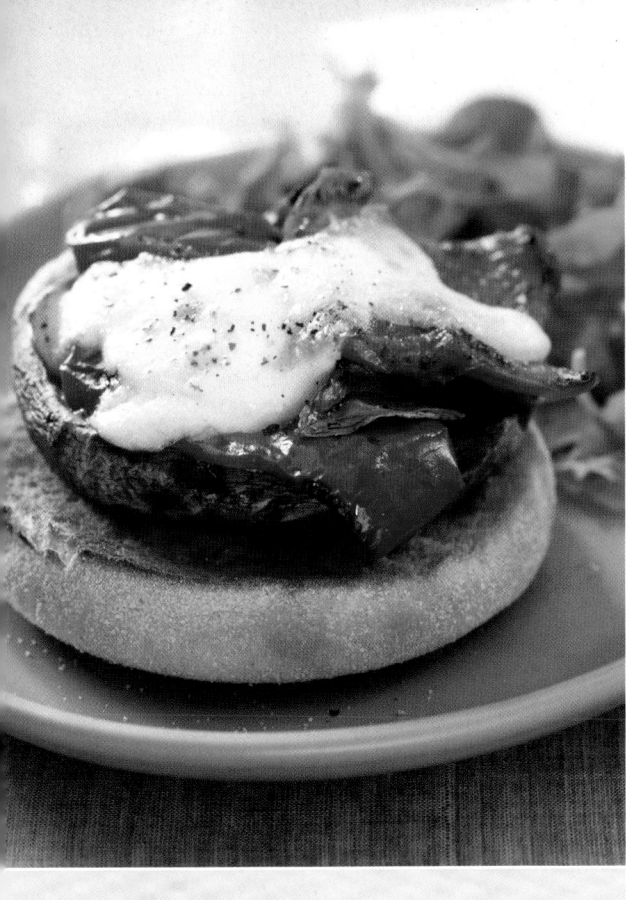

1

Light Bites

Mozzarella Mushrooms

Quick Crab Cakes

Camembert and Tomato Tarts

Sticky Chicken Thighs

Falafel, Rocket and Soured Cream Wraps

Mushroom, Spinach and Miso Soup

Throw-it-all-together Salad

Tomato Crostini with Feta and Basil

French Toast

Scrambled Eggs with Smoked Salmon

Croque Monsieur

Easy Pea Soup

Cheesy Tuna Melt

Fast Fish Soup

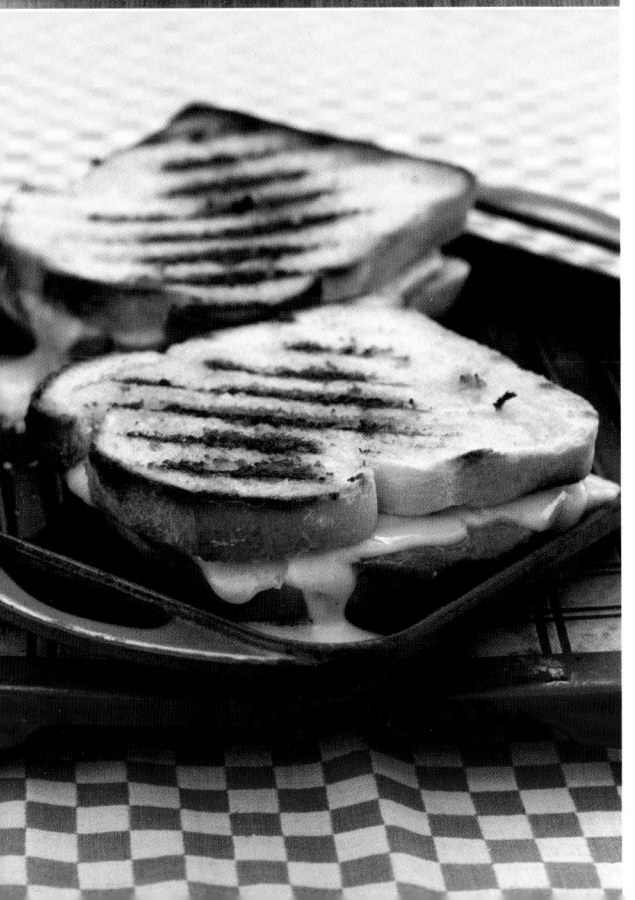

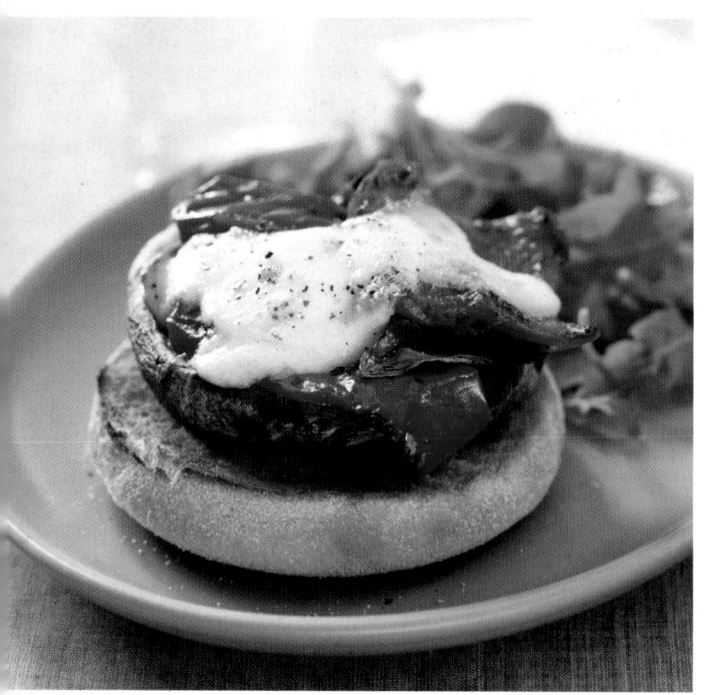

Mozzarella Mushrooms

8 large portobello mushrooms

8 slices marinated red pepper

8 fresh basil leaves

150g (5oz) mozzarella, cut into 8 slices

4 English muffins, halved

salt and ground black pepper

green salad to serve

1 Preheat the oven to 200°C (180°C fan oven) mark 6. Lay the mushrooms side by side in a roasting tin and season with salt and pepper. Top each mushroom with a slice of red pepper and a basil leaf. Lay a slice of mozzarella on top of each mushroom. Season again. Roast in the oven for 15–20 minutes until the mushrooms are tender and the cheese has melted.

2 Meanwhile, toast the muffin halves until golden. Put a mozzarella mushroom on top of each muffin half. Serve immediately with a green salad.

Serves 4	EASY		NUTRITIONAL INFORMATION	
	Preparation Time 2–3 minutes	Cooking Time 15–20 minutes	Per Serving 137 calories, 8.5g fat (of which 5g saturates), 5g carbohydrate, 0.4g salt	Vegetarian

Cook's Tips

Chillies vary enormously in strength, from quite mild to blisteringly hot, depending on the type of chilli and its ripeness. Taste a small piece first to check it's not too hot for you.

Be extremely careful when handling chillies not to touch or rub your eyes with your fingers, or they will sting. Wash knives immediately after handling chillies. As a precaution, use rubber gloves when preparing them, if you like.

Waste Not

Use leftover bread to make breadcrumbs and freeze – a great timesaver. You can use them from frozen.

200g (7oz) fresh crabmeat

2 spring onions, finely chopped

2 red chillies, seeded and finely chopped (see Cook's Tips)

finely grated zest of 1 lime

4 tbsp freshly chopped coriander

about 40g (1½oz) wholemeal breadcrumbs

1 tbsp groundnut oil

1 tbsp plain flour

salt and ground black pepper

thinly sliced red chilli, seeds removed, to garnish

1 lime, cut into wedges, and salad leaves to serve

Quick Crab Cakes

1 Put the crabmeat in a bowl, then mix with the spring onions, chillies, lime zest, coriander and seasoning. Add enough breadcrumbs to hold the mixture together, then form into four small patties.

2 Heat ½ tbsp groundnut oil in a pan. Dredge the patties with flour and fry on one side for 3 minutes. Add the remaining oil, then turn the patties over and fry for a further 2–3 minutes. Garnish the crab cakes with thinly sliced red chilli and serve with lime wedges to squeeze over them, and salad leaves.

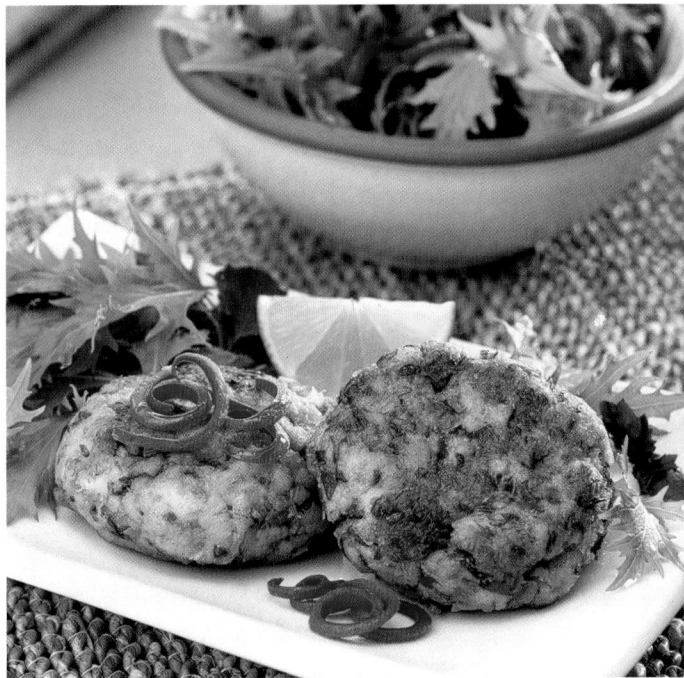

EASY		NUTRITIONAL INFORMATION		Serves
Preparation Time 15 minutes	**Cooking Time** 6 minutes	**Per Serving** 124 calories, 4g fat (of which 1g saturates), 12g carbohydrate, 0.9g salt	Dairy free	**4**

Cook's Tip

Originally from Provence in southern France, tapenade is a strongly flavoured paste made from black olives, capers, anchovies, garlic and olive oil.

Camembert and Tomato Tarts

½ x 375g pack ready-rolled puff pastry
2 tbsp tapenade (see Cook's Tip)
200g (7oz) cherry tomatoes, halved
75g (3oz) Camembert, sliced
salad to serve

1 Preheat the oven to 220°C (200°C fan oven) mark 7. Cut the puff pastry into four pieces. Score a border and prick the pastry inside the border with a fork. Put on to a baking sheet and cook for 8–10 minutes until risen.

2 Press down the centre of each tart slightly with the back of a fish slice, then spread with the tapenade. Top with the tomatoes and sliced Camembert. Put back into the oven for a further 7–8 minutes until golden brown. Serve warm with salad.

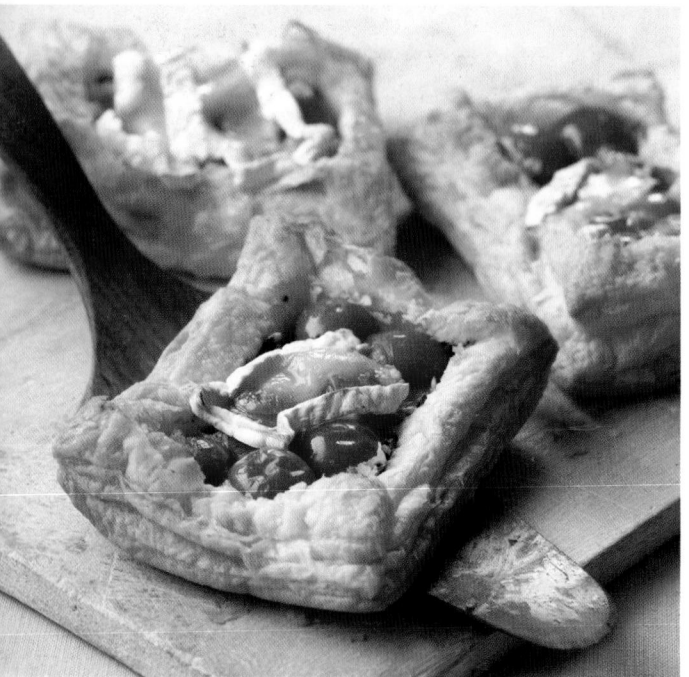

Serves 4	EASY		NUTRITIONAL INFORMATION
	Preparation Time 10 minutes	**Cooking Time** 15–20 minutes	**Per Serving** 253 calories, 17g fat (of which 4g saturates), 19g carbohydrate, 1.1g salt

Try Something Different

Try this with sausages instead of the chicken.

Italian marinade Mix 1 crushed garlic clove with 4 tbsp olive oil, the juice of 1 lemon and 1 tsp dried oregano. If you like, leave to marinate for 1–2 hours before cooking.

Oriental marinade Mix together 2 tbsp soy sauce, 1 tsp demerara sugar, 2 tbsp dry sherry or apple juice, 1 tsp finely chopped fresh root ginger and 1 crushed garlic clove.

Honey and mustard Mix together 2 tbsp grain mustard, 3 tbsp clear honey and the grated zest and juice of 1 lemon.

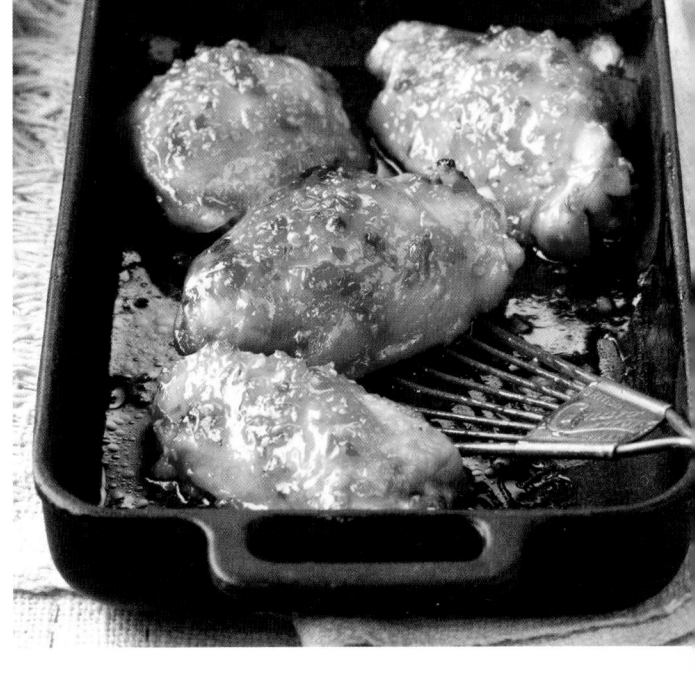

Sticky Chicken Thighs

1 garlic clove, crushed
1 tbsp clear honey
1 tbsp Thai sweet chilli sauce
4 chicken thighs
green salad to serve

1 Preheat the oven to 200°C (180°C fan oven) mark 6. Put the garlic into a bowl with the honey and chilli sauce and mix together. Add the chicken thighs and toss to coat.

2 Put into a roasting tin and roast for 15–20 minutes until the chicken is golden and cooked through. Serve with a crisp green salad.

EASY		NUTRITIONAL INFORMATION		Serves
Preparation Time 5 minutes	**Cooking Time** 20 minutes	**Per Serving** 218 calories, 12g fat (of which 3g saturates), 5g carbohydrate, 0.4g salt	Gluten free • Dairy free	**4**

Falafel, Rocket and Soured Cream Wraps

6 large flour tortillas
200g (7oz) soured cream
100g (3½oz) wild rocket
a small handful of fresh coriander, chopped
1 celery stick, finely chopped
180g pack ready-made falafel, roughly chopped or crumbled

1 Lay the tortillas on a board and spread each one with a little soured cream.

2 Divide the rocket among the wraps and sprinkle with coriander, celery and falafel.

3 Roll up as tightly as you can, then wrap each roll in clingfilm and chill for up to 3 hours or until ready to use. To serve, unwrap and cut each roll into quarters.

Serves	EASY	NUTRITIONAL INFORMATION	
6	**Preparation Time** 5 minutes, plus chilling	**Per Serving** 270 calories, 8.8g fat (of which 4.4g saturates), 42.1g carbohydrate, 0.5g salt	Vegetarian

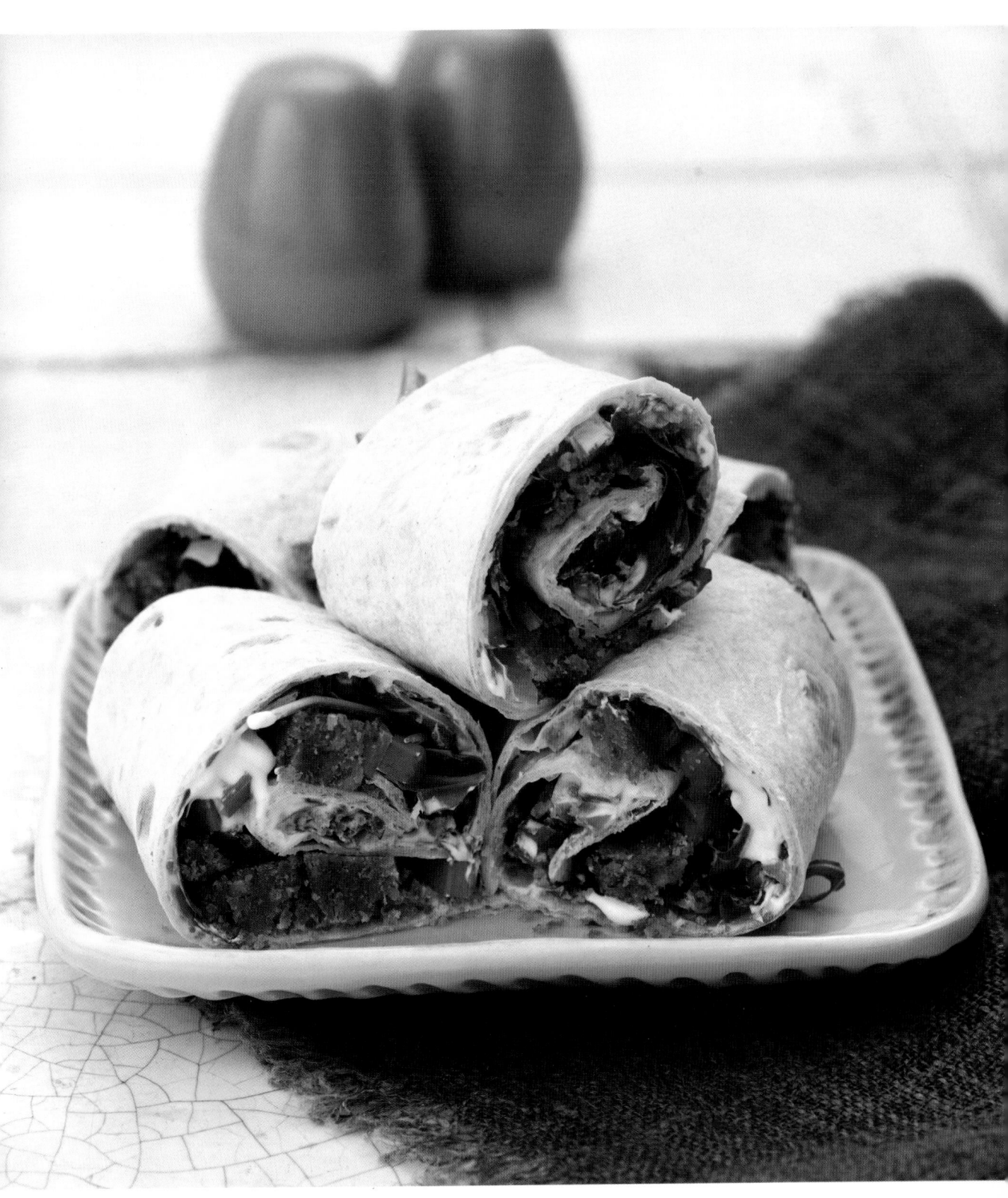

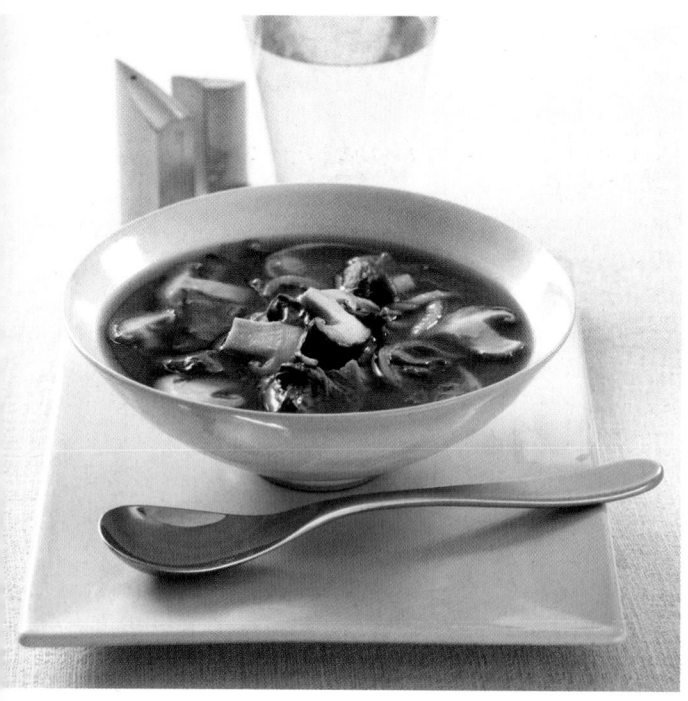

Cook's Tip

Miso (fermented barley and soya beans) contains beneficial live enzymes that can be destroyed by boiling. Miso is best added as a flavouring at the end of cooking. It's available from Asian shops, health-food shops and larger supermarkets.

Mushroom, Spinach and Miso Soup

1 tbsp vegetable oil

1 onion, finely sliced

125g (4oz) shiitake mushrooms, finely sliced

225g (8oz) baby spinach leaves

1.1 litres (2 pints) vegetable or chicken stock

4 tbsp mugi miso (see Cook's Tip)

1 Heat the oil in a large pan over a low heat. Add the onion and cook gently for 15 minutes or until soft.

2 Add the mushrooms and cook for 5 minutes, then stir in the spinach and stock. Heat for 3 minutes, then stir in the miso – don't boil, as miso is a live culture (see Cook's Tip). Spoon the soup into warmed bowls and serve hot.

Serves	EASY		NUTRITIONAL INFORMATION	
6	**Preparation Time** 5 minutes	**Cooking Time** 25 minutes	**Per Serving** 55 calories, 2g fat (of which trace saturates), 6g carbohydrate, 1.3g salt	Dairy free

Cook's Tips

Use leftover roast chicken or beef, or cooked ham for this recipe.

Use washed and prepared salad instead of Chinese leaves and watercress.

4 chargrilled chicken breasts, about 125g (4oz) each, torn into strips

2 carrots, cut into strips

½ cucumber, halved lengthways, seeded and cut into ribbons

a handful of fresh coriander leaves, roughly chopped

½ head of Chinese leaves, shredded

4 handfuls of watercress

4 spring onions, shredded

Throw-it-all-together Salad

For the dressing

5 tbsp peanut butter

2 tbsp sweet chilli sauce

juice of 1 lime

salt and ground black pepper

1 Put the chicken strips and all the salad ingredients into a large salad bowl.

2 To make the dressing, put the peanut butter, chilli sauce and lime juice in a small bowl and mix together well. Season with salt and pepper. If the dressing is too thick to pour, add 2–3 tbsp cold water, a tablespoon at a time, to thin it – use just enough water to make the dressing the correct consistency.

3 Drizzle the dressing over the salad, toss gently together and serve.

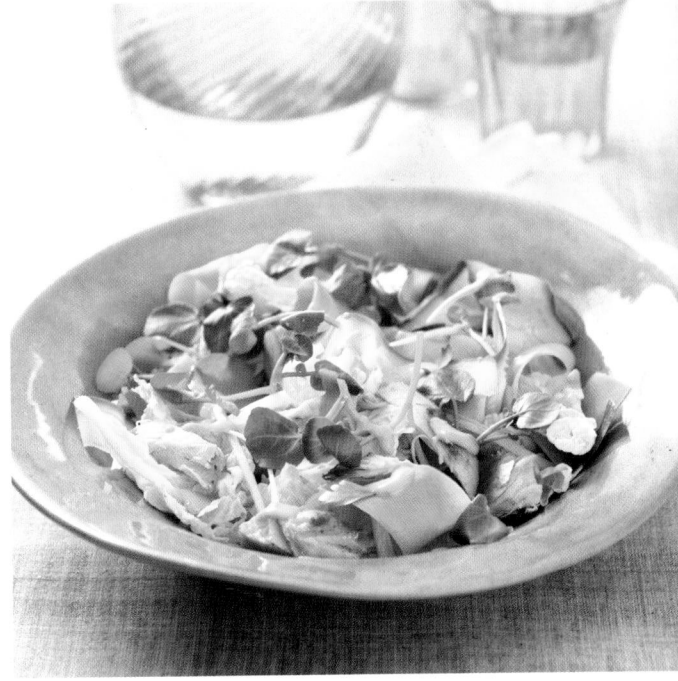

EASY	NUTRITIONAL INFORMATION		Serves
Preparation Time 10 minutes	**Per Serving** 215 calories, 9g fat (of which 2g saturates), 9g carbohydrate, 0.6g salt	Gluten free • Dairy free	**4**

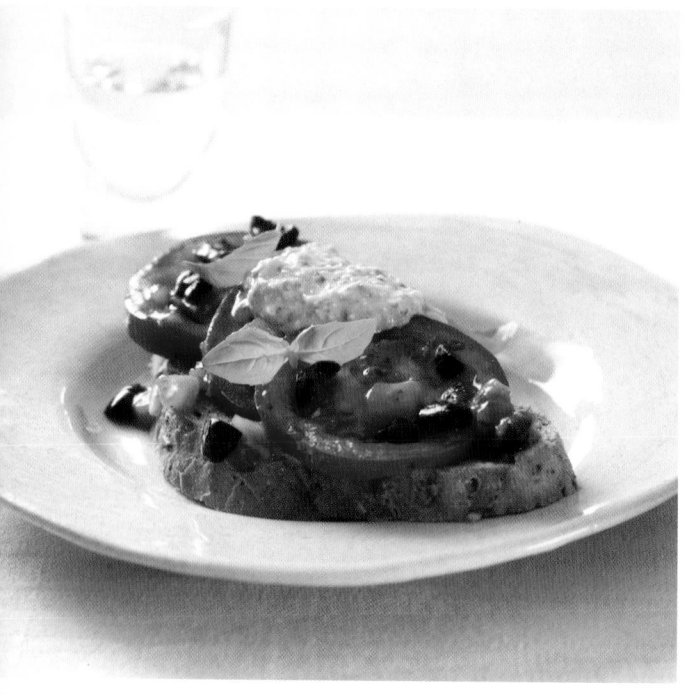

Tomato Crostini with Feta and Basil

1 small garlic clove, crushed

3 tbsp freshly chopped basil, plus extra basil leaves to garnish

25g (1oz) pinenuts

2 tbsp extra virgin olive oil

grated zest and juice of 1 lime

50g (2oz) feta cheese

4 large tomatoes, vine-ripened if possible, thickly sliced

150g carton fresh tomato salsa

50g (2oz) pitted black olives, roughly chopped

4 thick slices country-style bread

salt and ground black pepper

1 Whiz the garlic, basil, pinenuts, olive oil, lime zest and juice together in a food processor to form a smooth paste. Alternatively, use a mortar and pestle. Add the feta cheese and blend until smooth. Thin with 1 tbsp water if necessary. Season with salt and pepper.

2 Put the tomatoes, salsa and olives in a bowl and gently toss together.

3 Toast the bread. Divide the tomato mixture among the slices of toast and spoon the basil and feta mixture over the top. Garnish with basil leaves and serve.

Serves 4	EASY		NUTRITIONAL INFORMATION	
	Preparation Time 20 minutes	Cooking Time 3 minutes	Per Serving 242 calories, 17g fat (of which 3g saturates), 18g carbohydrate, 1.5g salt	Vegetarian

Cook's Tips

Use leftover bread for this tasty brunch dish.
For a savoury version, use white bread and omit the spice and sugar; serve with tomato ketchup, or with bacon and maple syrup.

2 medium eggs

150ml (¼ pint) semi-skimmed milk

a generous pinch of freshly grated nutmeg or ground cinnamon

4 slices white bread, or fruit bread, crusts removed and each slice cut into four fingers

50g (2oz) butter

vegetable oil for frying

1 tbsp golden caster sugar

French Toast

1 Beat the eggs, milk and nutmeg or cinnamon together in a shallow dish.

2 Dip the pieces of bread into the mixture, coating them well.

3 Heat half the butter with 1 tbsp oil in a heavy-based frying pan. When the butter is foaming, fry the egg-coated bread pieces in batches, until golden on both sides, adding more butter and oil as needed. Sprinkle with sugar to serve for brunch.

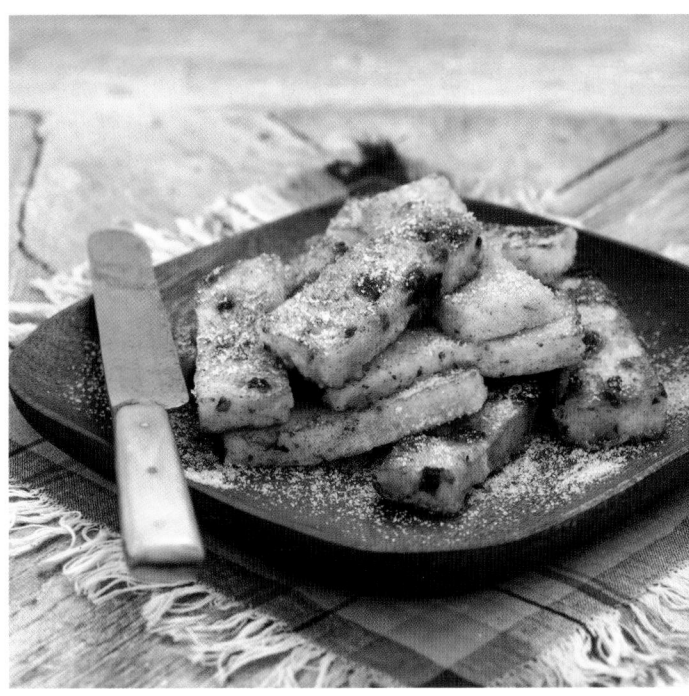

EASY		NUTRITIONAL INFORMATION		Serves
Preparation Time 5 minutes	**Cooking Time** 10 minutes	**Per Finger** 259 calories, 19.6g fat (of which 8.6g saturates), 15.2g carbohydrate, 0.7g salt	Vegetarian	**4**

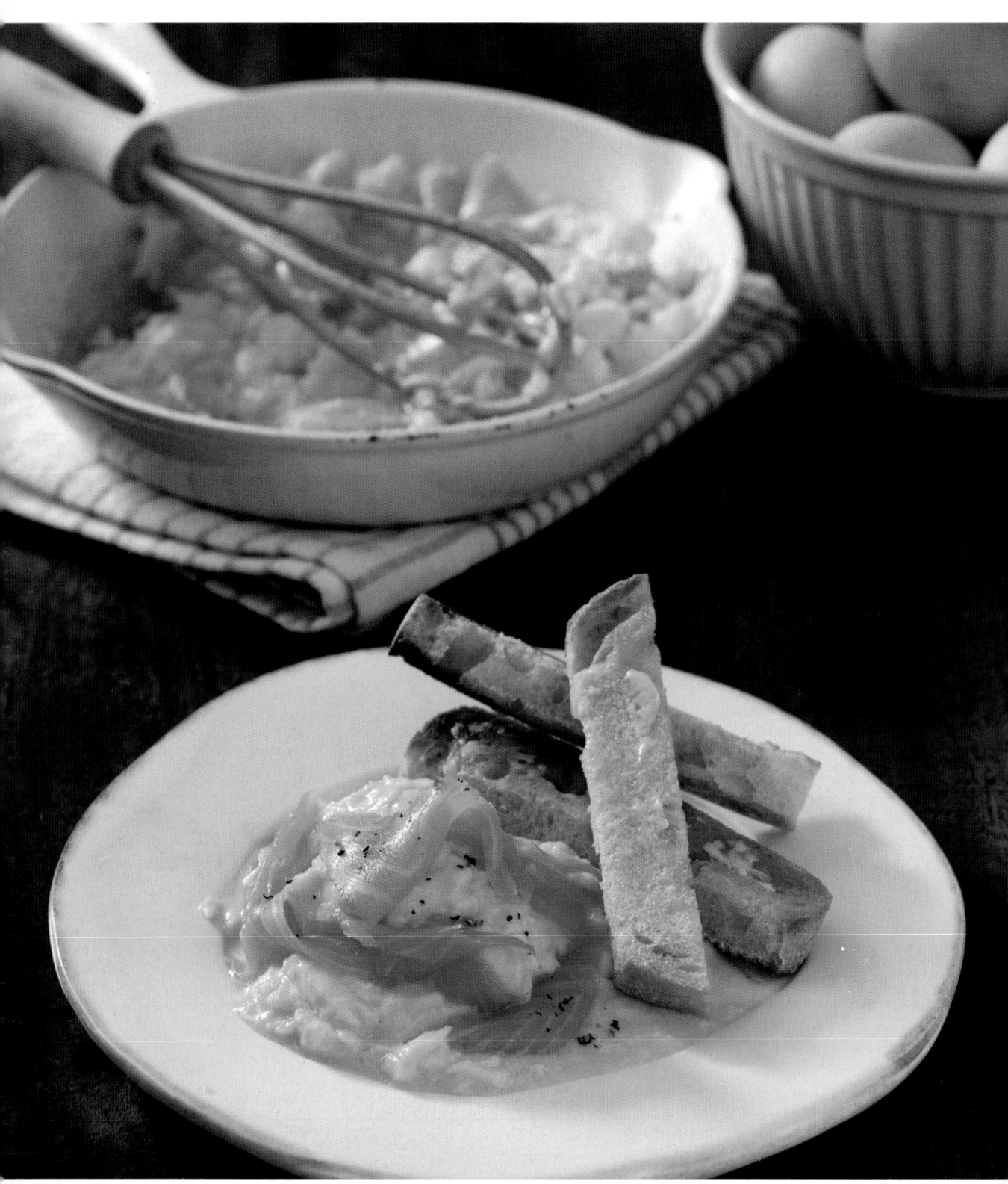

Scrambled Eggs with Smoked Salmon

6 large eggs

25g (1oz) butter, plus extra to spread

100g (3½oz) mascarpone

125g pack smoked salmon, sliced, or smoked salmon trimmings

6 slices sourdough or rye bread, toasted, buttered and cut into slim rectangles for soldiers

salt and ground black pepper

1 Crack the eggs into a jug and lightly beat together. Season well.

2 Melt the butter in a non-stick pan over a low heat. Add the eggs and stir constantly until the mixture thickens. Add the mascarpone and season well. Cook for 1–2 minutes longer, until the mixture just becomes firm, then fold in the smoked salmon. Serve at once with toasted bread soldiers.

EASY		NUTRITIONAL INFORMATION	Serves
Preparation Time 10 minutes	**Cooking Time** 5 minutes	**Per Serving** 457 calories, 33.9g fat (of which 17.3g saturates), 17.2g carbohydrate, 2.7g salt	**4**

Croque Monsieur

4 slices white bread
butter, softened, to spread, plus extra for frying
Dijon mustard, to taste
125g (4oz) Gruyère cheese
4 slices ham

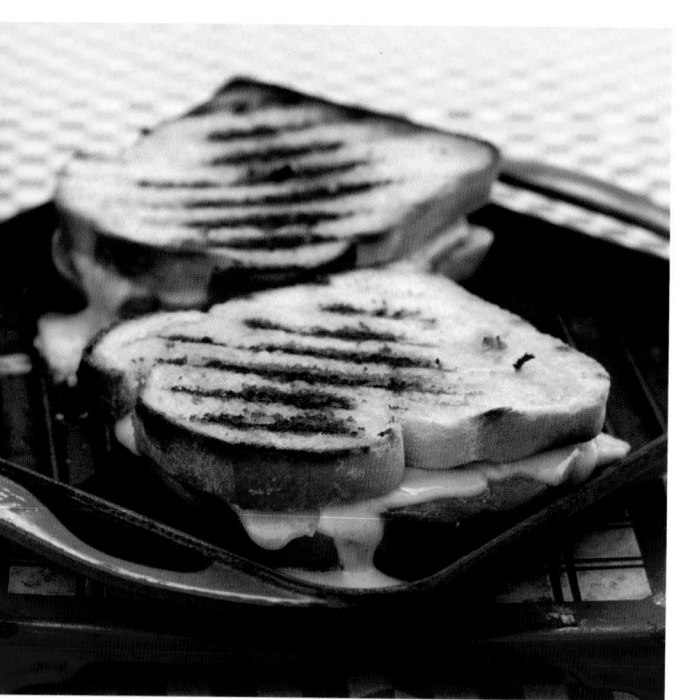

1 Spread each slice of bread on both sides with the butter. Then spread one side of two slices of bread with a little Dijon mustard.

2 Divide the cheese and ham between the two mustard-spread bread slices. Put the other slice of bread on top and press down.

3 Heat a griddle with a little butter until hot and fry the sandwiches for 2–3 minutes on each side until golden and crispy and the cheese starts to melt.

4 Slice in half and serve immediately.

Serves 2	EASY		NUTRITIONAL INFORMATION
	Preparation Time 5 minutes	Cooking Time 8 minutes	Per Serving 551 calories, 35.4g fat (of which 22.4g saturates), 27.2g carbohydrate, 3.6g salt

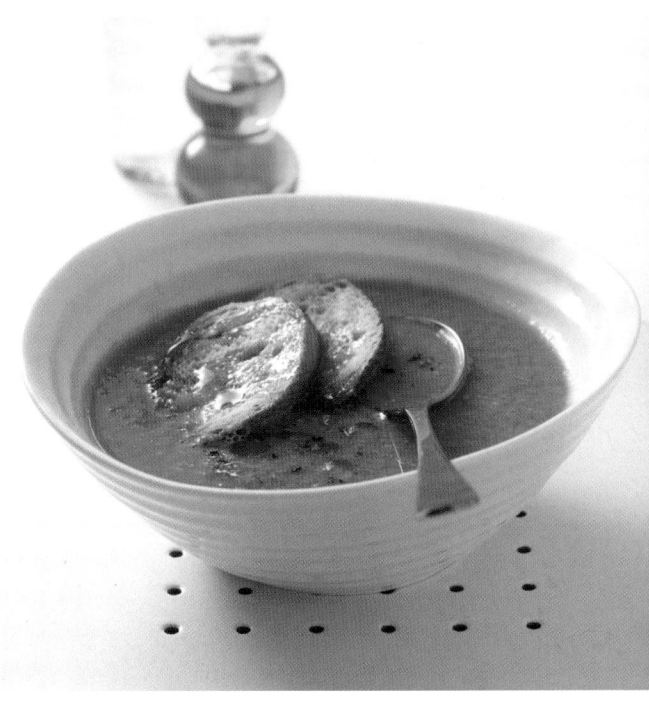

Easy Pea Soup

1 small baguette, thinly sliced

2 tbsp basil-infused olive oil, plus extra to drizzle

450g (1lb) frozen peas, thawed

600ml (1 pint) vegetable stock

salt and ground black pepper

1 Preheat the oven to 220°C (200°C fan oven) mark 7. To make the croûtons, put the baguette slices on a baking sheet, drizzle with 2 tbsp basil oil and cook in the oven for 10–15 minutes until golden.

2 Meanwhile, put the peas in a food processor or blender, add the stock and season with salt and pepper. Whiz for 2–3 minutes.

3 Pour the soup into a pan and bring to the boil, then reduce the heat and simmer for 10 minutes. Spoon into warmed bowls, add the croûtons, drizzle with extra oil and sprinkle with salt and pepper. Serve immediately.

EASY		NUTRITIONAL INFORMATION		Serves
Preparation Time 2 minutes, plus thawing	**Cooking Time** 15 minutes	**Per Serving** 408 calories, 9g fat (of which 2g saturates), 69g carbohydrate, 1.8g salt	Vegetarian • Dairy free	**6**

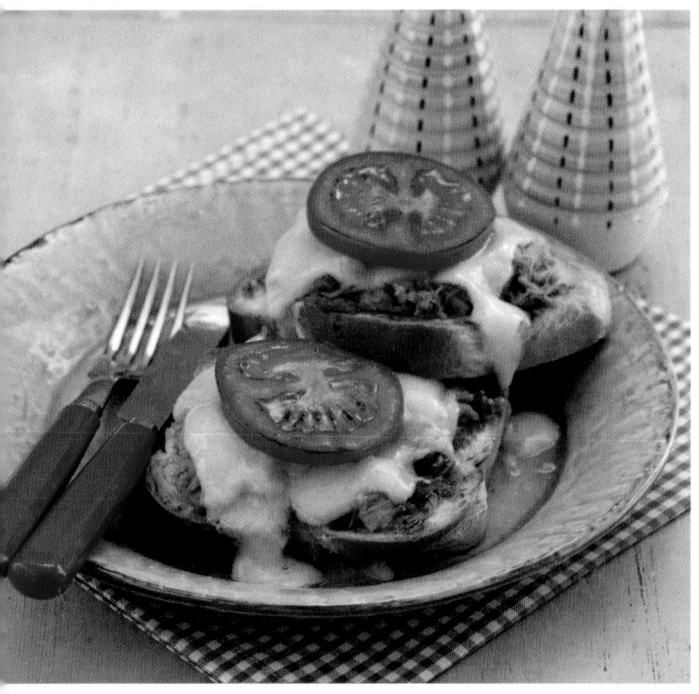

Cook's Tip

You can use any type of bread for this recipe.

Cheesy Tuna Melt

2 slices cholla bread
100g can tuna in sunflower oil, drained
75g (3oz) Gruyère cheese, sliced
1 tomato, sliced
salt and ground black pepper

1 Preheat the grill to high. Put the bread on a baking sheet and toast one side.

2 Turn the bread so that it is untoasted side up, then divide the tuna between the two pieces and add the cheese and tomato.

3 Grill until the cheese is bubbling and golden. Season with salt and pepper and serve immediately.

Serves 1	EASY		NUTRITIONAL INFORMATION
	Preparation Time 5 minutes	**Cooking Time** 5 minutes	**Per Serving** 747 calories, 35.6g fat (of which 18.1g saturates), 51.4g carbohydrate, 3.4g salt

Cook's Tip

Frozen seafood mix is a useful standby. Use it instead of the fish and shellfish in this recipe but take care not to overcook or it will become tough.

1 leek, finely sliced

4 fat garlic cloves, crushed

3 celery sticks, finely sliced

1 small fennel bulb, finely sliced

1 red chilli, seeded and finely chopped (see page 33)

3 tbsp olive oil

50ml (2fl oz) dry white wine

about 750g (1lb 10oz) mixed fish and shellfish, such as haddock, monkfish, salmon, raw shelled prawns and cleaned mussels

4 medium tomatoes, chopped

2 tbsp freshly chopped thyme

salt and ground black pepper

Fast Fish Soup

1 Put the leek in a large pan and add the garlic, celery, fennel, chilli and olive oil. Cook over a medium heat for 5 minutes or until the vegetables are soft and beginning to colour.

2 Stir in 1.1 litres (2 pints) boiling water and the wine. Bring to the boil, then simmer the soup, covered, for 5 minutes.

3 Meanwhile, cut the fish into large chunks. Add to the soup with the tomatoes and thyme. Continue simmering gently until the fish has just turned opaque. Add the prawns and simmer for 1 minute then add the mussels – if you're using them. As soon as all the mussels have opened, season the soup and ladle into warmed bowls. Discard any mussels that remain closed, then serve immediately.

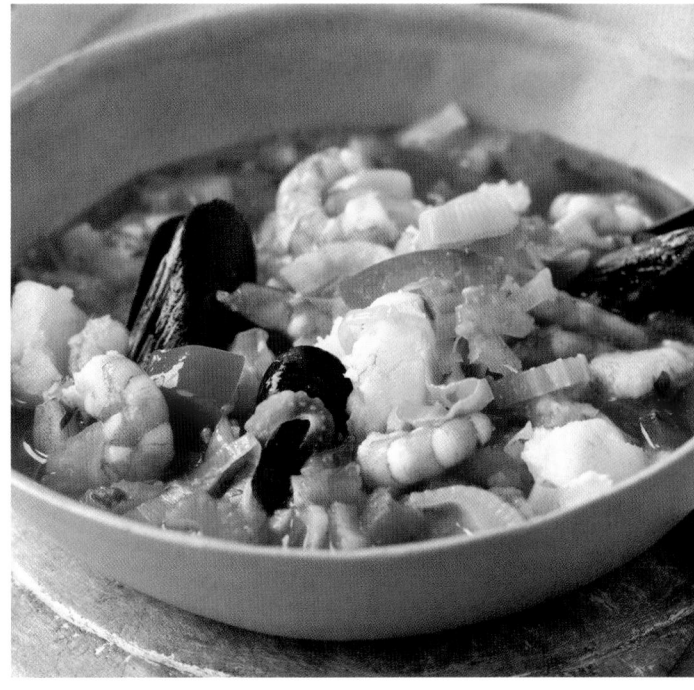

EASY		NUTRITIONAL INFORMATION		Serves
Preparation Time 10 minutes	**Cooking Time** 15 minutes	**Per Serving** 269 calories, 10g fat (of which 2g saturates), 6g carbohydrate, 0.6g salt	Gluten free • Dairy free	**4**

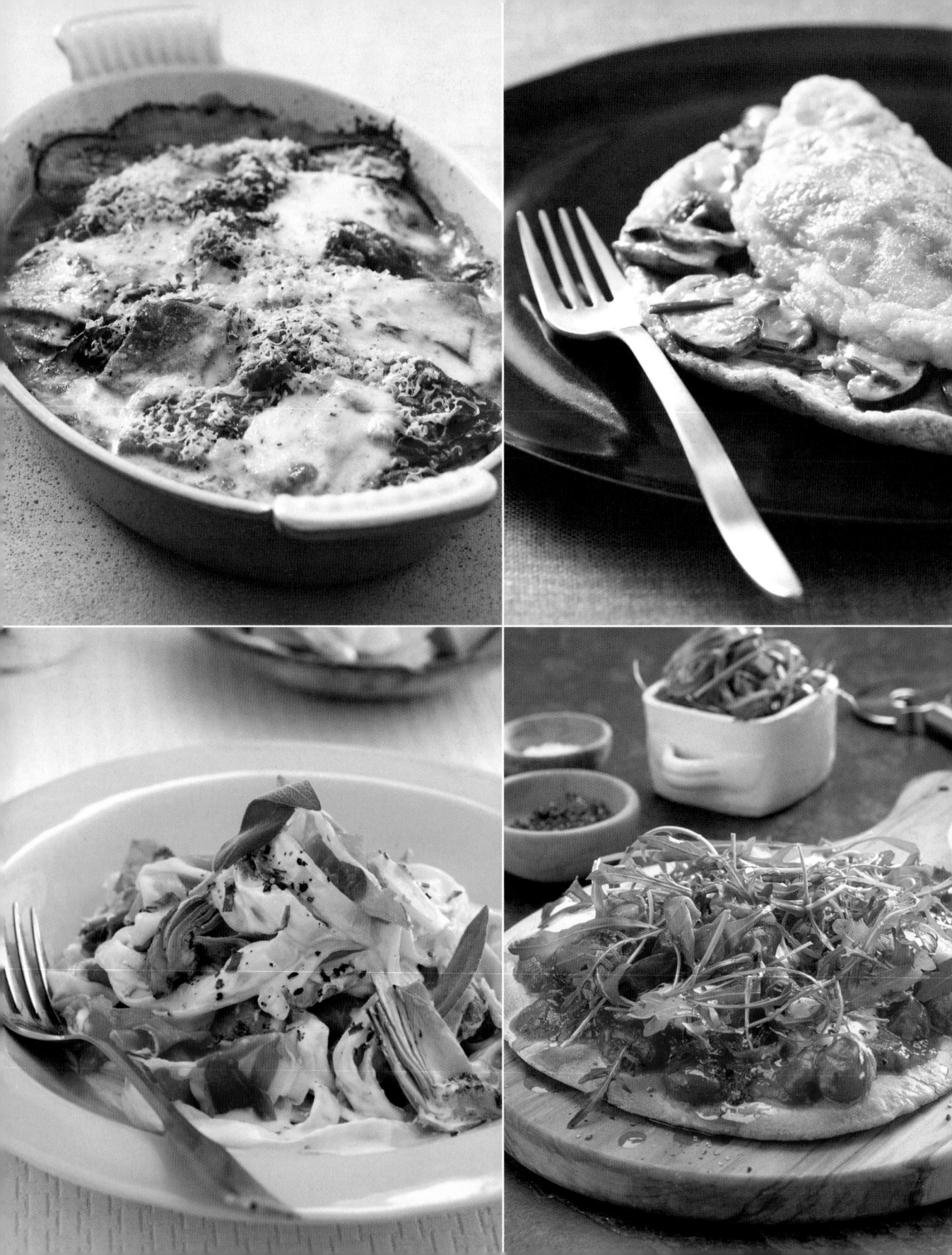

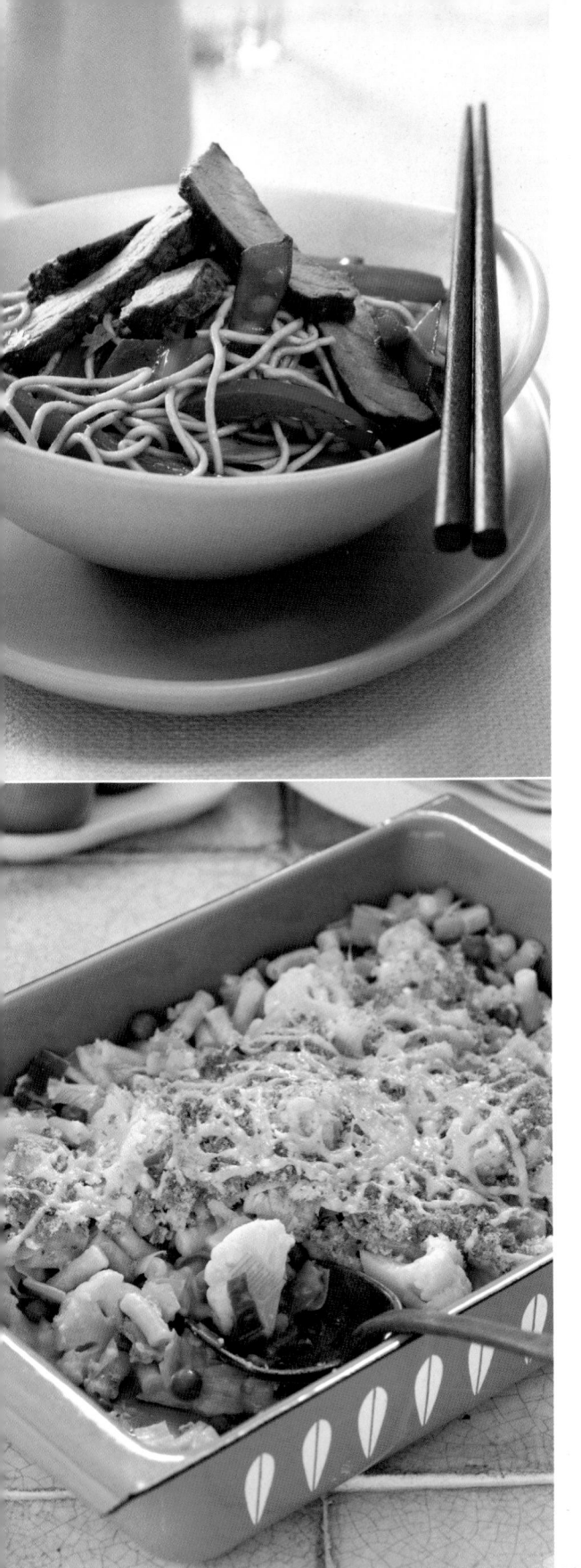

2

Midweek Suppers

Speedy Beef Noodles

250g (9oz) fine egg noodles
4 tbsp sesame oil, plus a little extra to brush
300g (11oz) beef fillet
4 tbsp chilli soy sauce
juice of 1 lime
2 red peppers, halved, seeded and cut into thin strips
200g (7oz) mangetouts, sliced
4 tbsp freshly chopped coriander

1 Put the noodles in a large bowl and cover with boiling water. Leave to soak for 4 minutes, then rinse under cold running water and set aside.

2 Meanwhile, brush a large frying pan or griddle with a little sesame oil and heat until hot. Fry the beef for 3–4 minutes on each side, or 4–5 minutes if you like it well done. Remove from the pan and keep warm.

3 Add the 4 tbsp sesame oil to the pan with the chilli soy sauce, lime juice, red peppers, mangetouts and coriander and stir to mix. Add the noodles and use two large spoons to toss them over the heat to combine with the sauce and warm through.

4 Cut the beef into thin slices and serve on a bed of noodles.

Serves	EASY		NUTRITIONAL INFORMATION	
4	Preparation Time 5 minutes	Cooking Time 10 minutes	Per Serving 510 calories, 19g fat (of which 5g saturates), 60g carbohydrate, 2.8g salt	Dairy free

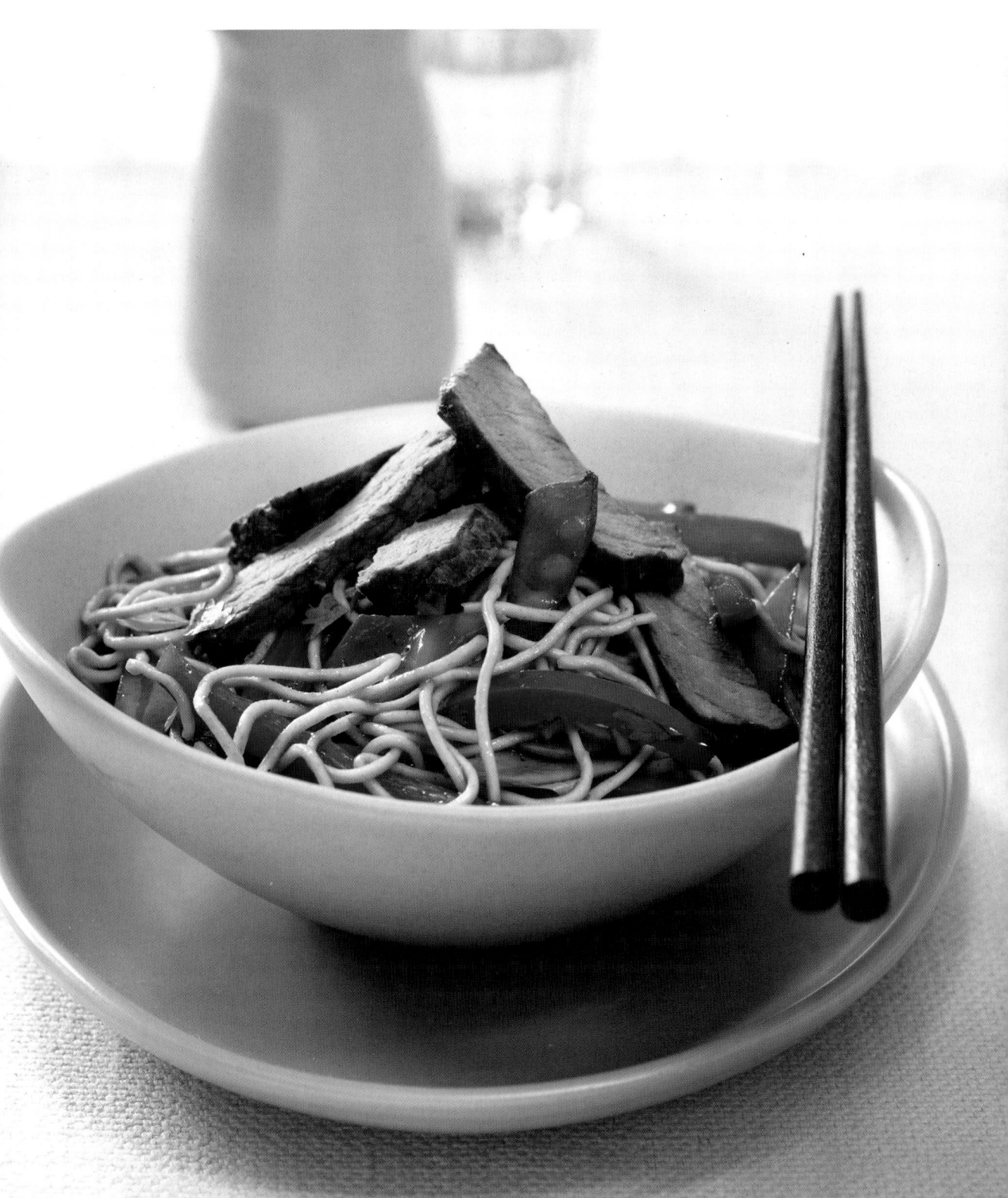

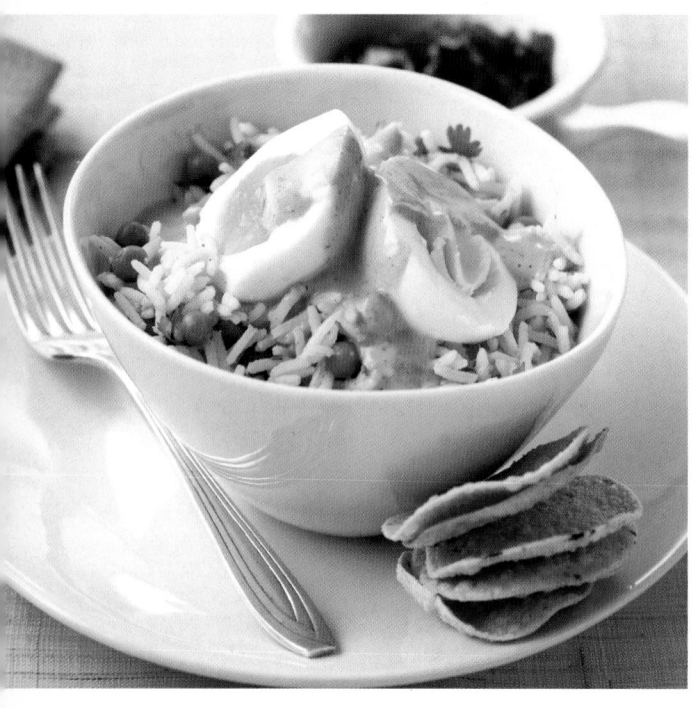

Spiced Egg Pilau

200g (7oz) basmati or wild rice
150g (5oz) frozen peas
4 medium eggs
200ml (7fl oz) coconut cream
1 tsp mild curry paste
1 tbsp sweet chilli sauce
1 tbsp smooth peanut butter
1 large bunch fresh coriander, roughly chopped
mini poppadums and mango chutney to serve

1 Put the rice into a pan with 450ml (³/₄pint) boiling water and cook according to the pack instructions until just tender. Add the frozen peas for the last 5 minutes of cooking time.

2 Meanwhile, put the eggs into a large pan of boiling water and simmer for 6 minutes, then drain and shell.

3 Put the coconut cream, curry paste, chilli sauce and peanut butter into a small pan and whisk together. Heat the sauce gently, stirring, without allowing it to boil.

4 Drain the rice and stir in the chopped coriander and 2 tbsp of the sauce.

5 Divide the rice among four bowls. Cut the eggs into halves and serve on the rice, spooning the remaining coconut sauce over the top. Serve with poppadums and chutney.

Serves 4	EASY		NUTRITIONAL INFORMATION	
	Preparation Time 5 minutes	**Cooking Time** 15 minutes	**Per Serving** 331 calories, 9g fat (of which 12g saturates), 50g carbohydrate, 0.6g salt	Vegetarian Gluten free • Dairy free

Waste Not

Use leftover cooked pasta, beans or potatoes: tip the pasta into a pan of boiling water and bring back to the boil for 30 seconds. Bring the beans or potatoes to room temperature, but there's no need to reboil them.

Pasta with Pesto and Beans

350g (12oz) dried pasta shapes

175g (6oz) fine green beans, roughly chopped

175g (6oz) small salad potatoes, such as Anya, thickly sliced

250g (9oz) fresh pesto sauce

freshly grated Parmesan to serve

1 Bring a large pan of water to the boil. Add the pasta, bring back to the boil and cook for 5 minutes.

2 Add the beans and potatoes to the pan and continue to boil for a further 7–8 minutes until the potatoes are just tender.

3 Drain the pasta, beans and potatoes in a colander, then tip everything back into the pan and stir in the pesto sauce. Serve scattered with freshly grated Parmesan.

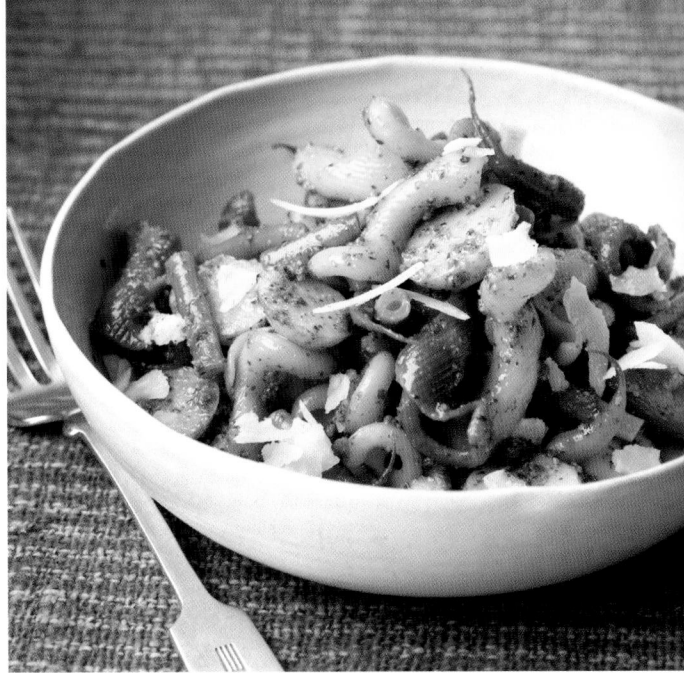

EASY		NUTRITIONAL INFORMATION		Serves
Preparation Time 5 minutes	**Cooking Time** 15 minutes	**Per Serving** 738 calories, 38g fat (of which 10g saturates), 74g carbohydrate, 1g salt	Vegetarian	**4**

Waste Not

Use leftover double cream with a squeeze of lemon juice instead of soured cream.

Chilli Bean Cake

3 tbsp olive oil

75g (3oz) wholemeal breadcrumbs

1 bunch of spring onions, finely chopped

1 orange pepper, seeded and chopped

1 small green chilli, seeded and finely chopped (see page 33)

1 garlic clove, crushed

1 tsp ground turmeric (optional)

400g can mixed beans, drained

3 tbsp mayonnaise

a small handful of fresh basil, chopped

salt and ground black pepper

soured cream, freshly chopped coriander, lime wedges and tomato salad to serve (optional)

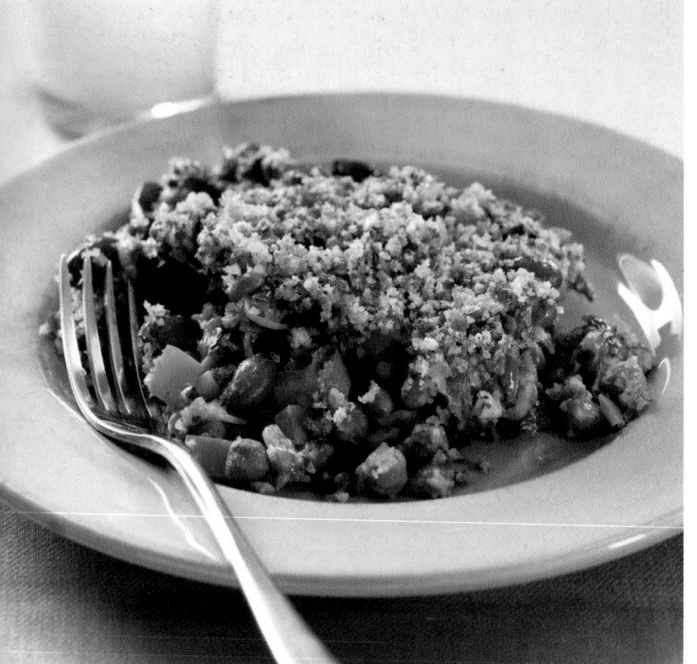

1 Heat 2 tbsp olive oil in a non-stick frying pan over a medium heat and fry the breadcrumbs until golden and beginning to crisp. Remove and set aside.

2 Using the same pan, add the remaining oil and fry the spring onions until soft and golden. Add the orange pepper, chilli, garlic and turmeric, if using. Cook, stirring, for 5 minutes.

3 Tip in the beans, mayonnaise, two-thirds of the fried breadcrumbs and the basil. Season with salt and pepper, then mash roughly with a fork. Press the mixture down to flatten. Sprinkle the remaining breadcrumbs over. Fry the bean cake over a medium heat for 4–5 minutes until the base is golden. Remove from the heat, cut into wedges and serve with soured cream, coriander, lime wedges and tomato salad if you like.

Serves 4	EASY		NUTRITIONAL INFORMATION	
	Preparation Time 10 minutes	**Cooking Time** 20 minutes	**Per Serving** 265 calories, 6g fat (of which 1g saturates), 41g carbohydrate, 2.1g salt	Vegetarian • Dairy free

Cook's Tip

Make the cheese sauce in the microwave: put the butter, flour and milk into a large microwave-proof bowl and whisk together. Cook in a 900W microwave on full power for 4 minutes, whisking every minute, until the sauce has thickened. Stir in the cheese until it melts. Stir in the mustard and season to taste.

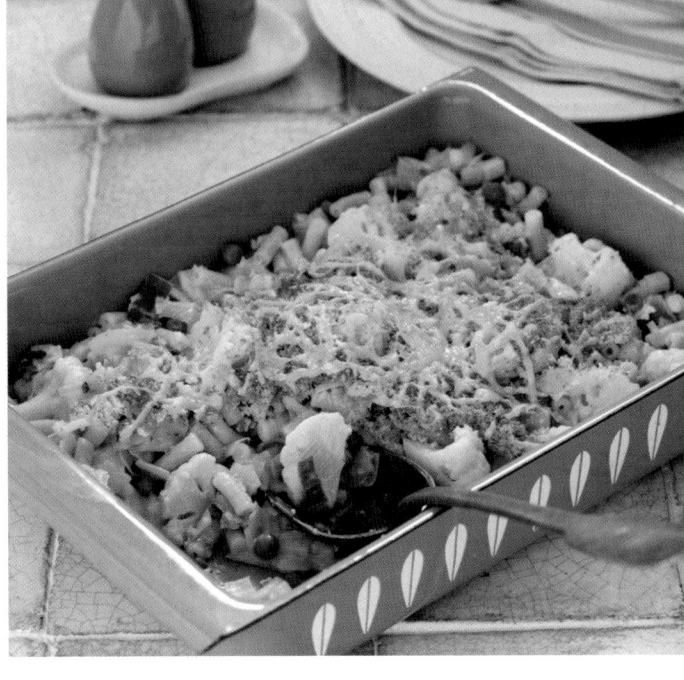

Cheese and Vegetable Bake

250g (9oz) macaroni
1 cauliflower, cut into florets
2 leeks, finely chopped
100g (3½oz) frozen peas
crusty bread to serve

For the cheese sauce
15g (½oz) butter
15g (½oz) plain flour
200ml (7fl oz) skimmed milk
75g (3oz) Parmesan, grated
2 tsp Dijon mustard
25g (1oz) wholemeal breadcrumbs
salt and ground black pepper

1 Cook the macaroni in a large pan of boiling water for 6 minutes, adding the cauliflower and leeks for the last 4 minutes, and the peas for the last 2 minutes.

2 Meanwhile, make the cheese sauce. Melt the butter in a pan and add the flour. Cook for 1–2 minutes, then take off the heat and gradually stir in the milk. Bring to the boil slowly, stirring until the sauce thickens. Stir in 50g (2oz) Parmesan and the mustard. Season with salt and pepper.

3 Preheat the grill to medium. Drain the pasta and the vegetables, and put back in the pan. Add the cheese sauce and mix well. Spoon into a large, shallow 2 litre (3½ pint) ovenproof dish and scatter the remaining Parmesan and the breadcrumbs over. Grill for 5 minutes or until golden and crisp. Serve hot with bread.

EASY		NUTRITIONAL INFORMATION		Serves
Preparation Time 15 minutes	**Cooking Time** 15 minutes	**Per Serving** 471 calories, 12.9g fat (of which 6.5g saturates), 66.8g carbohydrate, 0.8g salt	Vegetarian	**4**

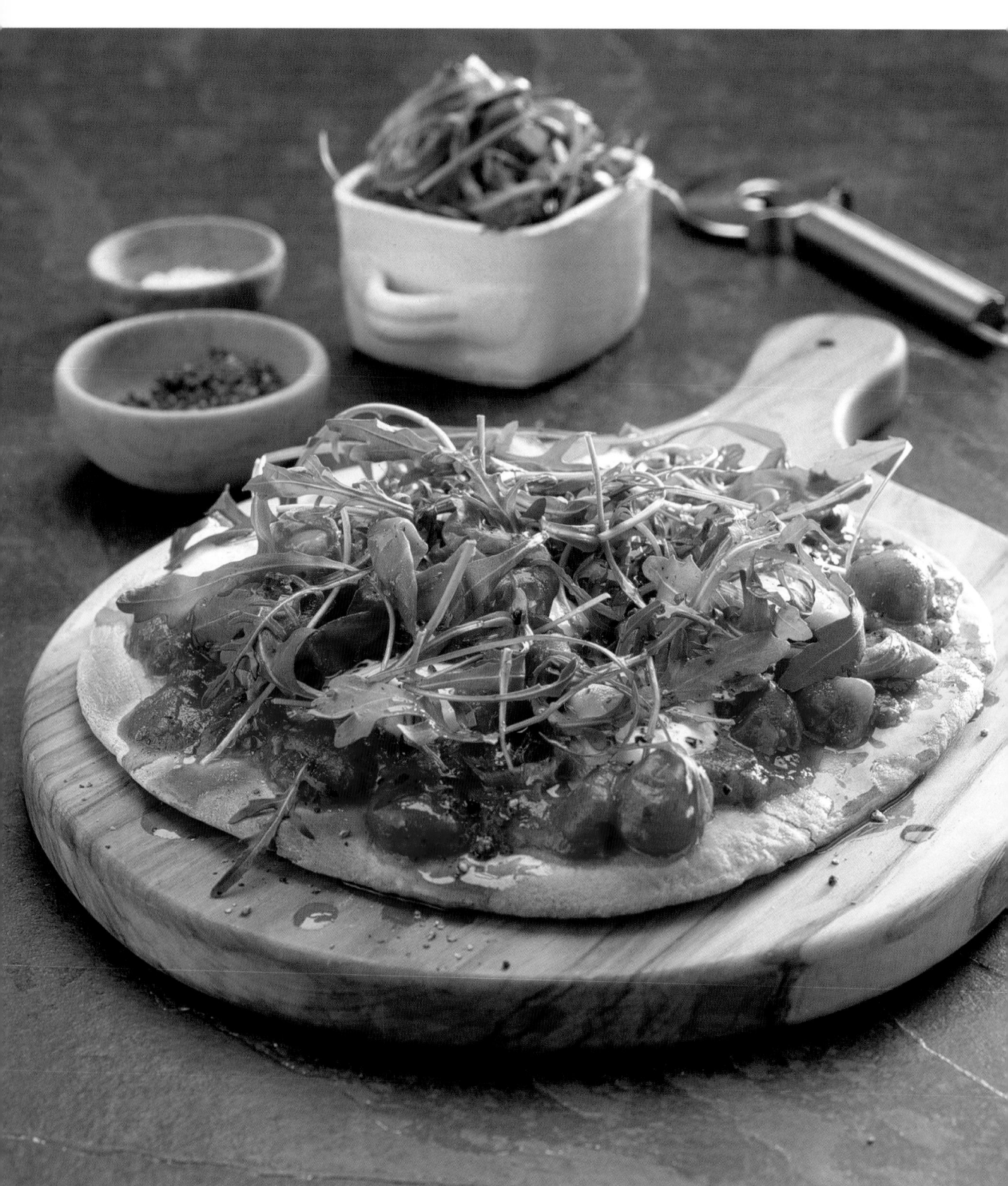

Mozzarella, Parma Ham and Rocket Pizza

a little plain flour to dust

290g pack pizza base mix

350g (12oz) fresh tomato and chilli pasta sauce

250g (9oz) buffalo mozzarella cheese, drained and roughly chopped

6 slices Parma ham, torn into strips

50g (2oz) rocket

a little extra virgin olive oil to drizzle

salt and ground black pepper

1 Preheat the oven to 200°C (180°C fan oven) mark 6 and lightly flour two large baking sheets. Mix up the pizza base according to the pack instructions. Divide the dough into two and knead each ball on a lightly floured surface for about 5 minutes, then roll them out to make two 23cm (9in) rounds. Put each on to the prepared baking sheet.

2 Divide the tomato sauce between the pizza bases and spread it over, leaving a small border around each edge. Scatter over the mozzarella pieces, then scatter with ham. Season well with salt and pepper.

3 Cook the pizzas for 15–18 minutes until golden. Slide on to a wooden board, top with rocket leaves and drizzle with olive oil. Cut in half to serve.

Cook's Tip

If you're short of time, buy two ready-made pizza bases.

EASY		NUTRITIONAL INFORMATION	Serves
Preparation Time 10 minutes	**Cooking Time** 15–18 minutes	**Per Serving** 508 calories, 19.1g fat (of which 10.5g saturates), 64.2g carbohydrate, 1.9g salt	**4**

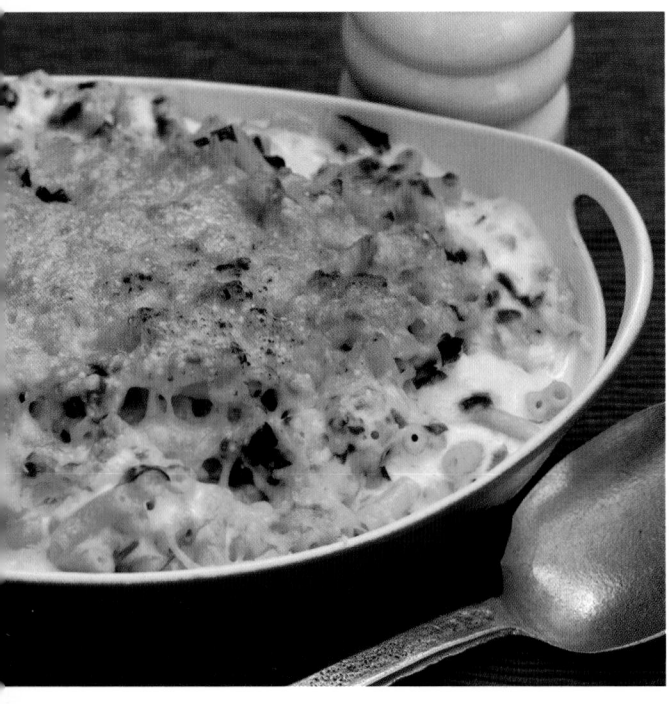

Fast Macaroni Cheese

500g (1lb 2oz) macaroni
500ml (18fl oz) crème fraîche
200g (7oz) freshly grated Parmesan
2 tbsp ready-made English or Dijon mustard
5 tbsp freshly chopped flat-leafed parsley
ground black pepper
green salad to serve

1 Bring a large pan of salted water to the boil and cook the macaroni according to the pack instructions. Drain and keep to one side.

2 Preheat the grill to high. Put the crème fraîche into a pan and heat gently. Stir in 175g (6oz) Parmesan, the mustard and parsley and season well with black pepper. Stir the pasta through the sauce, spoon into bowls and sprinkle with the remaining cheese. Grill until golden and serve immediately with salad.

Serves	EASY		NUTRITIONAL INFORMATION	
4	Preparation Time 5 minutes	Cooking Time 15 minutes	Per Serving 1137 calories, 69.2g fat (of which 44.4g saturates), 96.4g carbohydrate, 2g salt	Vegetarian

Mushroom Soufflé Omelette

50g (2oz) small chestnut mushrooms, sliced

3 tbsp crème fraîche

2 medium eggs, separated

15g (½oz) butter

5 fresh chives, roughly chopped

salt and ground black pepper

mixed salad to serve

1 Heat a non-stick frying pan, add the mushrooms and cook, stirring, for 3 minutes to brown slightly, then stir in the crème fraîche and turn off the heat.

2 Lightly beat the egg yolks in a bowl, add 2 tbsp cold water and season with salt and pepper.

3 Put the egg whites into a clean, grease-free bowl and whisk until stiff but not dry, then gently fold into the egg yolks with a large metal spoon. Do not overmix. Heat an 18cm (7in) non-stick frying pan over a medium heat. Add the butter, then the egg mixture, tilting the pan to cover the base. Cook for 3 minutes or until the underside is golden brown.

4 Meanwhile, preheat the grill. Gently reheat the mushrooms and add the chives. Slide the omelette pan under the grill (wrap a wooden handle in foil) for 1 minute or until the surface is just firm and puffy. Tip the mushroom mixture on top. Run a spatula underneath the omelette to loosen it, then carefully fold it and turn out on to a plate. Serve with salad.

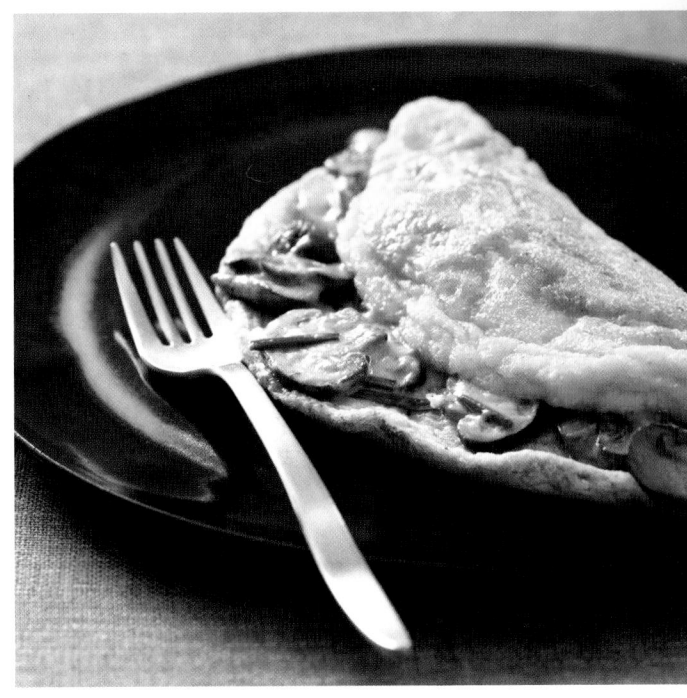

EASY		NUTRITIONAL INFORMATION		Serves
Preparation Time 5 minutes	**Cooking Time** 7–10 minutes	**Per Serving** 440 calories, 42g fat (of which 23g saturates), 2g carbohydrate, 0.6g salt	Vegetarian • Gluten free	**1**

Cook's Tip

Choose bags or bunches of fresh basil rather than using the leaves of plants sold in pots, as the leaves of herbs in packs or bunches are larger and have a stronger, more peppery flavour.

Aubergine Parmigiana

2 large aubergines, thinly sliced lengthways

2 tbsp olive oil, plus extra to brush

3 fat garlic cloves, thinly sliced

2 x 200ml cartons fresh napoletana sauce

4 ready-roasted red peppers, roughly chopped

20g (³/₄oz) fresh basil, roughly chopped (see Cook's Tip)

150g (5oz) Taleggio or Fontina cheese, coarsely grated

50g (2oz) Parmesan, coarsely grated

salt and ground black pepper

ciabatta to serve

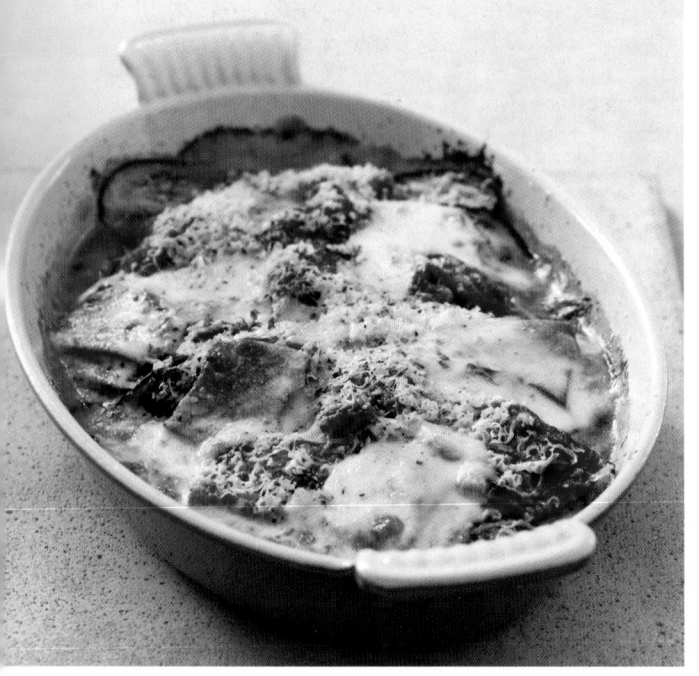

1 Preheat the oven to 200°C (180°C fan oven) mark 6 and preheat the grill to high. Put the aubergines on an oiled baking sheet. Brush with olive oil, scatter over the garlic and season with salt and pepper. Grill for 5–6 minutes until golden.

2 Spread a little napoletana sauce over the base of an oiled ovenproof dish, then cover with a layer of aubergine and peppers, packing the layers together as tightly as you can. Sprinkle a little basil and some of each cheese over the top. Repeat the layers, finishing with a layer of cheese. Season with pepper. Cook in the oven for 20 minutes or until golden. Serve hot with ciabatta.

Serves 4	EASY		NUTRITIONAL INFORMATION	
	Preparation Time 5 minutes	**Cooking Time** 25 minutes	**Per Serving** 370 calories, 25g fat (of which 11g saturates), 17g carbohydrate, 2.1g salt	Vegetarian • Gluten free

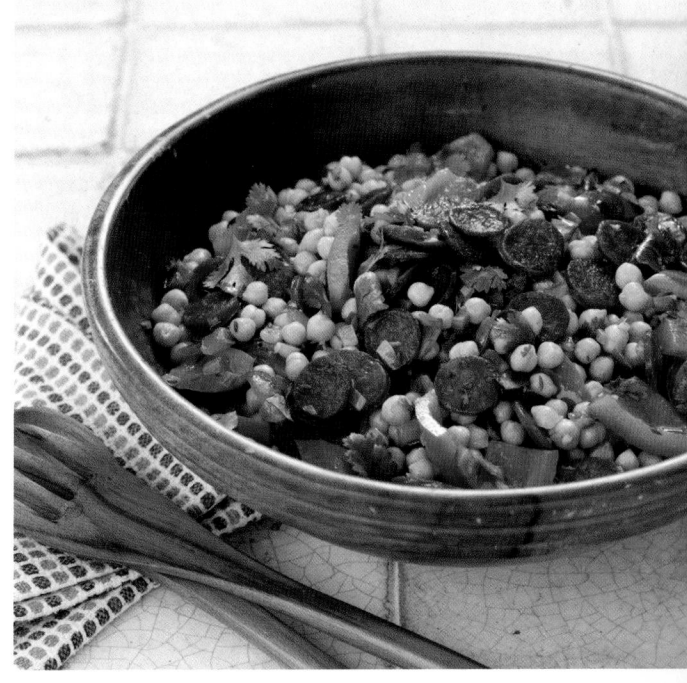

Warm Spicy Chorizo and Chickpea Salad

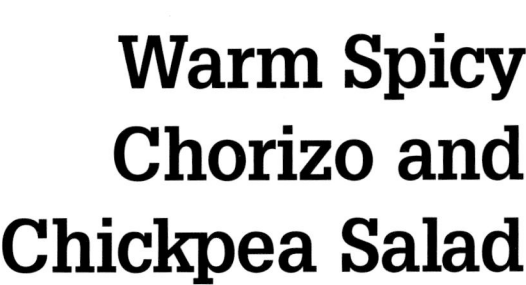

5 tbsp olive oil

200g (7oz) chorizo or spicy sausage, thinly sliced

225g (8oz) red onion, chopped

1 large red pepper, seeded and roughly chopped

3 garlic cloves, finely chopped

1 tsp cumin seeds

2 x 400g cans chickpeas, drained and rinsed

2 tbsp freshly chopped coriander

juice of 1 lemon

salt and ground black pepper

1 Heat 1 tbsp olive oil in a non-stick frying pan and cook the chorizo or spicy sausage over a medium heat for 1–2 minutes until lightly browned. Remove the chorizo with a slotted spoon and put to one side. Fry the onion in the chorizo oil for 8–10 minutes or until browned.

2 Add the red pepper, garlic, cumin and chickpeas to the onion and cook for a further 5 minutes, stirring frequently to prevent sticking. Remove the pan from the heat and add the chorizo.

3 Add the coriander, lemon juice and remaining olive oil. Season well and serve immediately.

EASY		NUTRITIONAL INFORMATION		Serves
Preparation Time 15 minutes	**Cooking Time** about 15 minutes	**Per Serving** 365 calories, 23.5g fat (of which 5.7g saturates), 27g carbohydrate, 1.3g salt	Dairy free	**6**

Creamy Parma Ham and Artichoke Tagliatelle

500g (1lb 2oz) tagliatelle

500ml (18fl oz) crème fraîche

280g jar roasted artichoke hearts, drained and each cut in half

80g pack Parma ham (6 slices), torn into strips

2 tbsp freshly chopped sage leaves, plus extra to garnish

40g (1½oz) Parmesan shavings

salt and ground black pepper

1 Bring a large pan of water to the boil. Add the pasta, cover and bring back to the boil, then remove the lid and simmer according to the pack instructions.

2 Drain well, reserving a little of the cooking water, then put the pasta back into the pan.

3 Add the crème fraîche to the pan with the artichoke hearts, Parma ham and sage, then stir everything together, thinning the mixture with a ladleful of cooking water. Season well.

4 Spoon into warmed bowls, top with Parmesan shavings and garnish each portion with a sage leaf.

Cook's Tip

Parmesan shavings can be bought in supermarkets. To make your own, use a vegetable peeler to pare off shavings from a block of Parmesan.

Serves	EASY		NUTRITIONAL INFORMATION
4	**Preparation Time** 5 minutes	**Cooking Time** 12 minutes	**Per Serving** 972 calories, 56.3g fat (of which 36.4g saturates), 96.5g carbohydrate, 1.1g salt [to come]

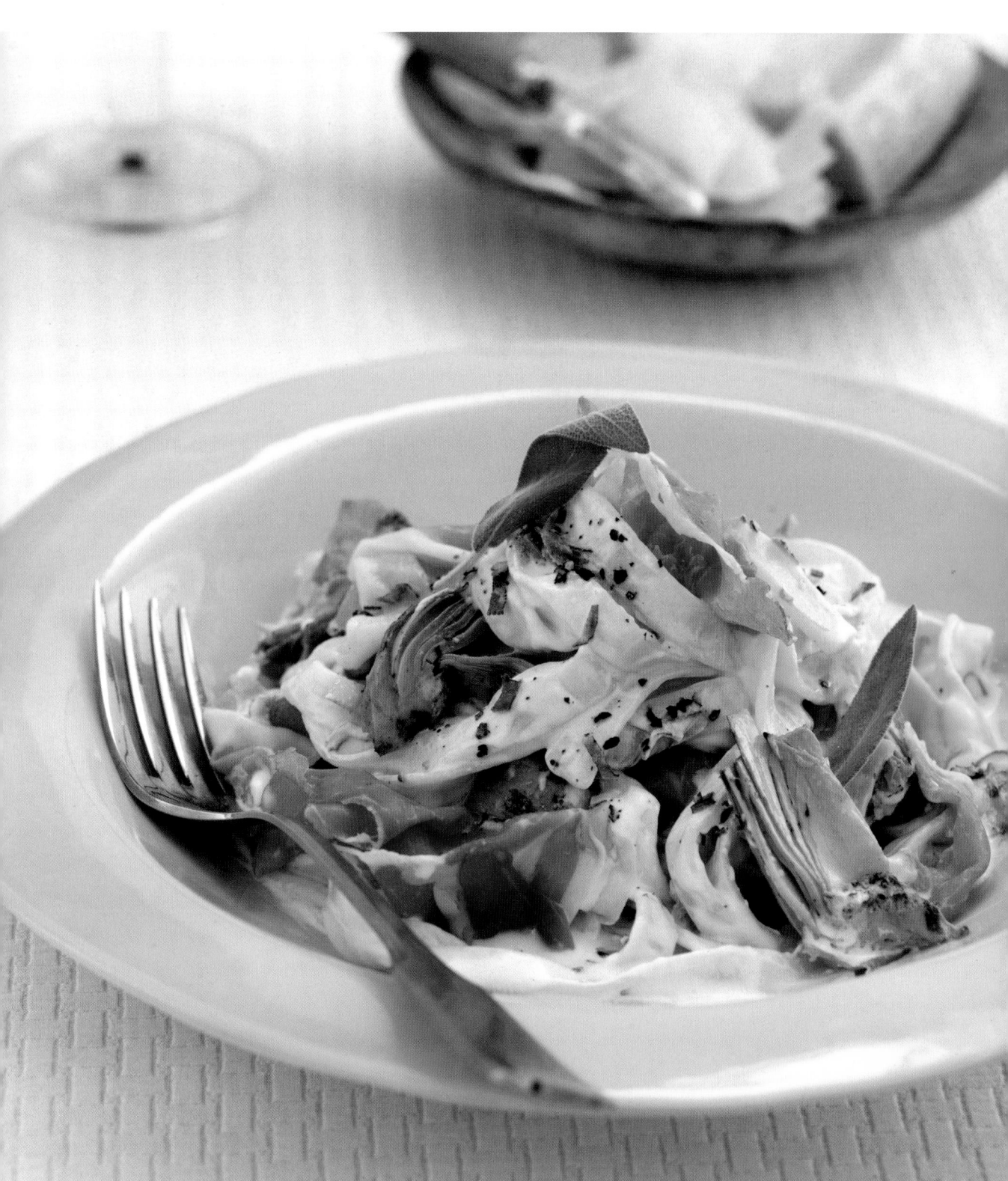

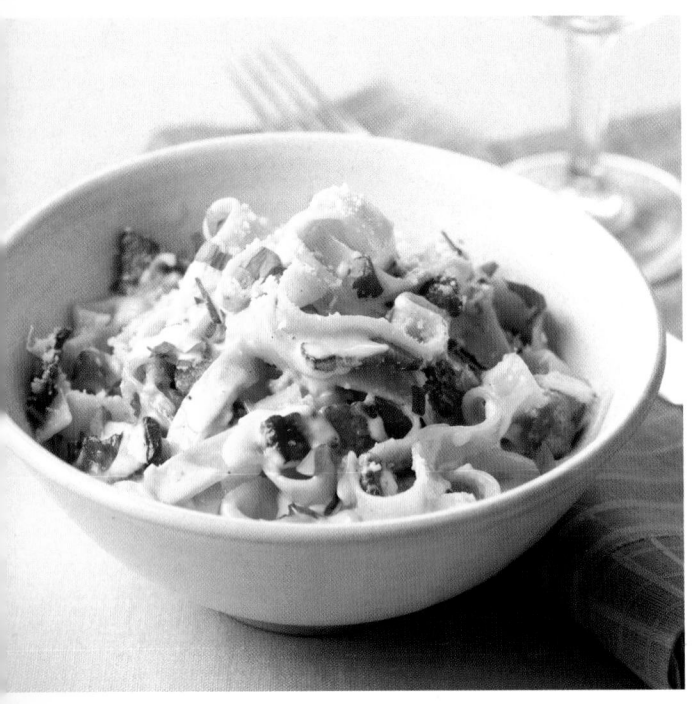

Quick and Easy Carbonara

350g (12oz) tagliatelle
150g (5oz) smoked bacon, chopped
1 tbsp olive oil
2 large egg yolks
150ml (¼ pint) double cream
50g (2oz) freshly grated Parmesan
2 tbsp freshly chopped parsley

1 Bring a large pan of water to the boil. Add the pasta, bring back to the boil and cook for 4 minutes or according to the pack instructions.

2 Meanwhile, fry the bacon in the olive oil for 4–5 minutes. Add to the drained pasta and keep hot.

3 Put the egg yolks in a bowl and add the cream. Whisk together. Add to the pasta with the Parmesan and parsley. Toss well and serve.

Serves 4	EASY		NUTRITIONAL INFORMATION
	Preparation Time 5 minutes	**Cooking Time** 10 minutes	**Per Serving** 688 calories, 39g fat (of which 19g saturates), 65g carbohydrate, 1.6g salt

Cook's Tip

Adding the reserved pasta cooking water stops the pasta absorbing too much of the crème fraîche.

500g (1lb 2oz) dried linguine pasta

a little olive oil

1 fat garlic clove, crushed

200ml (7fl oz) half-fat crème fraîche

225g (8oz) hot-smoked salmon, flaked

200g (7oz) peas

two handfuls of basil, roughly torn, to garnish

salt and ground black pepper

Simple Salmon Pasta

1 Cook the pasta in a large pan of boiling salted water according to the pack instructions, then drain, reserving a couple of tablespoons of the cooking water.

2 Meanwhile, heat the olive oil in a large pan, add the garlic and fry gently until golden. Add the crème fraîche, the flaked salmon and peas and stir in. Cook for 1–2 minutes until warmed through, then add the reserved water from the pasta.

3 Toss the pasta into the sauce, season with salt and pepper and serve garnished with the torn basil.

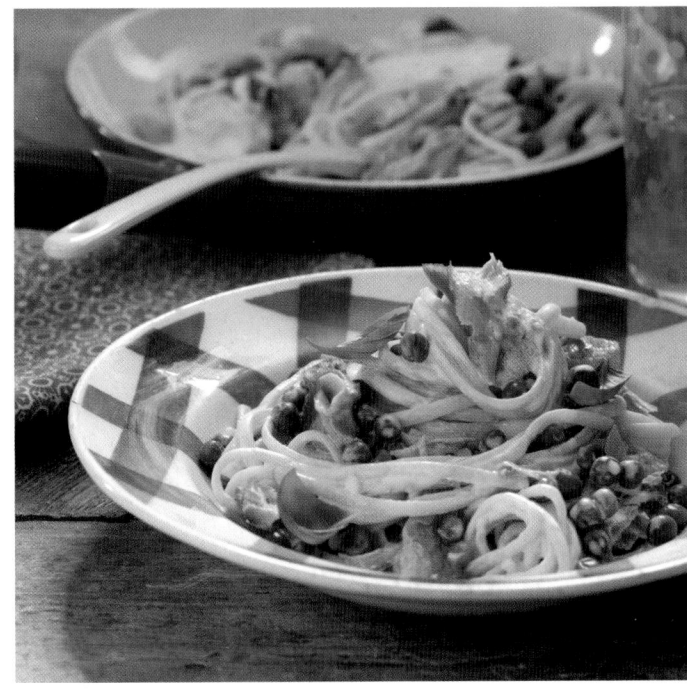

EASY		NUTRITIONAL INFORMATION	Serves
Preparation Time 2 minutes	**Cooking Time** 8 minutes	**Per Serving** 630 calories, 13g fat (of which 5.9g saturates), 100.5g carbohydrate, 2.7g salt	**4**

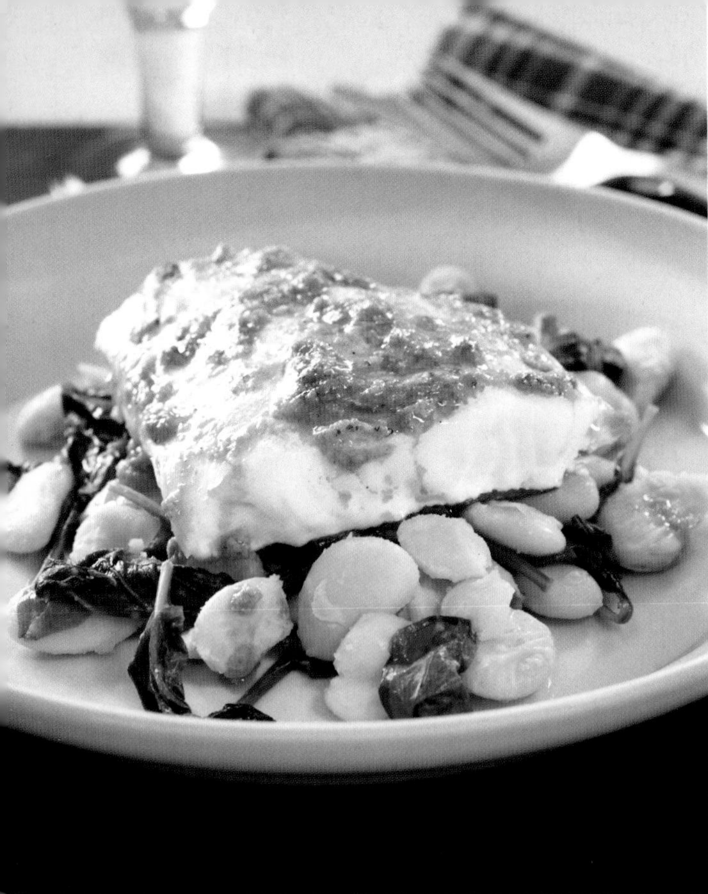

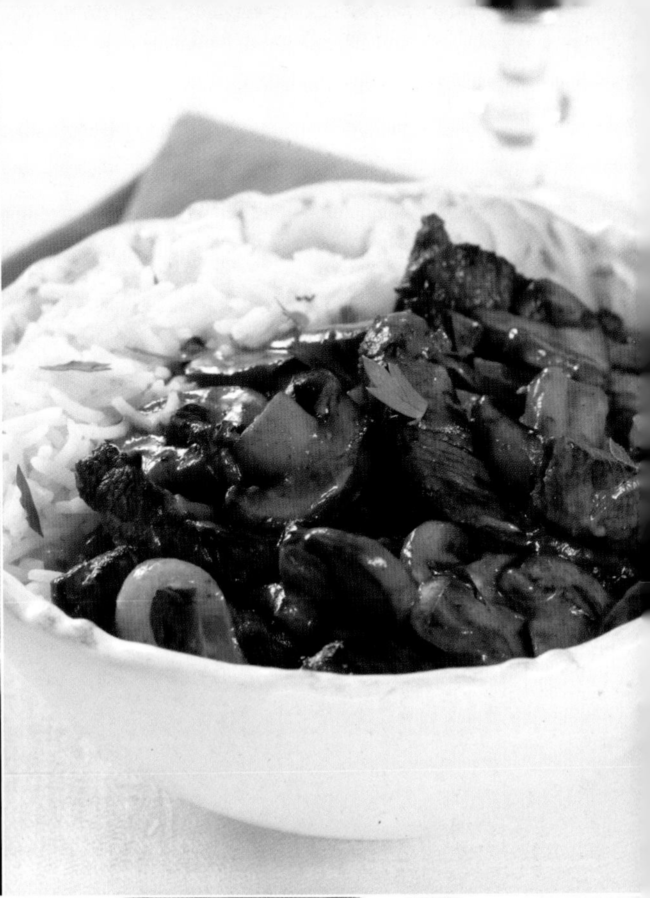

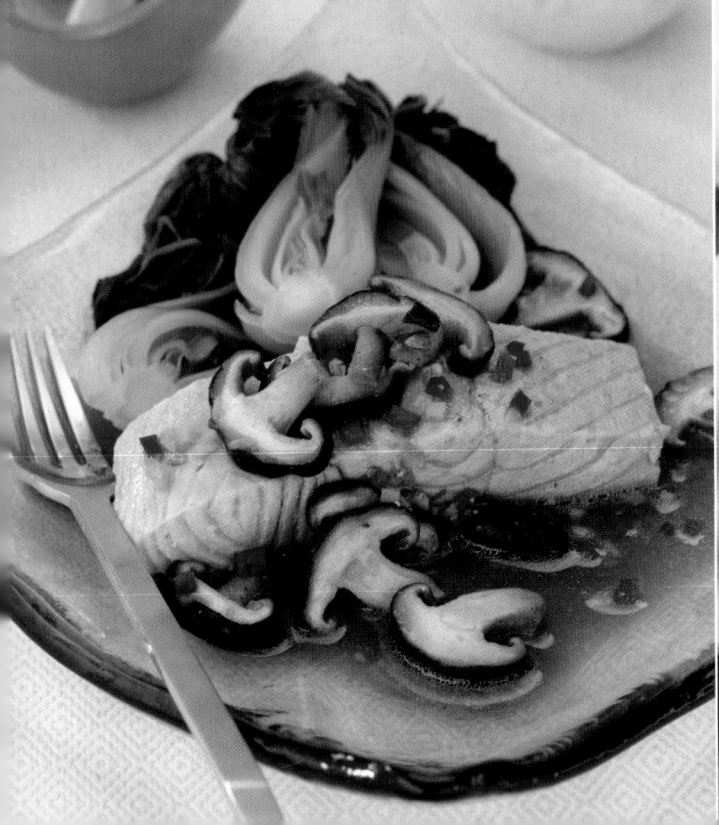
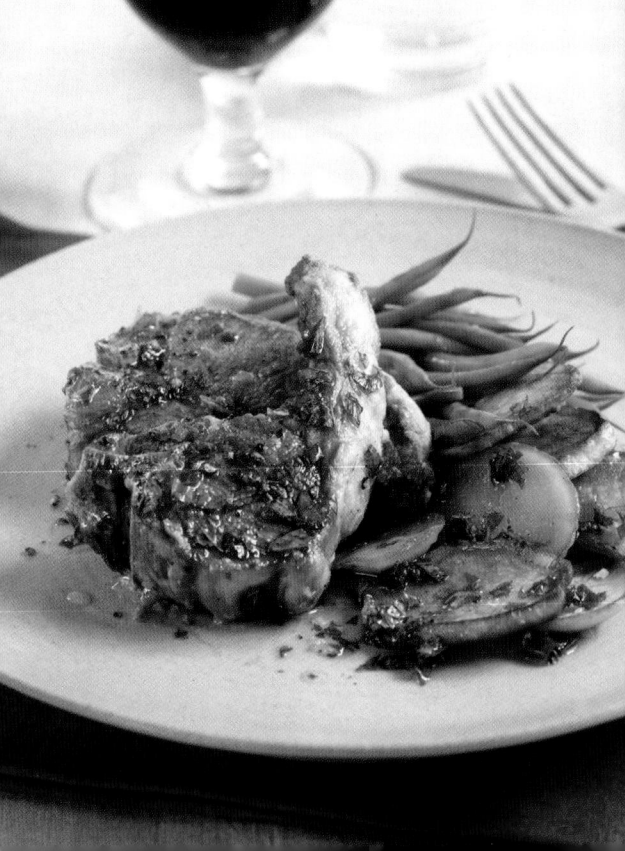

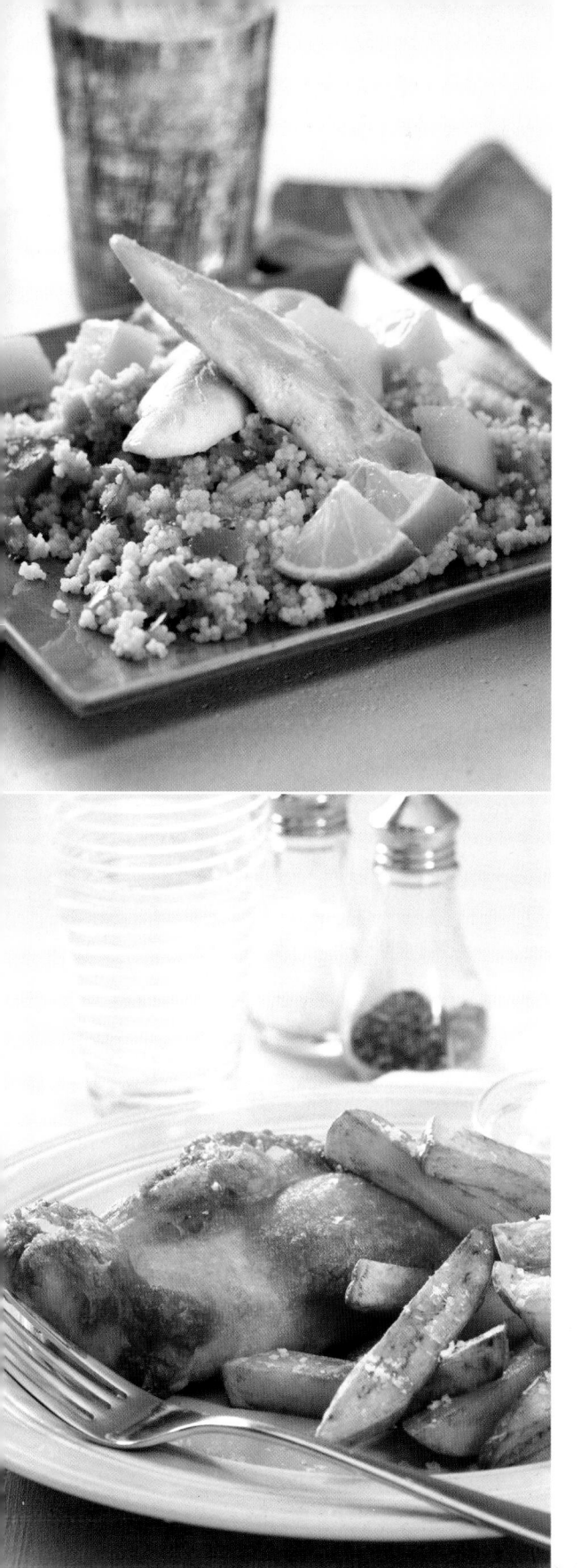

3

Meat and Fish in Minutes

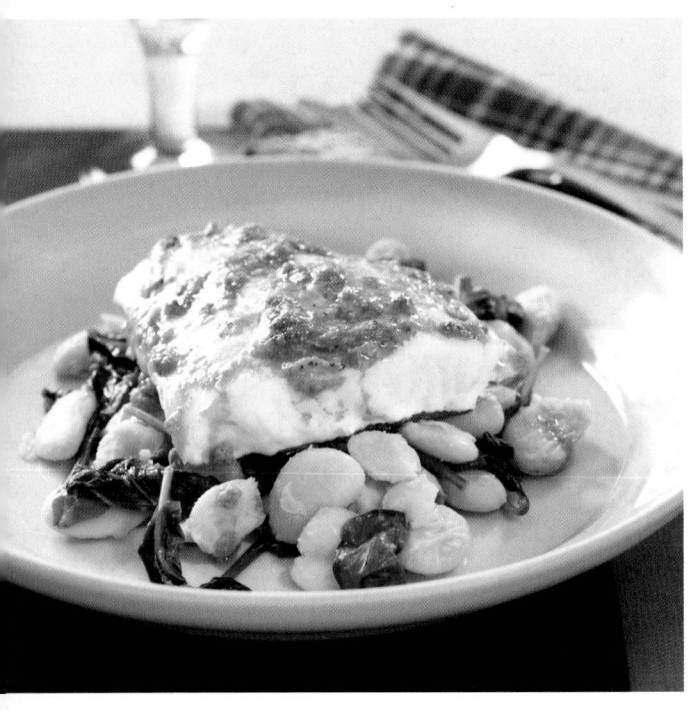

Pesto Cod with Butter Beans

4 cod fillets, about 150g (5oz) each

4 tbsp red pepper pesto

2 tbsp olive oil

2 x 400g cans butter beans, drained and rinsed

2 garlic cloves, crushed

225g (8oz) fresh spinach

a squeeze of lemon juice

salt and ground black pepper

1 Preheat the grill to medium. Spread each cod fillet evenly with 1 tbsp red pesto and grill for 10–15 minutes until the flesh is opaque and just cooked.

2 Meanwhile, heat the olive oil in a pan and add the butter beans and garlic. Cook for 10 minutes, stirring occasionally and mashing the beans lightly as they warm through. Season with salt and pepper.

3 About 2–3 minutes before serving, add the spinach to the pan and allow it to wilt. Spoon the butter beans on to four warmed plates and top with the cod and any juices from grilling. Squeeze a little lemon juice over each piece of fish and serve immediately.

Serves 4	EASY		NUTRITIONAL INFORMATION	
	Preparation Time 5 minutes	**Cooking Time** 15 minutes	**Per Serving** 403 calories, 16g fat (of which 3g saturates), 24g carbohydrate, 2.5g salt	Gluten free

Quick Fish and Chips

4 litres (7 pints) sunflower oil for deep-frying

125g (4oz) self-raising flour

¼ tsp baking powder

¼ tsp salt

1 medium egg

150ml (¼ pint) sparkling mineral water

2 hake fillets, about 125g (4oz) each

450g (1lb) Desirée potatoes, cut into 1cm (½in) chips

salt, vinegar and garlic mayonnaise to serve

1 Heat the oil in a deep-fryer to 190°C (test by frying a small cube of bread; it should brown in 20 seconds).

2 Whiz the flour, baking powder, salt, egg and water in a food processor until combined into a batter. Remove the blade from the food processor. Alternatively, put the ingredients in a bowl and beat everything together until smooth. Drop one of the fish fillets into the batter to coat it.

3 Put half the chips in the deep-fryer, then add the battered fish. Fry for 6 minutes or until just cooked, then remove and drain well on kitchen paper. Keep warm if not serving immediately.

4 Drop the remaining fillet into the batter to coat, then repeat step 3 with the remaining chips. Serve with salt, vinegar and garlic mayonnaise.

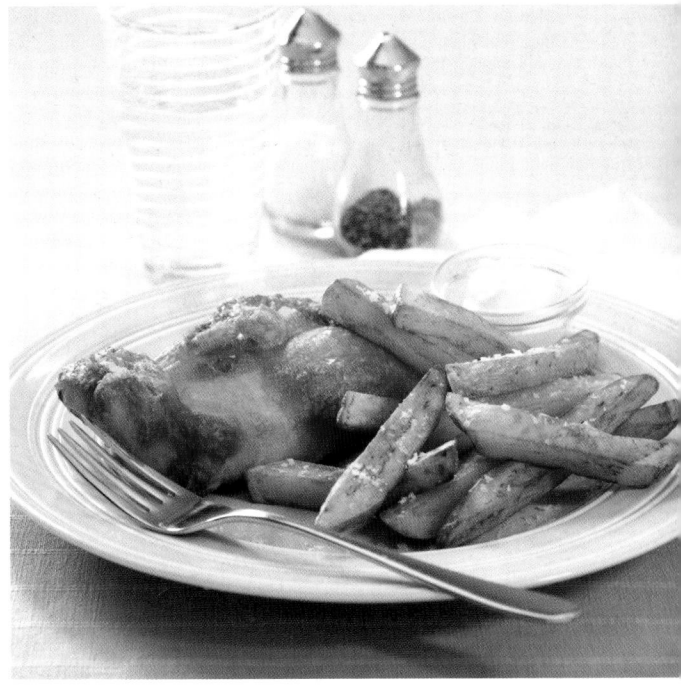

EASY		NUTRITIONAL INFORMATION		Serves
Preparation Time 15 minutes	**Cooking Time** 12 minutes	**Per Serving** 1186 calories, 79g fat (of which 18g saturates), 73g carbohydrate, 3.2g salt	Dairy free	**2**

Quick Steak Supper

2 sirloin steaks

3 tsp olive oil

4 large mushrooms, sliced

1 red onion, sliced

1 tbsp Dijon mustard

25g (1oz) butter

2 ciabattas, halved lengthways, then quartered, to make eight pieces

salt and ground black pepper

green salad to serve

1 Heat a griddle or large frying pan until very hot. Rub the steaks with 1 tsp olive oil, season with salt and pepper and fry for about 2 minutes on each side if you like your steak rare, or 4 minutes each side for medium. Remove from the pan and leave to 'rest'.

2 Heat the remaining olive oil in the pan. Add the mushrooms and red onion. Fry, stirring, for 5 minutes or until softened. Stir in the Dijon mustard and butter, and take off the heat.

3 Toast the ciabatta pieces on both sides. Thinly slice the steaks and divide among four pieces of ciabatta. Top with the mushrooms, onion and remaining ciabatta and serve with a green salad.

Try Something Different

Instead of ciabatta, serve the steak with tagliatelle or other pasta.

Serves	EASY		NUTRITIONAL INFORMATION
4	**Preparation Time** 10 minutes	**Cooking Time** 10 minutes	**Per Serving** 452 calories, 17g fat (of which 6g saturates), 44g carbohydrate, 1.6g salt

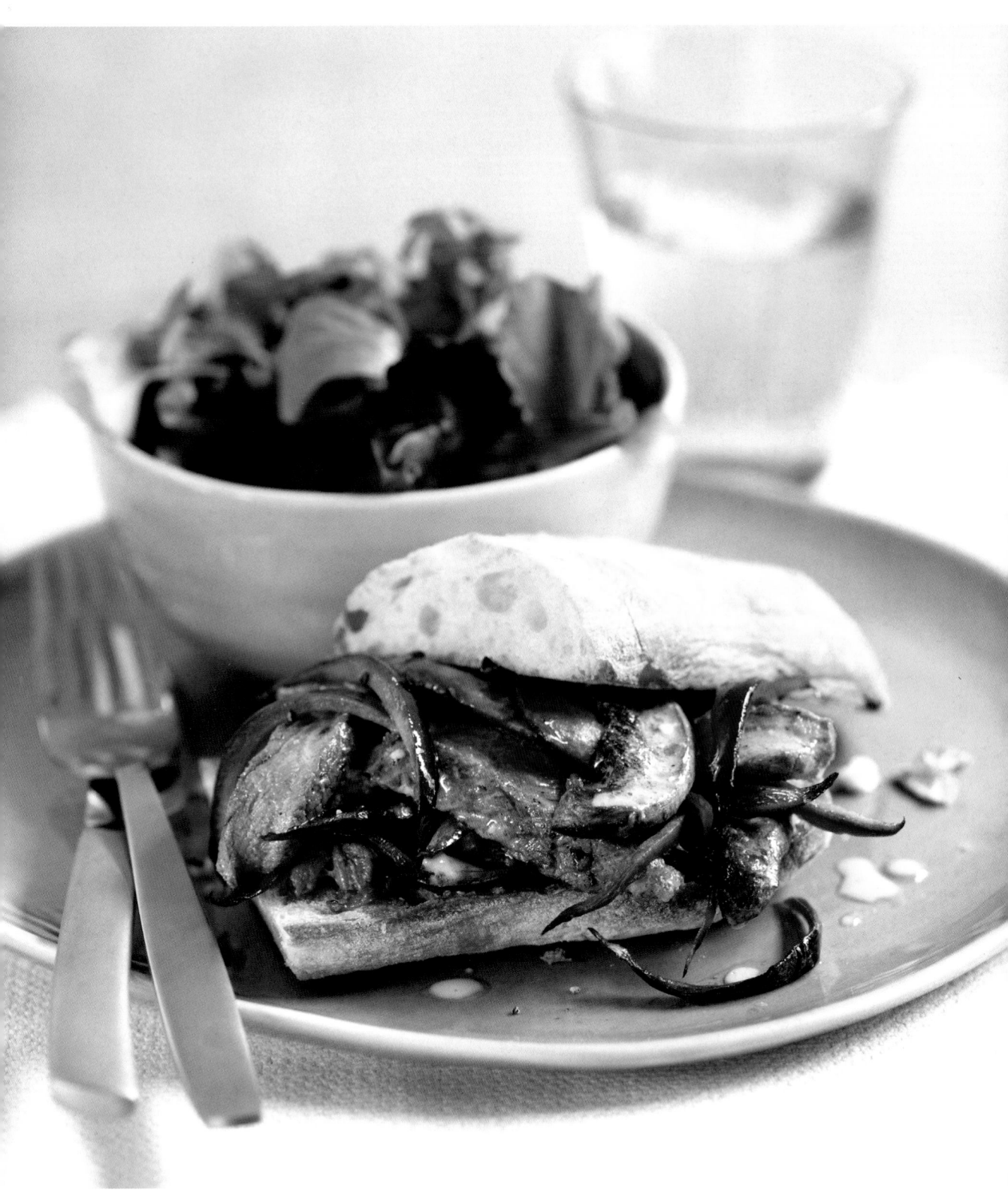

Calf's Liver with Fried Sage and Balsamic Vinegar

15g (½oz) butter plus a little olive oil for frying

12 sage leaves

4 thin slices calf's liver

1–2 tbsp balsamic vinegar

rice, with freshly chopped parsley stirred through, or grilled polenta to serve

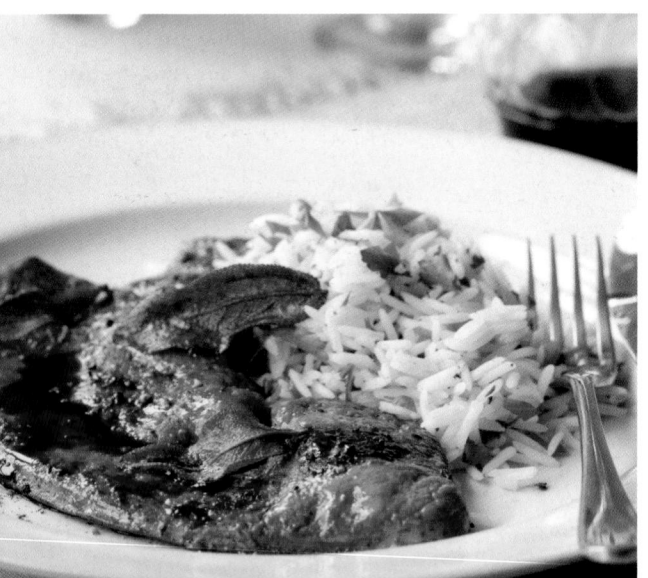

1 Melt the butter with a little olive oil in a heavy-based frying pan and when hot add the sage leaves. Cook briefly for 1 minute or so until crisp. Remove, put in a single layer in a shallow dish and keep warm in the oven.

2 Add a little extra oil to the pan, put in two slices of calf's liver and cook quickly for 30 seconds on each side over a high heat. Remove and put on a plate while you quickly cook the remaining two slices.

3 Put all four slices back in the pan, splash the balsamic vinegar over the top and cook for another minute or so. Top with the crispy sage leaves. Serve immediately with rice or polenta.

Serves 4	EASY		NUTRITIONAL INFORMATION	
	Preparation Time 5 minutes	**Cooking Time** 5 minutes	**Per Serving** 88 calories, 6g fat (of which 3g saturates), trace carbohydrate, 0.1g salt	Gluten free • Dairy free

Try Something Different

Use mango instead of the papaya. Make sure it's ripe before you buy it – give it a gentle squeeze to check.
Try the spice rub and fruity relish with pork chops, or with meaty fish such as salmon or tuna steaks.

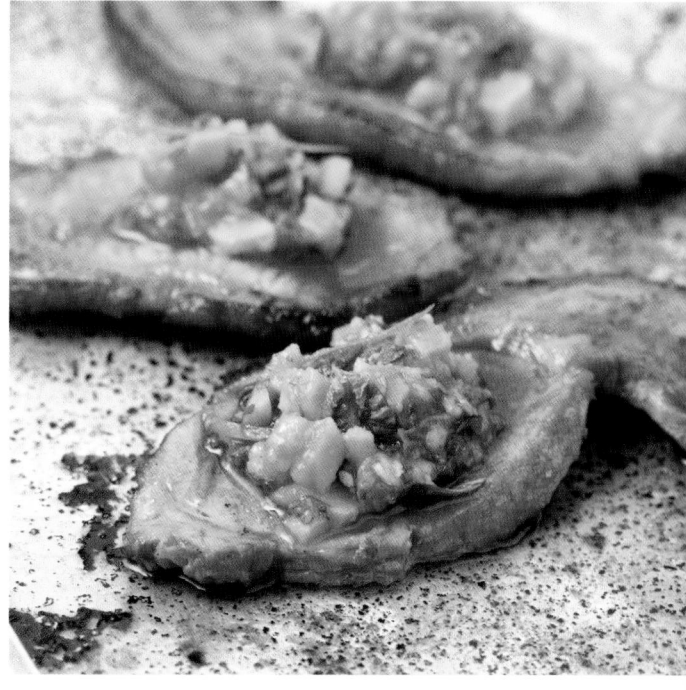

Cumin-spiced Gammon

a large pinch of ground cumin
a large pinch of paprika
2 tbsp olive oil
2 tsp light muscovado sugar
8 thin smoked gammon steaks, about 125g (4oz) each
2 large ripe papayas
grated zest and juice of 2 limes
1/2 red chilli, seeded and finely chopped (see page 33)
20g (3/4oz) fresh mint, finely chopped
green vegetables to serve

1 Preheat the grill to medium-high. In a small bowl, mix together the cumin, paprika, olive oil and half the sugar. Put the gammon on to a non-stick baking sheet, then brush the spiced oil over each side.

2 Grill the gammon for about 5 minutes on each side, basting once or twice with the juices.

3 Meanwhile, cut each papaya in half, then deseed and peel. Roughly chop half the flesh and put into a bowl. Purée the remaining fruit with the lime juice. Add to the bowl with the lime zest, chilli, mint and remaining sugar. Spoon the mixture on top of the gammon and serve immediately with vegetables.

EASY		NUTRITIONAL INFORMATION		Serves
Preparation Time 10 minutes	**Cooking Time** 10 minutes	**Per Serving** 492 calories, 18g fat (of which 5g saturates), 3g carbohydrate, 13.8g salt	Gluten free • Dairy free	**4**

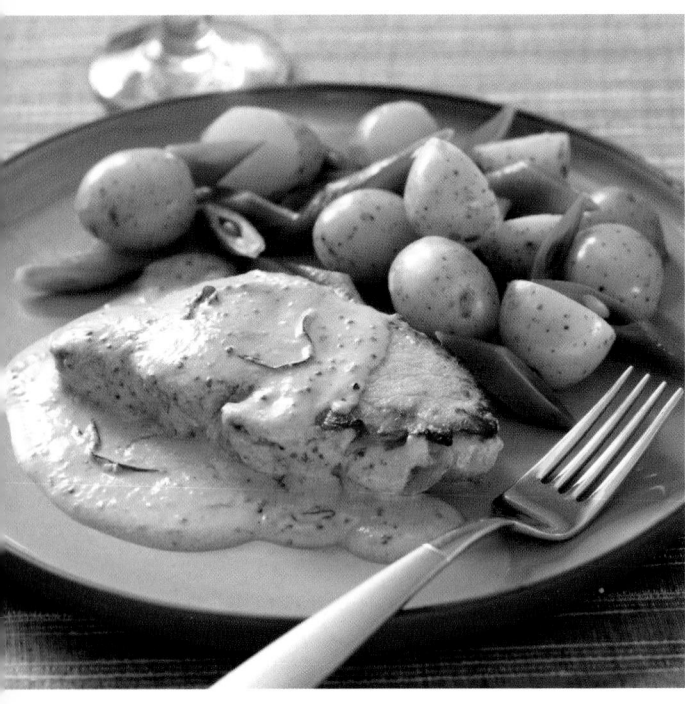

Flash-in-the-pan Pork

700g (1½lb) new potatoes, scrubbed, halved if large

175g (6oz) runner beans, sliced

4 pork escalopes, about 150g (5oz) each

1 tbsp sunflower or olive oil

150ml (¼ pint) hot chicken stock

150ml (¼ pint) apple cider

2 tbsp wholegrain mustard

150g (5oz) Greek yogurt

4 fresh tarragon stems, leaves only

a squeeze of lemon juice

salt and ground black pepper

1 Cook the new potatoes in a large pan of boiling salted water for 10 minutes. Add the beans and cook for a further 5 minutes or until tender. Drain.

2 Meanwhile, season the escalopes with salt and pepper, then heat the oil in a large non-stick frying pan over a medium heat. Cook the pork for 3 minutes on each side or until browned. Remove from the pan and keep warm. Add the stock, cider and mustard to the pan and increase the heat to reduce the liquid by half.

3 Just before serving, reduce the heat and add the yogurt, tarragon leaves and lemon juice. Put the pork back into the pan to coat with the sauce and warm through. Serve with the potatoes and beans.

Serves 4	EASY		NUTRITIONAL INFORMATION	
	Preparation Time 5 minutes	**Cooking Time** 15 minutes	**Per Serving** 346 calories, 12g fat (of which 4g saturates), 32g carbohydrate, 0.6g salt	Gluten free

Waste Not

Use leftover roast chicken.

125g (4oz) couscous

1 ripe mango, peeled, stoned and cut into
2.5cm (1in) chunks

1 tbsp lemon or lime juice

125g tub fresh tomato salsa

3 tbsp mango chutney

3 tbsp orange juice

2 tbsp freshly chopped coriander, plus extra to garnish

200g (7oz) chargrilled chicken fillets, sliced

salt and ground black pepper

lime wedges to garnish

Chicken with Spicy Couscous

1 Put the couscous in a large bowl and pour 300ml
(½ pint) boiling water over. Season well with salt and
pepper, then leave to stand for 15 minutes.

2 Put the mango chunks on a plate and sprinkle with
the lemon or lime juice.

3 In a small bowl, mix together the tomato salsa,
mango chutney, orange juice and coriander.

4 Drain the couscous if necessary, fluff the grains with
a fork, then stir in the salsa mixture and check the
seasoning. Turn out on to a large serving dish and
arrange the chicken and mango on top.

5 Just before serving garnish with lime wedges.

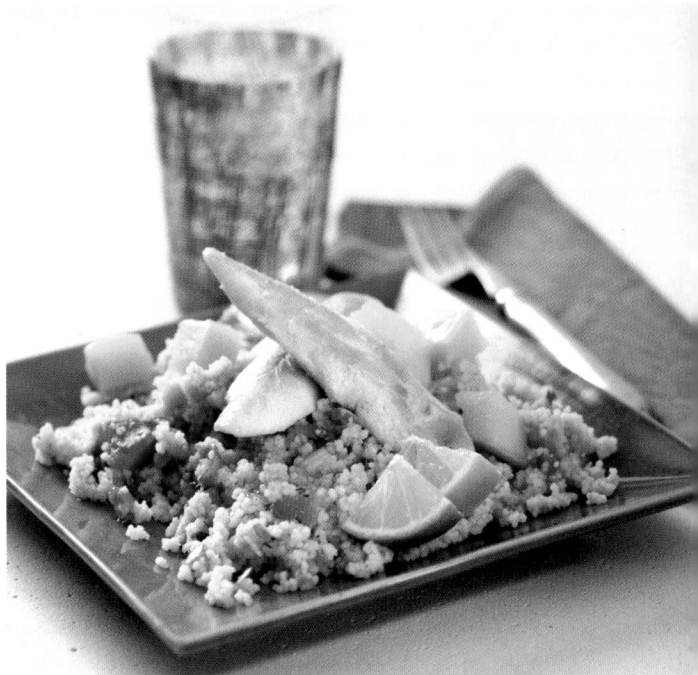

EASY		NUTRITIONAL INFORMATION	Serves
Preparation Time 15 minutes	**Cooking Time** 15 minutes, plus 15 minutes soaking	**Per Serving** 187 calories, 4g fat (of which 1g saturates), 24g carbohydrate, 0.1g salt	**4**

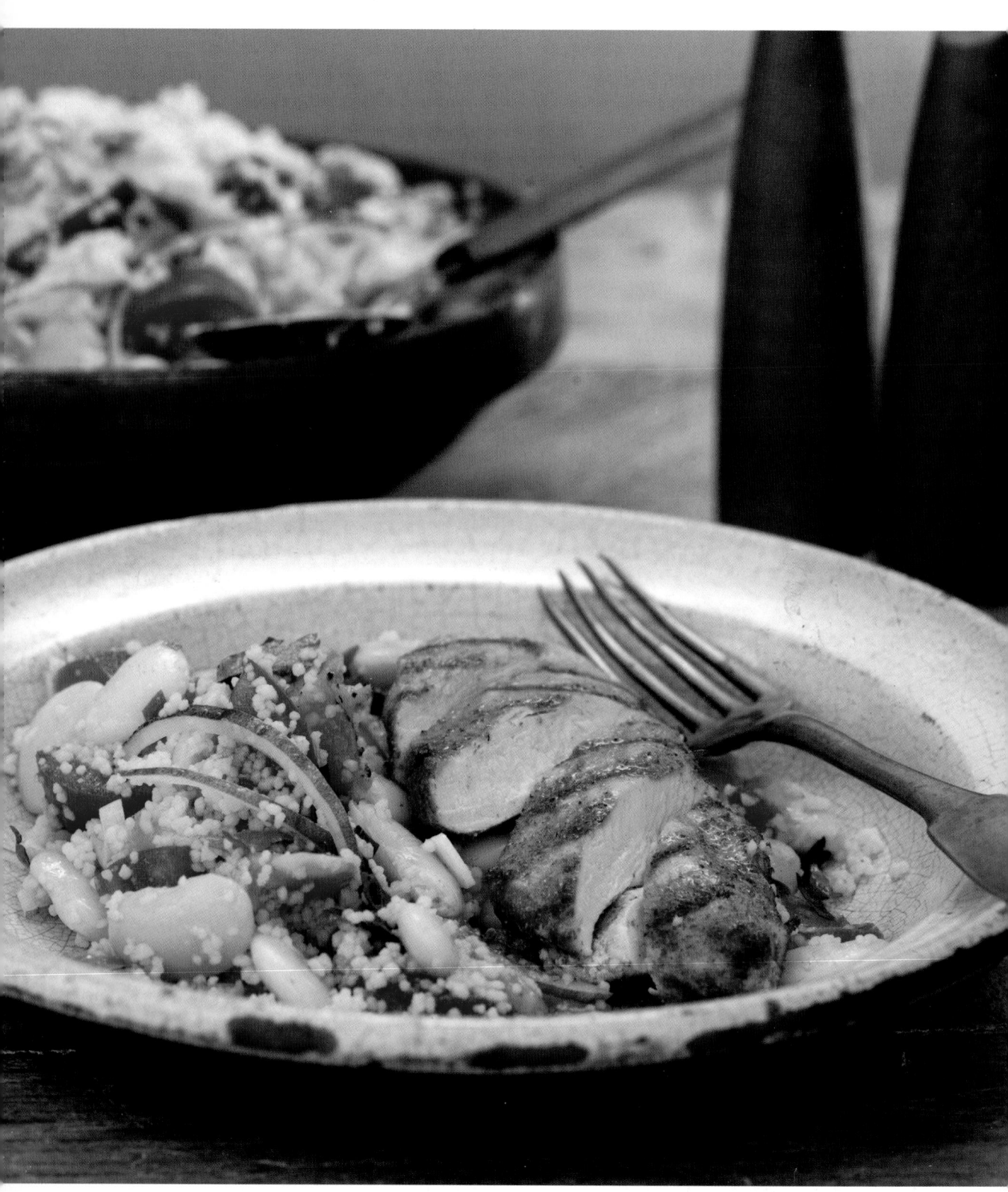

Spiced Chicken with Garlic Butter Beans

4 skinless chicken breasts, about 100g (3½oz) each

1 tbsp olive oil

1 tsp ground coriander

1 tsp ground cumin

100g (3½oz) couscous

3 tbsp extra virgin olive oil

1 garlic clove, sliced

2 x 400g cans butter beans, drained and rinsed

juice of 1 lemon

1 small red onion, thinly sliced

50g (2oz) marinated roasted peppers, drained

2 medium tomatoes, seeded and chopped

1 tbsp freshly chopped coriander

1 tbsp freshly chopped flat-leafed parsley

salt and ground black pepper

1 Put the chicken on a board, cover with clingfilm and flatten lightly with a rolling pin. Put the olive oil into a large bowl with the ground coriander and cumin. Mix together, then add the chicken and turn to coat.

2 Heat a large frying pan and cook the chicken for 5–7 minutes on each side until golden and the juices run clear when pierced with a sharp knife.

3 While the chicken is cooking, put the couscous into a bowl and add 100ml (3½fl oz) boiling water. Cover with clingfilm and set aside.

4 Put the extra virgin olive oil in a small pan with the garlic and butter beans and warm through for 3–4 minutes over a low heat. Stir in the lemon juice and season with salt and pepper.

5 Fluff up the couscous with a fork and tip in the warm butter beans. Add the onion, peppers, tomatoes and herbs and stir together. Slice each chicken breast into four pieces and arrange alongside the bean salad. Serve with a green salad and lemon wedges to squeeze over.

EASY		NUTRITIONAL INFORMATION		Serves
Preparation Time 10 minutes	**Cooking Time** 15 minutes	**Per Serving** 443 calories, 16.1g fat (of which 2.9g saturates), 42.1g carbohydrate, 2g salt	Dairy free	**4**

Cook's Tip

Smoked fish is quite salty so always taste the sauce before seasoning with any extra salt.

Simple Smoked Haddock

25g (1oz) unsalted butter

1 tbsp olive oil

1 garlic clove, thinly sliced

4 thick smoked haddock or cod fillets, about 175g (6oz) each

a small handful of freshly chopped parsley (optional)

finely grated zest of 1 small lemon, plus lemon wedges to serve (optional)

romanesco, cauliflower or broccoli to serve

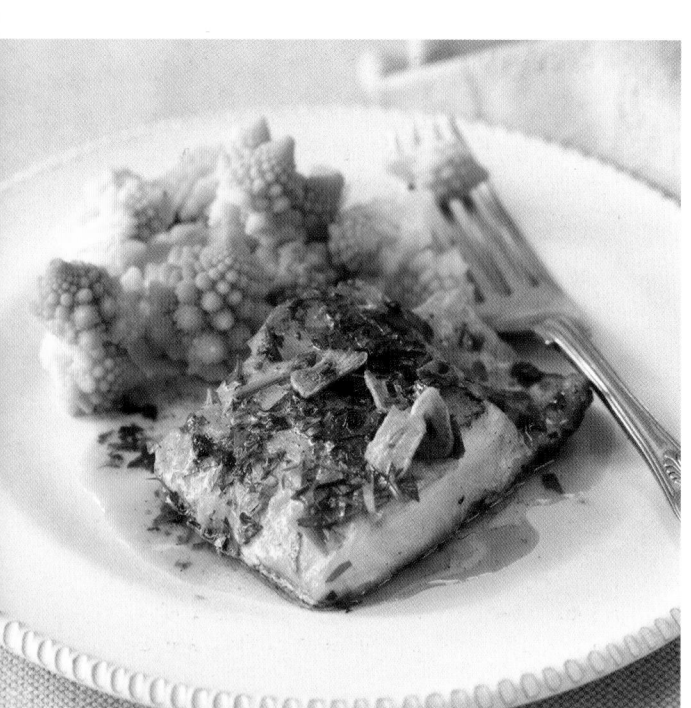

1 Heat the butter, olive oil and garlic in a large non-stick pan until the mixture starts to foam and sizzle. Put the fish into the pan, skin side down, and fry over a high heat for 10 minutes – this will give a golden crust underneath the fish.

2 Turn the fish over and scatter the parsley, if using, and lemon zest over it, then fry for a further 30 seconds. Put each cooked fillet on to a plate and spoon some of the buttery juices over. Serve with lemon wedges, if using, and steamed romanesco, cauliflower or broccoli.

Serves 4	EASY		NUTRITIONAL INFORMATION	
	Preparation Time 10 minutes	**Cooking Time** 10 minutes	**Per Serving** 217 calories, 9g fat (of which 4g saturates), 1g carbohydrate, 3.4g salt	Gluten free

Get Ahead

To freeze Complete the recipe, transfer to a freezerproof container, cool, label and freeze for up to three months.
To use Thaw overnight in the fridge. Put in a pan, cover and bring to the boil; reduce the heat to low and simmer until piping hot.

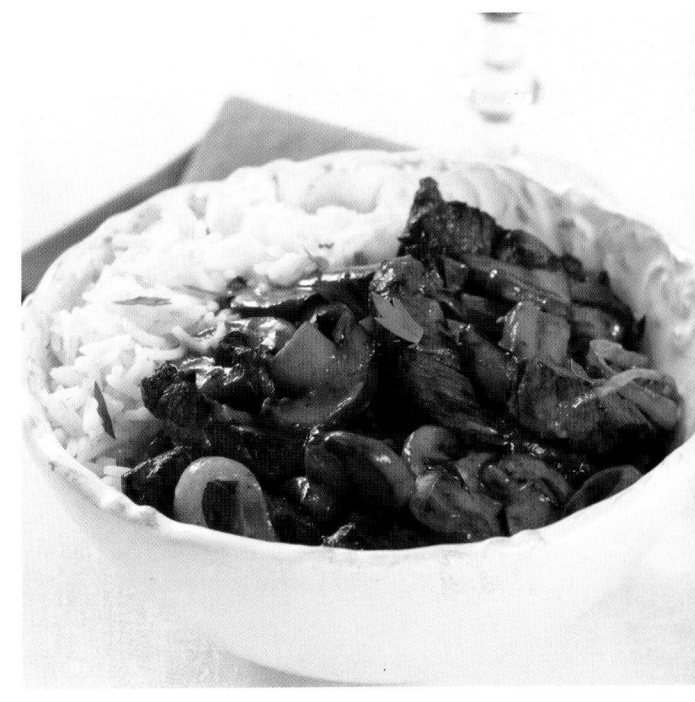

Quick Beef Stroganoff

700g (1½lb) rump or fillet steak, trimmed
50g (2oz) unsalted butter or 4 tbsp olive oil
1 onion, thinly sliced
225g (8oz) brown-cap mushrooms, sliced
3 tbsp brandy
1 tsp French mustard
200ml (7fl oz) crème fraîche
100ml (3½fl oz) double cream
3 tbsp freshly chopped flat-leafed parsley
salt and ground black pepper
rice or noodles to serve

1 Cut the steak into strips about 5mm (¼in) wide and 5cm (2in) long.

2 Heat half the butter or olive oil in a large heavy frying pan over a medium heat. Add the onion and cook gently for 10 minutes or until soft and golden. Remove with a slotted spoon and set aside. Add the mushrooms to the pan and cook, stirring, for 2–3 minutes until golden brown. Remove and set aside.

3 Increase the heat and quickly fry the meat, in two or three batches, for 2–3 minutes, stirring constantly to ensure even browning. Add the brandy and allow it to bubble to reduce.

4 Put the meat, onion and mushrooms back into the pan. Reduce the heat and stir in the mustard, crème fraîche and cream. Heat through, stir in most of the parsley and season with salt and pepper. Serve with rice or noodles, with the remaining parsley scattered over the top.

EASY		NUTRITIONAL INFORMATION		Serves
Preparation Time 10 minutes	**Cooking Time** 20 minutes	**Per Serving** 750 calories, 60g fat (of which 35g saturates), 3g carbohydrate, 0.5g salt	Gluten free	**4**

Italian Sausage Stew

25g (1oz) dried porcini mushrooms

2 tbsp olive oil

1 onion, sliced

2 garlic cloves, chopped

1 small red chilli, seeded and finely chopped (see page 33)

2 fresh rosemary stalks

300g (11oz) whole rustic Italian salami sausages, such as salami Milano, cut into 1cm (½in) slices

400g can chopped tomatoes

200ml (7fl oz) red wine

1 tsp salt

175g (6oz) quick-cook or instant polenta

50g (2oz) butter

50g (2oz) freshly grated Parmesan, plus extra shavings to serve (optional)

75g (3oz) Fontina cheese, cubed

ground black pepper

1 Put the mushrooms in a small bowl, pour over 100ml (3½fl oz) boiling water and soften in the microwave on full power for 3½ minutes, or leave to soak for 20 minutes. Set aside to cool.

2 Heat the olive oil in a large frying pan over a low heat, add the onion, garlic and chilli and cook gently for 5 minutes. Add the leaves from one rosemary stalk to the pan, stirring.

3 Add the salami and fry for 2 minutes on each side or until browned. Drain and chop the soaked mushrooms and add to the pan. Add the tomatoes and wine, then season with pepper. Simmer, uncovered, for 5 minutes.

4 Pour 750ml (1¼ pints) boiling water into a pan and add the salt. Bring back to the boil, pour in the polenta in a steady stream, stirring, and cook according to the pack instructions. Add the butter and both cheeses and mix together well.

5 To serve, divide the polenta among four serving plates and top with the Parmesan shavings, if you like. Spoon some sausage stew alongside each serving of polenta and garnish each with a rosemary sprig. Serve immediately.

Serves 4	EASY		NUTRITIONAL INFORMATION
	Preparation Time 10 minutes, plus soaking	**Cooking Time** 15 minutes	**Per Serving** 443 calories, 35g fat (of which 12g saturates), 6g carbohydrate, 3.4g salt

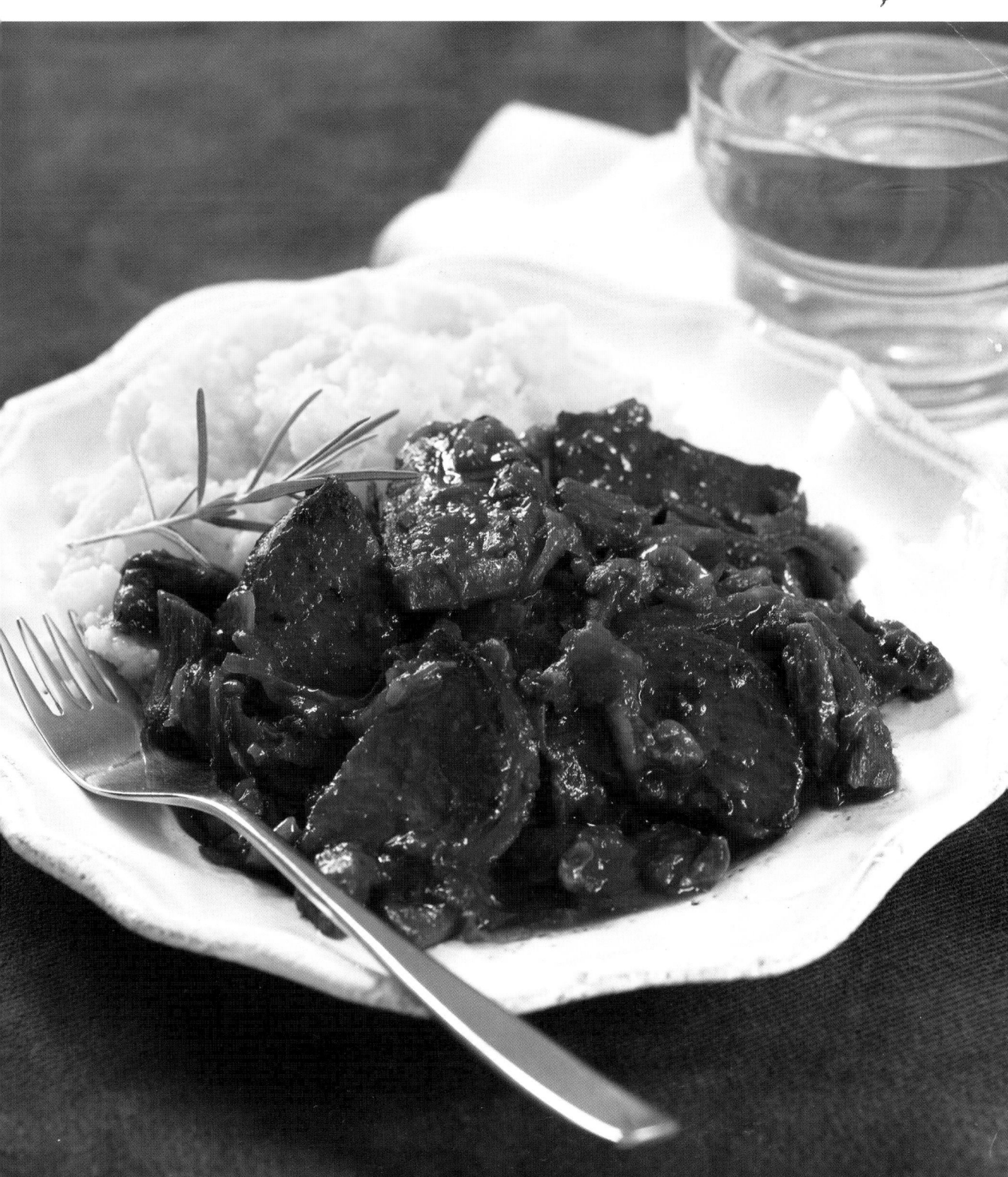

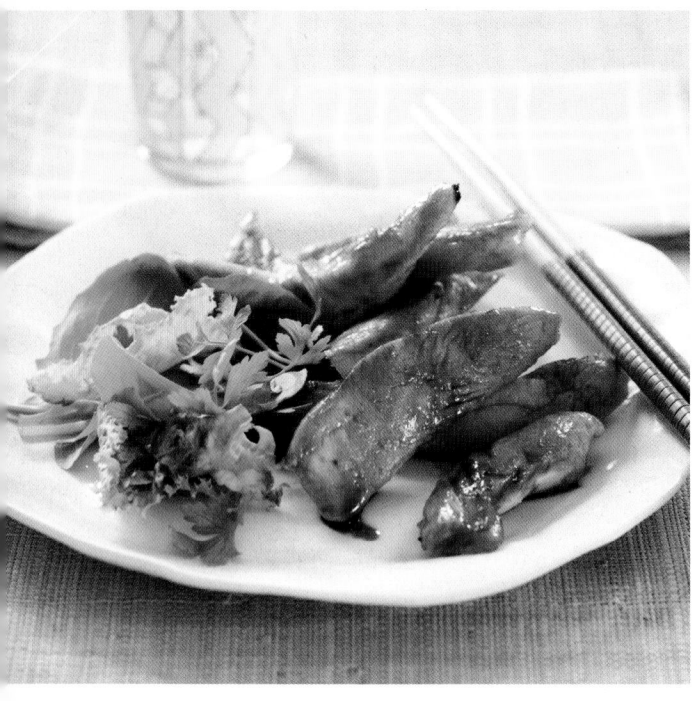

Try Something Different

Use limes instead of lemons. Knead them on the worktop for 30 seconds before squeezing so they yield as much juice as possible.

Lemon Chicken

4 small skinless chicken breasts, about 125g (4oz) each, cut into chunky strips

juice of 2 lemons

2 tbsp olive oil

4–6 tbsp demerara sugar

salt

green salad to serve

1 Put the chicken strips into a large bowl and season with salt. Add the lemon juice and olive oil and stir to mix.

2 Preheat the grill to medium. Spread the chicken out on a large baking sheet and sprinkle over half the sugar. Grill for 3–4 minutes until caramelised, then turn the chicken over, sprinkle with the remaining sugar and grill until the chicken is cooked through and golden.

3 Divide the chicken among four plates and serve with a green salad.

Serves 4	EASY		NUTRITIONAL INFORMATION	
	Preparation Time 2 minutes	**Cooking Time** 6–8 minutes	**Per Serving** 231 calories, 7g fat (of which 1g saturates), 13g carbohydrate, 0.2g salt	Gluten free • Dairy free

Cook's Tips

Make your own mint sauce: finely chop 20g (³/₄oz) fresh mint and mix with 1 tbsp each olive oil and white wine vinegar.

Make your own garlic-infused oil: gently heat 2 tbsp olive oil with peeled, sliced garlic for 5 minutes and use immediately. Do not store.

Lamb Chops with Crispy Garlic Potatoes

2 tbsp mint sauce (see Cook's Tips)

8 small lamb chops

3 medium potatoes, peeled and cut into 5mm (¹/₄in) slices

2 tbsp garlic-infused olive oil (see Cook's Tips)

1 tbsp olive oil

salt and ground black pepper

steamed green beans to serve

1 Spread the mint sauce over the lamb chops and leave to marinate while you prepare the potatoes.

2 Boil the potatoes in a pan of lightly salted water for 2 minutes or until just starting to soften. Drain, tip back into the pan, season with salt and pepper and toss with the garlic oil.

3 Meanwhile, heat the olive oil in a large frying pan and fry the chops for 4–5 minutes on each side until just cooked, adding a splash of boiling water to the pan to make a sauce. Remove the chops and sauce from the pan and keep warm.

4 Add the potatoes to the pan. Fry over a medium heat for 10–12 minutes until crisp and golden. Divide the potatoes, chops and sauce among four plates and serve with green beans.

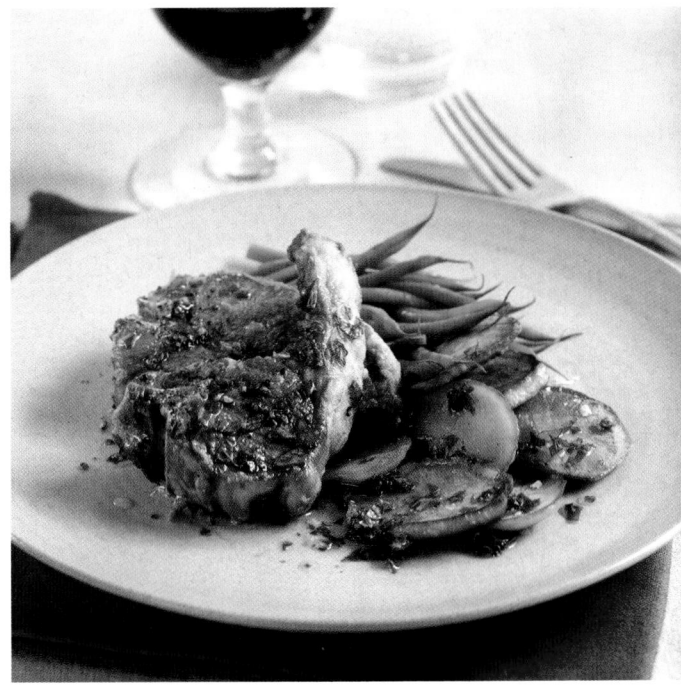

EASY		NUTRITIONAL INFORMATION		Serves
Preparation Time 10 minutes	**Cooking Time** 20 minutes	**Per Serving** 835 calories, 45g fat (of which 19g saturates), 22g carbohydrate, 0.7g salt	Gluten free • Dairy free	**4**

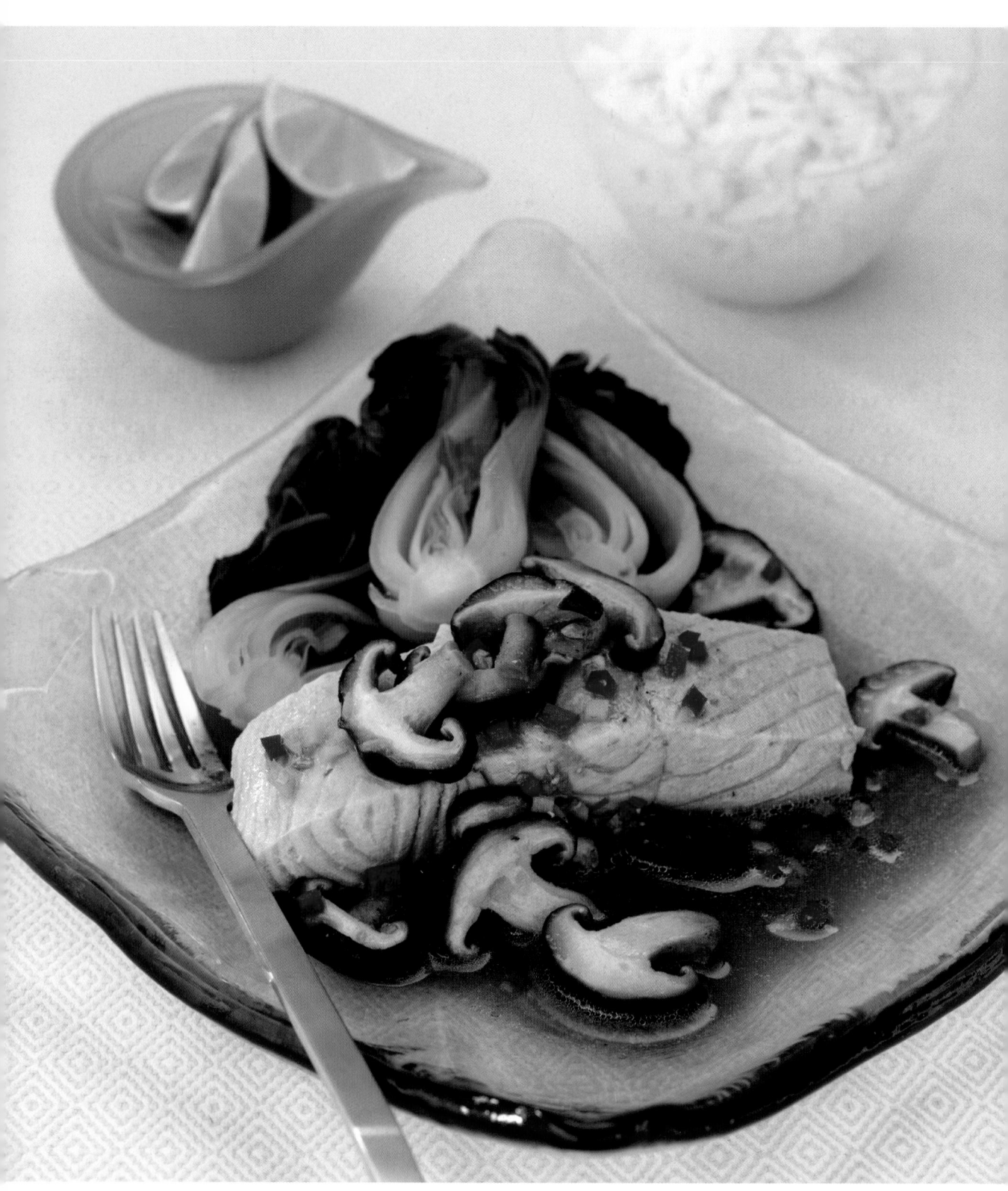

Cook's Tip

Thai fish sauce is widely used in South-east Asian cooking and is made from fermented anchovies. It adds a salty flavour to food and is called nam pla in Thailand.

Poached Thai Salmon

200g (7oz) Thai jasmine rice

1 tbsp sesame oil

1 red chilli, seeded and finely chopped (see page 33)

5cm (2in) piece fresh root ginger, peeled and finely chopped

1 garlic clove, crushed

1–2 tbsp miso paste (see page 38)

2 tsp Thai fish sauce

4 skinless salmon fillets, about 150g (5oz) each

150g (5oz) fresh shiitake mushrooms, sliced

250g (9oz) pak choi, roughly chopped

100g (3½oz) baby leaf spinach

1 lime, quartered

1 Put the rice into a small pan with 400ml (14fl oz) boiling water. Cover, bring to the boil, then reduce the heat to low. Cook according to the pack instructions.

2 Heat the sesame oil in a large shallow pan or wok, add the chilli, ginger and garlic and cook for 1–2 minutes. Add the miso paste and fish sauce, then pour over 500ml (18fl oz) hot water.

3 Add the salmon and mushrooms, then cover and simmer for 7–8 minutes until fish is just cooked. Steam the pak choi and spinach over boiling water for 4–5 minutes. Serve the salmon with some of the sauce, with the rice, vegetables and lime wedges to squeeze over.

EASY		NUTRITIONAL INFORMATION		Serves
Preparation Time 10 minutes	**Cooking Time** 15 minutes	**Per Serving** 484 calories, 19.1g fat (of which 3.4g saturates), 42.1g carbohydrate, 1.8g salt	Gluten free • Dairy free	**4**

Crispy Crumbed Fish

50g (2oz) fresh breadcrumbs

a small handful of freshly chopped flat-leafed parsley

2 tbsp capers, chopped

grated zest of 1 lemon

4 haddock or pollack fillets, about 150g (5oz) each

½ tbsp Dijon mustard

juice of ½ lemon

salt and ground black pepper

new potatoes and mixed salad to serve

1 Preheat the oven to 180°C (160°C fan oven) mark 4. Put the breadcrumbs into a bowl with the parsley, capers and lemon zest. Mix well, then set aside.

2 Put the fish fillets on to a baking tray. Mix the mustard and half the lemon juice in a bowl with a little salt and pepper, then spread over the top of each piece of fish. Spoon the breadcrumb mixture over the top – don't worry if some falls off.

3 Cook in the oven for 10–15 minutes until the fish is cooked and the breadcrumbs are golden. Pour the remaining lemon juice over the top and serve with new potatoes and a mixed salad.

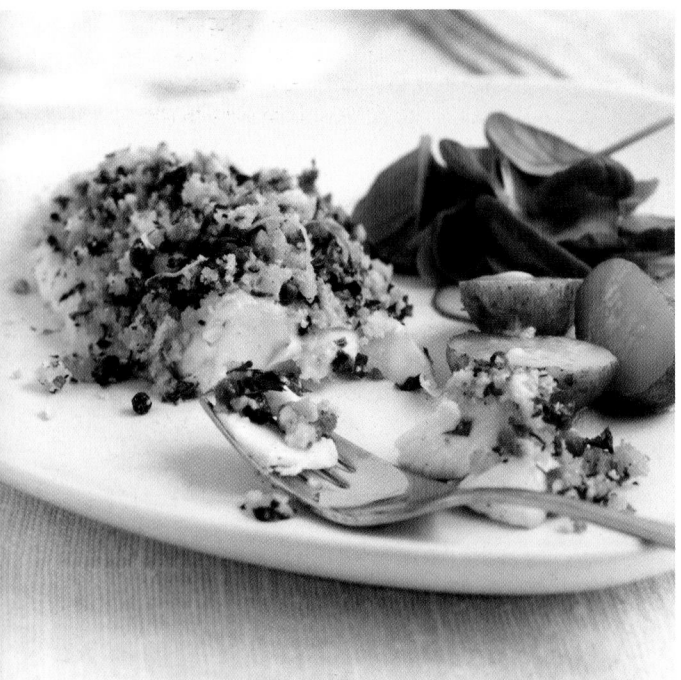

Serves 4	EASY		NUTRITIONAL INFORMATION	
	Preparation Time 5 minutes	**Cooking Time** 10–15 minutes	**Per Serving** 171 calories, 1g fat (of which trace saturates), 10g carbohydrate, 0.8g salt	Dairy free

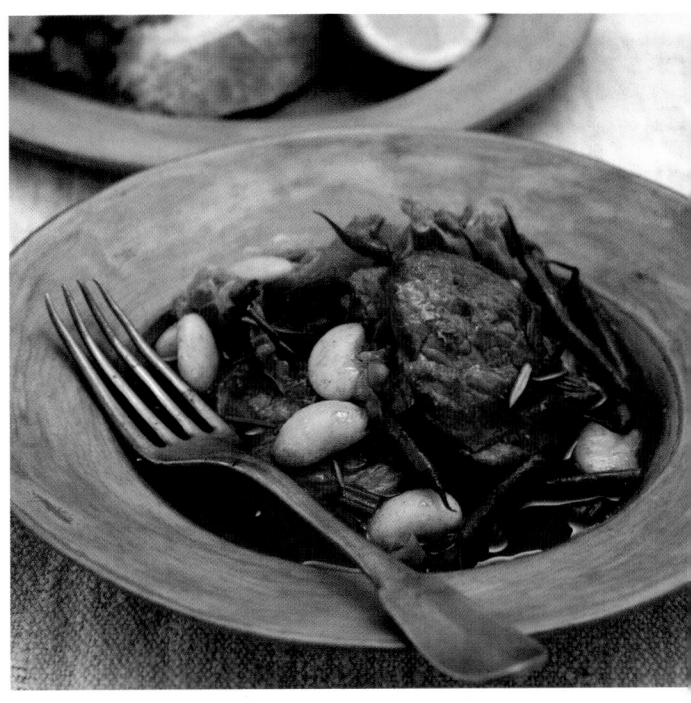

Spanish-style Pork

500g (1lb 2oz) pork fillet, trimmed and sliced
2 tbsp olive oil
1 Spanish onion, chopped
2 celery sticks, finely chopped
2 tsp smoked paprika
1 tbsp tomato purée
750ml (1¼ pints) hot chicken stock
400g can butter beans, drained and rinsed
¼ Savoy cabbage, finely shredded
200g (7oz) green beans, trimmed and halved
salt and ground black pepper
1 tbsp freshly chopped rosemary to garnish
lemon wedges and crusty bread to serve

1 Lay the pork out on a board, cover with clingfilm and flatten slightly with a rolling pin. Heat 1 tbsp olive oil in a frying pan and fry the pork over a medium to high heat until browned. Remove from the pan and set aside.

2 Heat the remaining oil and gently fry the onion and celery for 10 minutes or until softened. Stir in the paprika and tomato purée, and cook for 1 minute. Stir in the stock, butter beans and cabbage. Season with salt and pepper.

3 Return the pork to the pan and bring to the boil, then simmer for 10 minutes, adding the green beans for the last 4 minutes. Garnish with rosemary and serve with lemon wedges and crusty bread on the side.

EASY		NUTRITIONAL INFORMATION		Serves
Preparation Time 15 minutes	**Cooking Time** 25 minutes	**Per Serving** 349 calories, 11.9g fat (of which 2.7g saturates), 26.1g carbohydrate, 1.2g salt	Gluten free • Dairy free	**4**

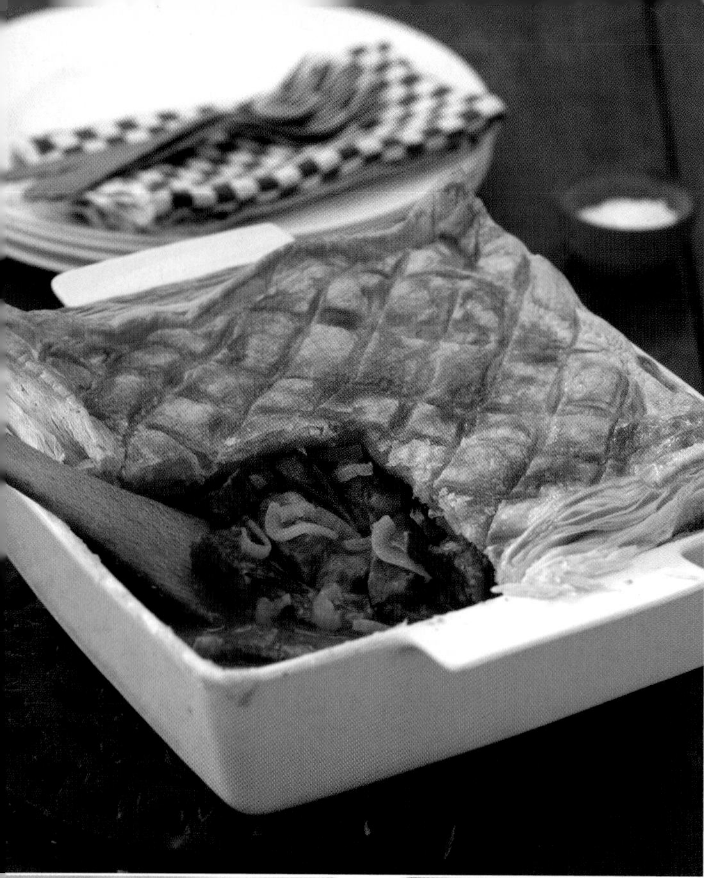

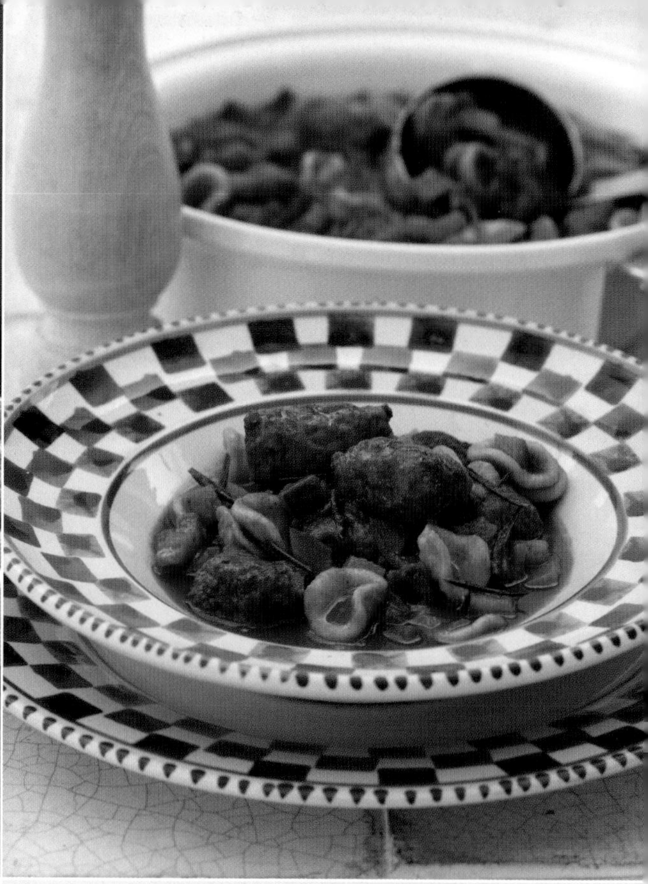

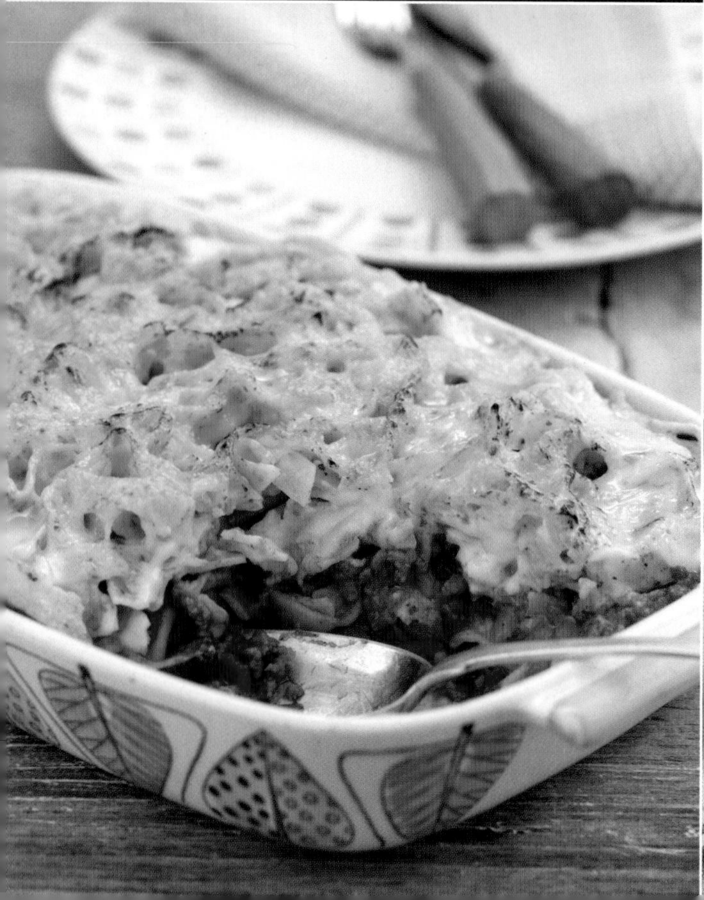

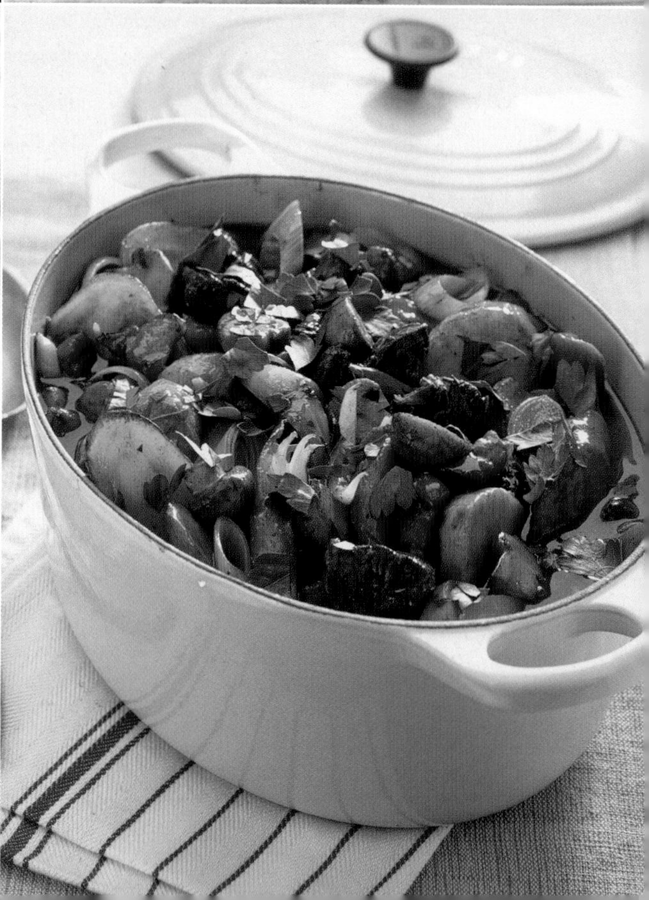

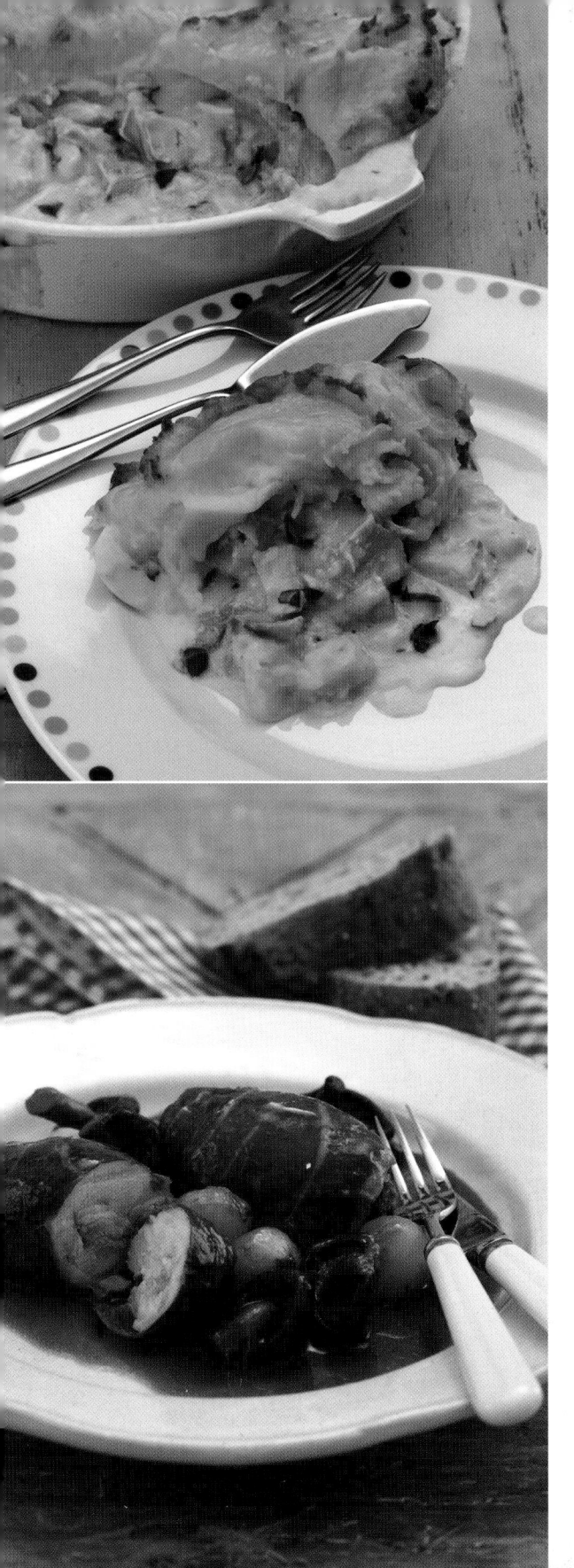

4

Cook Once, Eat Twice

Tagliatelle Bake

Braised Beef

Mushroom and Roasted Potato Bake

Moroccan Chicken with Chickpeas

Lamb and Leek Hotpot

Chunky One-pot Bolognese

Luxury Smoked Fish Pie

Winter Hotpot

Chicken in Red Wine

Steak and Onion Puff Pie

Braised Lamb Shanks with Cannellini Beans

Perfect Roast Chicken

Italian Lamb

Get Ahead

This dish is ideal for freezing for an easy meal another day. Double the quantities and make another meal for four or make two meals for two people and freeze.

Complete the recipe to the end of step 2, then layer the mince and pasta in a freezerproof, heatproof container. Cool and freeze for up to three months.

To use Thaw overnight in the fridge. Bake in the oven at 190°C (170°C fan oven) mark 5 for 25 minutes, then place under a hot grill for 2–3 minutes until bubbling.

Alternatively, make double the meat mixture, freeze half and serve with spaghetti or flour tortillas.

Tagliatelle Bake

1 tbsp olive oil

1 large onion, finely chopped

450g (1lb) minced beef

2 garlic cloves, crushed

290g jar marinated vegetables

2 x 400g cans chopped tomatoes

1 tsp dried marjoram

375g (12oz) fresh garlic and herb tagliatelle

330g jar ready-made cheese sauce

4 tbsp milk

75g (3oz) Cheddar cheese, grated

salt

mixed salad to serve

1 Heat the olive oil in a pan. Add the onion and fry until soft. Add the beef and fry, stirring, until the meat is brown. Add the garlic, marinated vegetables, tomatoes and marjoram. Simmer for 25 minutes or until the meat is tender.

2 Cook the tagliatelle in a pan of boiling salted water according to the pack instructions. Drain, put back into the pan and stir in the cheese sauce and milk. Heat through for 3 minutes.

3 Preheat the grill. Put alternate layers of mince and pasta in a heatproof dish and top with the cheese. Cook under the hot grill until bubbling. Serve with a mixed salad.

Serves 4	EASY		NUTRITIONAL INFORMATION
	Preparation Time 5 minutes	**Cooking Time** 45 minutes	**Per Serving** 935 calories, 42.1g fat (of which 19g saturates), 97.1g carbohydrate, 1.6g salt

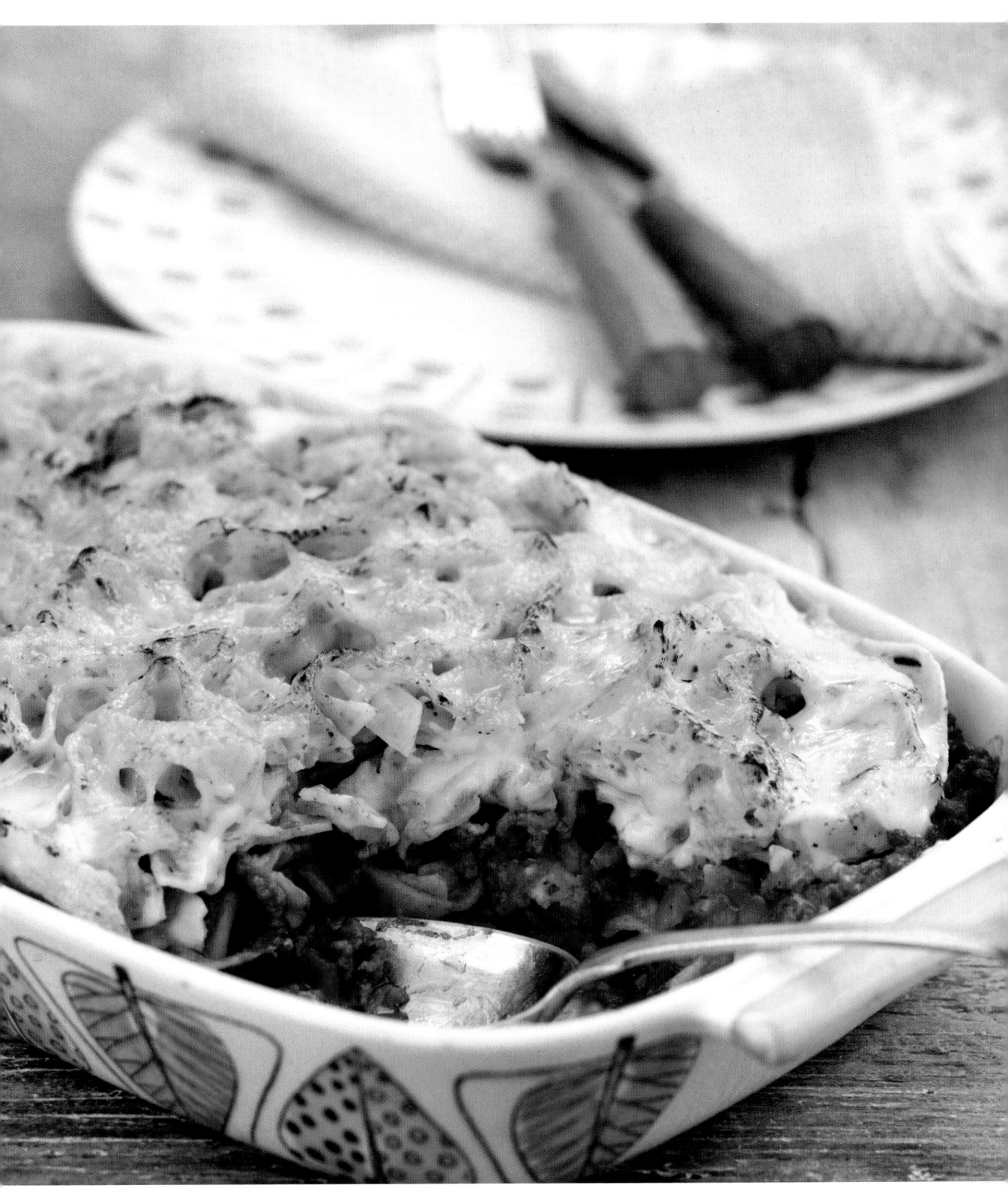

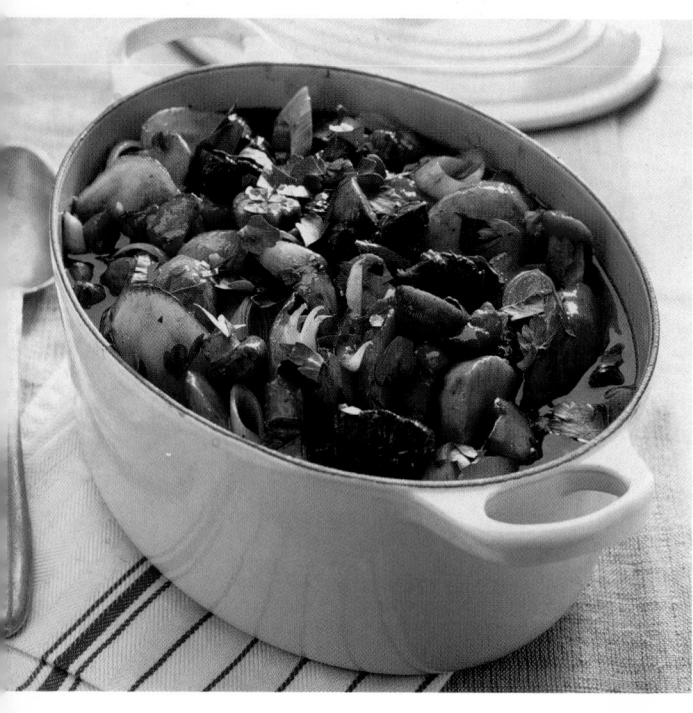

Get Ahead

This dish is ideal for freezing for an easy meal another day. Double the quantities and make another meal for four or make two meals for two people and freeze.

Complete the recipe, then transfer to a freezerproof container, cool and freeze for up to three months.

To use Thaw overnight at cool room temperature. Preheat the oven to 180°C (160°C fan oven) mark 4. Bring to the boil on the hob, cover tightly and reheat in the oven for about 30 minutes or until piping hot.

Alternatively, top the cooked beef with a puff pastry lid (see page 103) and bake in a preheated oven at 220°C (200°C fan oven) mark 7 for 30 minutes until the pastry is risen and golden.

Braised Beef

175g (6oz) smoked pancetta or smoked streaky bacon, cut into cubes

2 medium leeks, thickly sliced

1 tbsp olive oil

450g (1lb) braising steak, cut into 5cm (2in) pieces

1 large onion, finely chopped

2 carrots, thickly sliced

2 parsnips, thickly sliced

1 tbsp plain flour

300ml (½ pint) red wine

1–2 tbsp redcurrant jelly

125g (4oz) chestnut mushrooms, halved

freshly chopped flat-leafed parsley to garnish

salt and ground black pepper

mashed potato to serve

1 Preheat the oven to 170°C (150°C fan oven) mark 3. Fry the pancetta or bacon in a shallow flameproof casserole for 2–3 minutes until golden. Add the leeks. Cook for 2 minutes or until the leeks are beginning to colour. Remove with a slotted spoon and set aside.

2 Heat the olive oil in the casserole and fry the beef in batches for 2–3 minutes until golden on all sides. Remove and set aside. Add the onion and fry over a low heat for 5 minutes or until golden. Stir in the carrots and parsnips and fry for 1–2 minutes.

3 Put the beef back into the casserole and stir in the flour to soak up the juices. Gradually add the red wine and 300ml (½ pint) water, then stir in the redcurrant jelly. Season with salt and pepper and bring to the boil. Cover with a tight-fitting lid and cook in the oven for 2 hours.

4 Stir in the leeks, pancetta and mushrooms, re-cover and cook for a further 1 hour. Scatter with parsley and serve with mashed potato.

Serves 4	EASY		NUTRITIONAL INFORMATION	
	Preparation Time 20 minutes	**Cooking Time** about 3½ hours	**Per Serving** 554 calories, 25.3g fat (of which 8.6g saturates), 33g carbohydrate, 1.7g salt	Dairy free

Get Ahead

This dish is ideal for freezing. Freeze leftover portions separately or double the quantities and freeze half for another day.

Complete the recipe to the end of step 4, then cool and freeze for up to one month.

To use Thaw overnight at cool room temperature. Preheat the oven to 200°C (180°C fan oven) mark 6. Bake for 40–45 minutes until golden and bubbling.

Mushroom and Roasted Potato Bake

900g (2lb) small potatoes, peeled and quartered

6 tbsp olive oil

225g (8oz) onions, roughly chopped

450g (1lb) mixed fresh mushrooms, such as shiitake and brown-cap, roughly chopped

2 garlic cloves, crushed

2 tbsp tomato purée

4 tbsp sun-dried tomato paste

25g (1oz) dried porcini mushrooms, rinsed (optional)

2 tsp freshly chopped thyme

300ml (½ pint) each of dry white wine and vegetable stock

300ml (½ pint) double cream

400g (14oz) large fresh spinach leaves, roughly chopped

175g (6oz) Gruyère cheese

125g (4oz) Parmesan, grated

300ml (½ pint) Greek yogurt

2 medium eggs, beaten

salt and ground black pepper

1 Preheat the oven to 200°C (180°C fan oven) mark 6. Toss the potatoes with 4 tbsp olive oil in a roasting tin and cook for 40 minutes or until tender.

2 Heat the remaining oil in a large heavy-based pan. Add the onions and cook for 10 minutes or until soft, then add the fresh mushrooms and garlic and cook over a high heat for 5 minutes. Stir in the tomato purée and tomato paste, the porcini mushrooms, if using, and the thyme and wine. Bring to the boil and simmer for 2 minutes. Add the stock and cream and bubble for 20 minutes or until well reduced and syrupy. Pour into a 2.4 litre (4¼ pint) ovenproof dish. Stir in the potatoes, spinach, Gruyère and half the Parmesan. Season well with salt and pepper.

3 Combine the yogurt with the eggs and season. Spoon over the vegetable mixture and sprinkle with the remaining Parmesan.

4 Cook in the oven for 30–35 minutes until golden and bubbling. Serve hot.

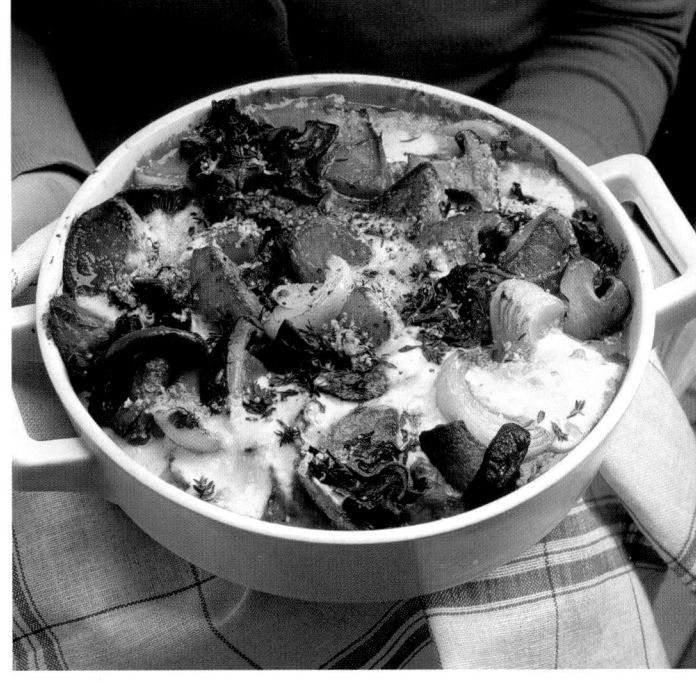

EASY	NUTRITIONAL INFORMATION		Serves
Preparation Time 15 minutes	**Cooking Time** 1¼ hours	**Per Serving** 809 calories, 62.6g fat (of which 30.6g saturates), 33.1g carbohydrate, 1.7g salt	Vegetarian Gluten free

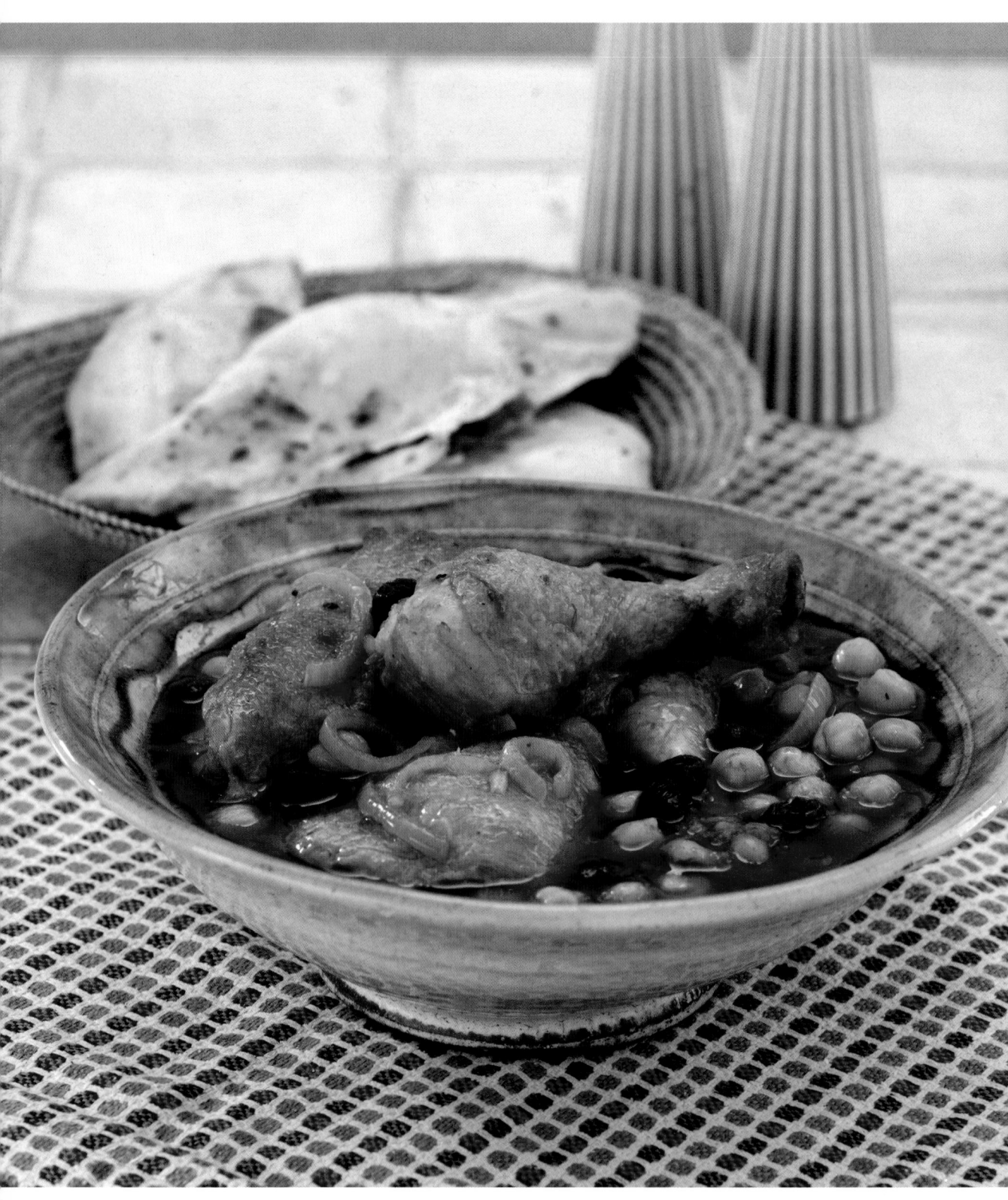

Moroccan Chicken with Chickpeas

12 chicken pieces, including thighs, drumsticks and breast

25g (1oz) butter

1 large onion, sliced

2 garlic cloves, crushed

2 tbsp harissa paste

a generous pinch of saffron

1 tsp salt

1 cinnamon stick

600ml (1 pint) chicken stock

75g (3oz) raisins

2 x 400g cans chickpeas, drained and rinsed

ground black pepper

plain naan or pitta bread to serve

1 Heat a large, wide non-stick pan. Add the chicken pieces and fry until well browned all over. Add the butter and, when melted, add the onion and garlic. Cook, stirring, for 5 minutes.

2 Add the harissa, saffron, salt and cinnamon stick, then season well with pepper. Pour in the stock and bring to the boil. Reduce the heat, cover and simmer gently for 25–30 minutes.

3 Add the raisins and chickpeas and bring to the boil. Simmer uncovered for 5–10 minutes.

4 Serve with warm flat bread such as plain naan or pitta.

Get Ahead

This dish is ideal for freezing. Freeze leftover portions separately.

Complete the recipe, then cool quickly. Put in a sealable container and freeze for up to three months.

To use Thaw overnight in the fridge. Put in a pan, cover and bring to the boil. Reduce the heat to low, then reheat for 40 minutes or until the chicken is hot right through.

Instead of bread, serve with couscous or brown rice.

EASY		NUTRITIONAL INFORMATION	Serves
Preparation Time 10 minutes	**Cooking Time** 50 minutes	**Per Serving** 440 calories, 18.1g fat (of which 5.9g saturates), 32.7g carbohydrate, 1g salt	6

Get Ahead

This dish is ideal for freezing. Freeze leftover portions separately.

Complete the recipe, then carefully transfer to a freezerproof, heatproof container. Cool and freeze for up to three months.

To use Thaw overnight at cool room temperature. Bake in the oven at 190°C (170°C fan oven) mark 5 for 30 minutes, until bubbling.

50g (2oz) butter

400g (14oz) leeks, sliced

1 onion, chopped

800g (1lb 12oz) casserole lamb, cubed

1 tbsp plain flour

1 tbsp olive oil

2 garlic cloves, crushed

800g (1lb 12oz) waxy potatoes such as Desirée, peeled and sliced

3 tbsp freshly chopped parsley

1 tsp freshly chopped thyme

600ml (1 pint) lamb stock

150ml (¼ pint) double cream

salt and ground black pepper

Lamb and Leek Hotpot

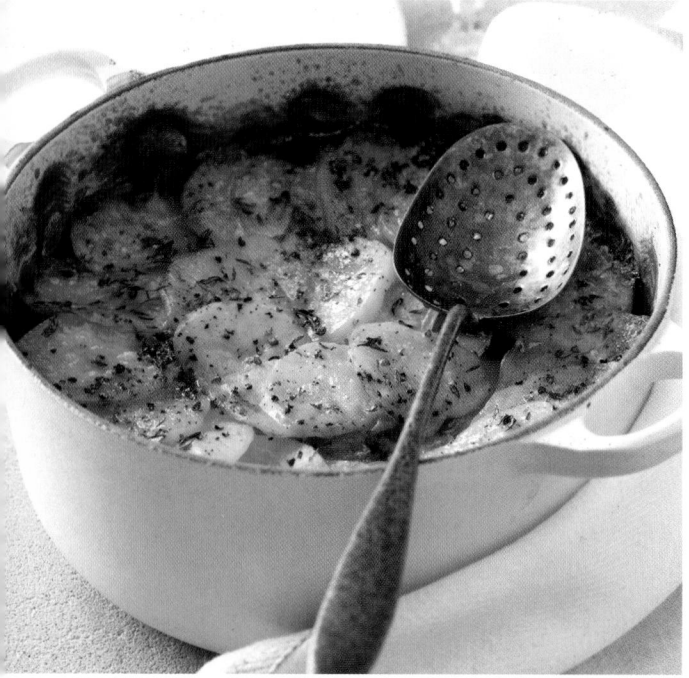

1 Melt half the butter in a 3.5 litre (6¼ pint) flameproof casserole dish over a low heat. Add the leeks and onion, stir to coat, then cover and cook for 10 minutes. Remove and put to one side.

2 Toss the lamb with the flour. Add the olive oil to the casserole and heat, then brown the meat in batches with the garlic and plenty of salt and pepper. Remove and set aside.

3 Preheat the oven to 170°C (150°C fan oven) mark 3. Put half the potatoes in a layer in the casserole and season with salt and pepper. Add the meat, then spoon the leek mixture on top. Arrange a layer of overlapping potatoes on top of that, sprinkle with the parsley and thyme, then pour in the stock.

4 Bring the casserole to the boil, cover, then cook in the oven for about 1 hour 50 minutes. Remove the lid, dot with the remaining butter and add the cream. Cook uncovered for 30–40 minutes until the potatoes are golden brown.

Serves 6	EASY		NUTRITIONAL INFORMATION
	Preparation Time 20 minutes	**Cooking Time** 2 hours 50 minutes	**Per Serving** 549 calories, 37g fat (of which 20g saturates), 25g carbohydrate, 0.5g salt

Get Ahead

This dish is ideal for freezing. Freeze leftover portions separately.

Complete the recipe to the end of step 4. Add the pasta and cook for 10 minutes – it will continue to cook right through when you reheat the Bolognese. Cool, put in a freezerproof container and freeze for up to three months.

To use Thaw overnight at cool room temperature, put in a pan and add 150ml (¼ pint) water. Bring to the boil, then simmer gently for 10 minutes or until the sauce is hot and the pasta is cooked.

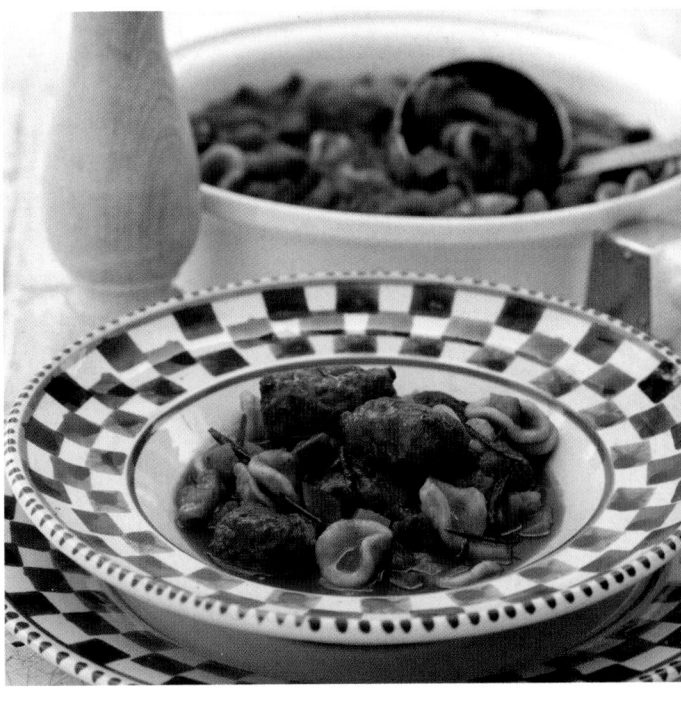

Chunky One-pot Bolognese

3 tbsp olive oil

2 large red onions, finely diced

a few fresh rosemary sprigs

1 large aubergine, finely diced

8 plump coarse sausages

350ml (12fl oz) full-bodied red wine

700g (1½lb) passata

4 tbsp sun-dried tomato paste

300ml (½ pint) hot vegetable stock

175g (6oz) small dried pasta, such as orecchiette

salt and ground black pepper

1 Heat 2 tbsp olive oil in a large, shallow non-stick pan. Add the onions and rosemary and cook over a gentle heat for 10 minutes or until soft and golden.

2 Add the aubergine and remaining oil and cook over a medium heat for 8–10 minutes until soft and golden.

3 Meanwhile, pull the skin off the sausages and divide each into four rough chunks. Tip the aubergine mixture on to a plate and add the sausage chunks to the hot pan. You won't need any extra oil.

4 Stir the sausage pieces over a high heat for 6–8 minutes until golden and beginning to turn crisp at the edges. Pour in the wine and allow to bubble for 6–8 minutes until only a little liquid remains. Put the aubergine mixture back into the pan, along with the passata, tomato paste and stock.

5 Stir the pasta into the liquid, cover, then simmer for 20 minutes or until the pasta is cooked. Taste and season with salt and pepper if necessary.

EASY		NUTRITIONAL INFORMATION		Serves
Preparation Time 15 minutes	**Cooking Time** about 1 hour	**Per Serving** 506 calories, 31g fat (of which 11g saturates), 40g carbohydrate, 1.5g salt	Dairy free	**6**

Luxury Smoked Fish Pie

1.1kg (2½lb) Desirée potatoes, peeled and cut into rough chunks

450ml (¾ pint) milk

125g (4oz) butter

125g (4oz) Cheddar cheese, grated

75ml (2½fl oz) dry white wine

150ml (¼ pint) fish stock

450g (1lb) skinless smoked haddock fillet, undyed if possible, cut into wide strips

350g (12oz) skinless salmon fillet, cut into wide strips

40g (1½oz) plain flour

75ml (2½fl oz) double cream

1 tbsp capers, drained, rinsed and chopped

1½ tbsp freshly chopped flat-leafed parsley

2 medium eggs, hard-boiled

salt and ground black pepper

1 Preheat the oven to 180°C (160°C fan oven) mark 4. Put the potatoes into a pan of salted water, bring to the boil, cover and simmer until tender.

2 Warm 100ml (3½fl oz) milk. Drain the potatoes, then put back in the pan over a low heat for 2 minutes. Mash until smooth. Stir in 75g (3oz) butter, half the cheese and the warmed milk; season with salt and pepper. Cover and put to one side.

3 Meanwhile, bring the wine, stock and remaining milk to the boil in a large wide pan. Add the haddock and salmon. Return the liquid to the boil, then reduce the heat to poach the fish gently for 5 minutes or until it flakes easily. Lift the fish with a draining spoon into a 1.4 litre (2½ pint) deep ovenproof dish and flake with a fork if necessary. Put the cooking liquid to one side.

4 Melt the remaining butter in another pan, add the flour and stir until smooth, then cook for 2 minutes. Gradually add the fish liquid, whisking until smooth. Bring to the boil, stirring, and cook for 2 minutes or until thickened. Stir in the cream, capers and parsley, and season with salt and pepper to taste.

5 Shell the eggs and chop roughly. Scatter over the fish then pour the sauce over. Spoon the potato mixture on top and sprinkle with the remaining cheese.

6 Bake the pie for 35–40 minutes until golden and bubbling at the edges. Serve hot.

Get Ahead

Double the ingredient quantities and make two pies, each to serve four people, then freeze one for another day. **Complete the recipe** to the end of step 4. Cool the sauce quickly, then complete step 5. Freeze for up to three months. **To use** Thaw overnight at cool room temperature. Bake at 190°C (170°C fan oven) mark 5 for 50–60 minutes until golden and bubbling at the edges.

Serves 4	EASY		NUTRITIONAL INFORMATION
	Preparation Time 30 minutes	**Cooking Time** 1 hour 20 minutes	**Per Serving** 1057 calories, 62.8g fat (of which 33.5g saturates), 66.1g carbohydrate, 3.8g salt

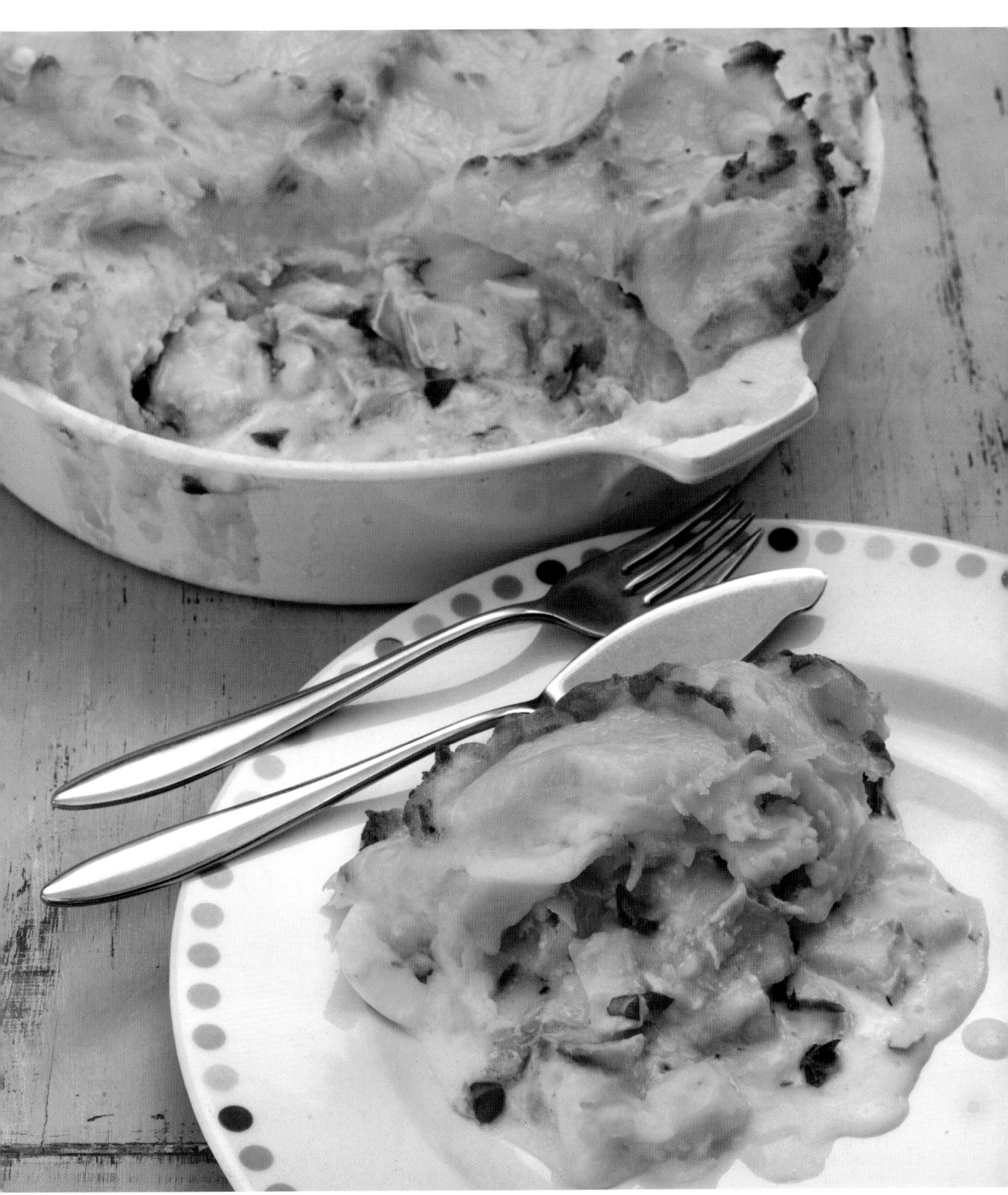

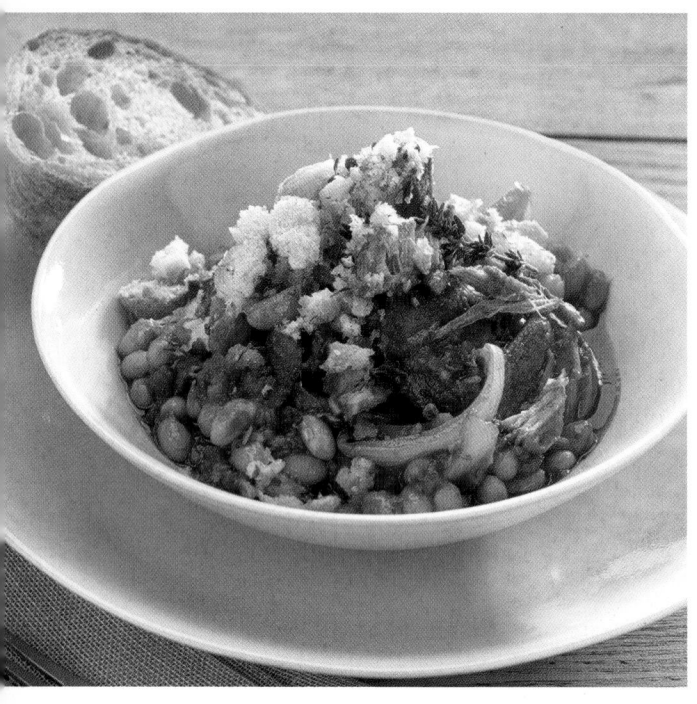

Get Ahead

This dish is ideal for freezing for an easy meal another day. The recipe will make two meals for four people.
Complete the recipe to the end of step 4. Cool quickly, cover and freeze for up to three months.
To use Thaw overnight at cool room temperature. Add 150ml (¼ pint) stock and bring to the boil. Cover and reheat at 180°C (160°C fan oven) mark 4 for 25 minutes; complete the recipe.

Cook's Tip

Marinate the pork for at least 8 hours, or overnight: put it in a large bowl with 6 garlic cloves, 2 tbsp olive oil, 2 tbsp red wine vinegar, 4 tbsp soft brown sugar, a few drops of chilli sauce and 2 tsp each of dried thyme and oregano. Season, mix well, then cover and leave in the fridge.

Winter Hotpot

1.4kg (3lb) boned shoulder of pork, cut into 2.5cm (1in) cubes, marinated (see Cook's Tip)

5 tbsp olive oil

450g (1lb) onions, halved and sliced

2 tbsp tomato purée

2 x 400g cans haricot beans, drained, liquid reserved

2 x 400g cans chopped tomatoes

300ml (½ pint) red wine

4 bay leaves

25g (1oz) butter

125g (4oz) white breadcrumbs from French bread or ciabatta

1 tsp dried oregano

125g (4oz) Gruyère cheese, grated

salt and ground black pepper

fresh thyme sprigs to garnish

1 Drain the pork, putting the marinade to one side. Preheat the oven to 180°C (160°C fan oven) mark 4.

2 Heat 3 tbsp olive oil in a large flameproof casserole and fry the pork in batches until well browned on all sides. Set aside. Add the remaining oil and cook the onions for 10 minutes over a high heat, stirring occasionally, until they are soft and caramelised. Add the tomato purée and cook for 1 minute. Put the meat back into the casserole with the bean liquid, tomatoes, wine, bay leaves and the reserved marinade. Bring to the boil, stirring, then cover and cook in the oven for 2 hours or until the pork is very tender.

3 About 20 minutes before the end of the cooking time, stir in the beans. Increase the oven temperature to 200°C (180°C fan oven) mark 6 and move the pork to a lower shelf. Heat the butter in a roasting tin, add the breadcrumbs and oregano and season. Brown on the top shelf for 10 minutes. Sprinkle the hotpot with the breadcrumbs and grated cheese. Garnish with thyme sprigs and serve.

Serves 8	EASY		NUTRITIONAL INFORMATION
	Preparation Time 20 minutes, plus at least 8 hours marinating	**Cooking Time** 2 hours 20 minutes	**Per Serving** 547 calories, 22.6g fat (of which 8.7g saturates), 30.8g carbohydrate, 1.9g salt

Get Ahead

This dish is ideal for freezing for an easy meal another day. Double the quantities and make another meal for four or make two meals for two people and freeze.

Complete the recipe, cool quickly, then put into a freezerproof container and freeze for up to three months.

To use Thaw overnight at cool room temperature, then put back into a pan. Bring slowly to the boil, then simmer gently for 10–15 minutes until piping hot.

Cook's Tips

If you can't buy prosciutto, thinly cut smoked streaky bacon will work just as well.

Use button mushrooms if you can't find shiitake.

Chicken in Red Wine

8 slices prosciutto

8 large boned and skinned chicken thighs

1 tbsp olive oil

1 fat garlic clove, crushed

about 12 shallots or button onions, peeled

225g (8oz) fresh shiitake mushrooms

1 tbsp plain flour

300ml (½ pint) red wine

300ml (½ pint) hot chicken stock

1 tbsp Worcestershire sauce

1 bay leaf

salt and ground black pepper

crusty bread to serve

1 Wrap a slice of prosciutto around each chicken thigh. Heat the olive oil in a large non-stick frying pan and fry the chicken pieces in batches for 8–10 minutes until golden all over. Transfer to a plate and set aside.

2 Add the garlic and shallots or button onions and fry over a gentle heat for 5 minutes or until the shallots are beginning to soften and turn golden. Stir in the mushrooms and flour and cook over a gentle heat for 1–2 minutes.

3 Put the chicken back in the pan and add the wine, stock, Worcestershire sauce and bay leaf. Season lightly with salt and pepper, bring to the boil for 5 minutes, then cover and simmer over a low heat for 45 minutes or until the chicken is tender. Serve with crusty bread.

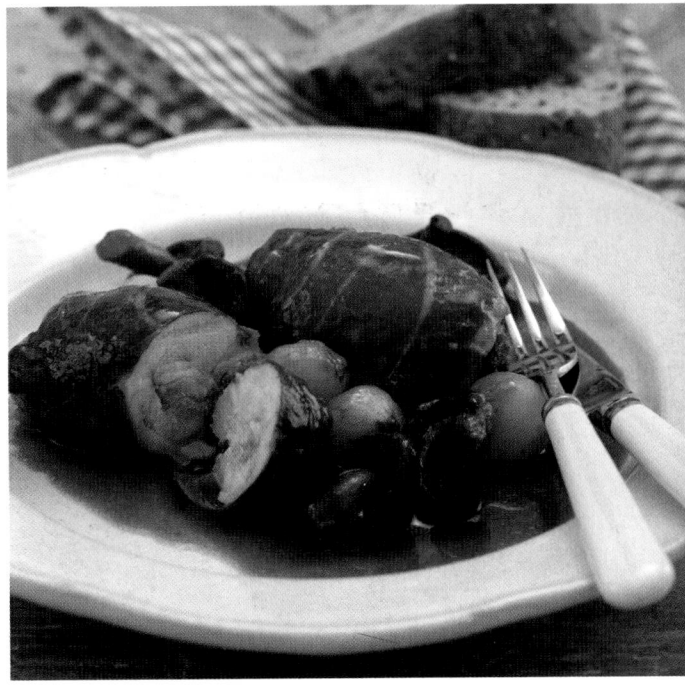

EASY		NUTRITIONAL INFORMATION		Serves
Preparation Time 15 minutes	**Cooking Time** 1 hour 10 minutes	**Per Serving** 358 calories, 13.5g fat (of which 3.8g saturates), 8.1g carbohydrate, 1.1g salt [to come	Dairy free	**4**

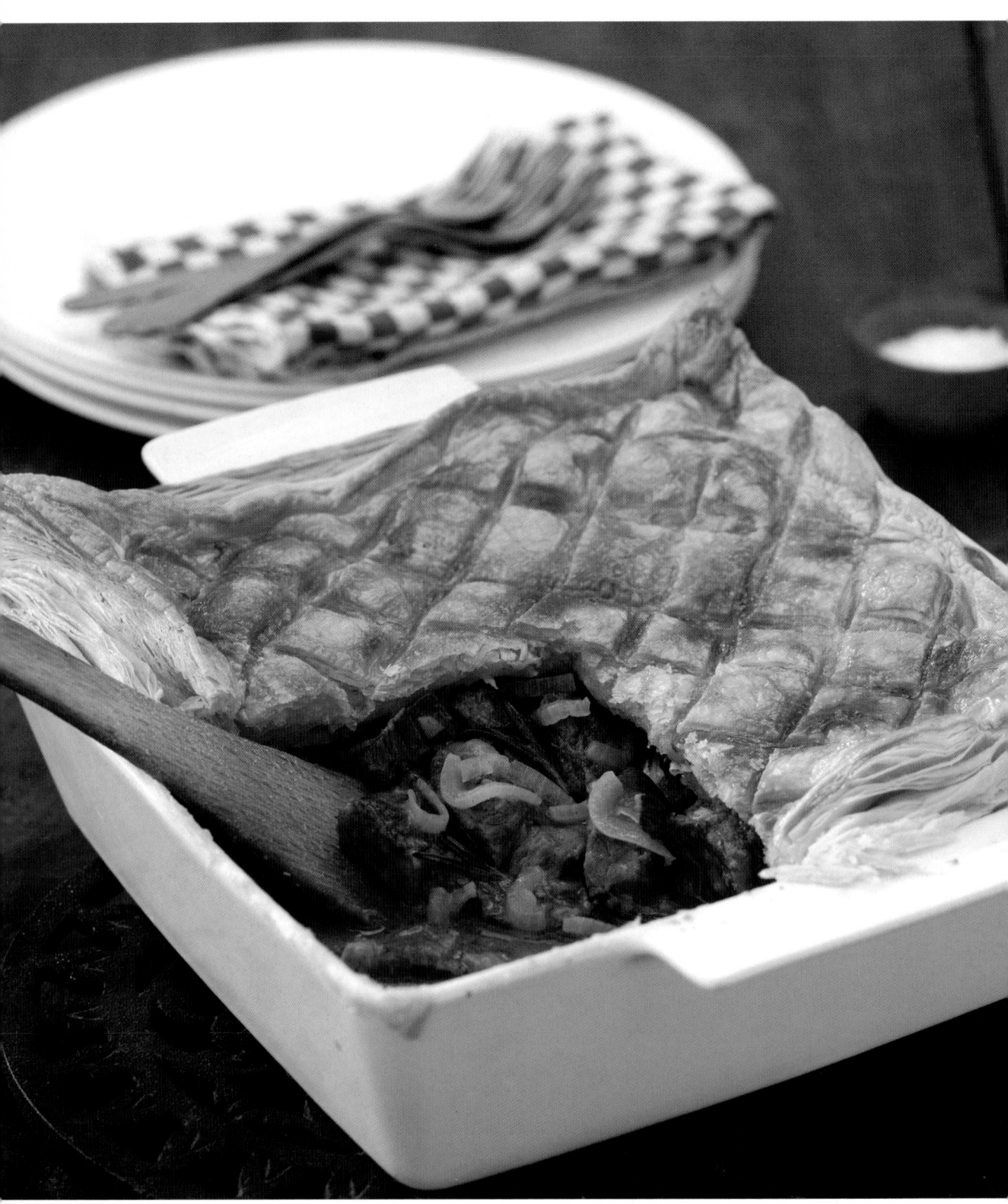

Steak and Onion Puff Pie

3 tbsp vegetable oil

2 onions, sliced

900g (2lb) casserole beef, cut into chunks

3 tbsp plain flour

500ml (18fl oz) hot beef stock

2 fresh rosemary sprigs, bruised

flour to dust

500g pack puff pastry

1 medium egg, beaten, to glaze

salt and ground black pepper

1 Preheat the oven to 170°C (150°C fan oven) mark 3. Heat 1 tbsp oil in a large flameproof casserole and sauté the onions for 10 minutes or until golden. Lift out and set aside.

2 Sear the meat in the same casserole, in batches, using more oil as necessary, until brown all over. Lift out each batch as soon as it is browned and put to one side.

3 Add the flour to the casserole and cook for 1–2 minutes to brown. Return the onions and beef to the casserole and add the stock and rosemary. Season well with salt and pepper. Cover and bring to the boil, then cook in the oven for 1½ hours or until the meat is tender.

4 About 30 minutes before the end of the cooking time, lightly dust a worksurface with flour and roll out the pastry. Cut out a lid using a 1.1 litre (2 pint) pie dish as a template, or use four 300ml (½ pint) dishes. Put on a baking sheet and chill.

5 Remove the casserole from the oven, then increase the heat to 220°C (200°C fan oven) mark 7. Pour the casserole into the pie dish (or individual dishes), brush the edge with water and put on the lid. Press down lightly to seal. Lightly score the top and brush over with the egg. Put the dish back on the baking sheet and bake for 30 minutes or until the pastry is risen and golden. Serve immediately.

Get Ahead

Double the ingredient quantities and make two pies, each to serve four people, freezing one for another day.
Complete the recipe to the end of step 3, then cool the casserole quickly. Roll out the pastry as step 4, then put the beef mixture into a pie dish. Brush the dish edge with water, then put on the pastry and press down lightly to seal. Score the pastry. Cover with clingfilm and freeze for up to three months.
To use Thaw overnight at cool room temperature or in the fridge. Lightly score the pastry, brush with beaten egg and cook at 220°C (200°C fan oven) mark 7 for 35 minutes or until the pastry is brown and the filling piping hot.

EASY		NUTRITIONAL INFORMATION	Serves
Preparation Time 30 minutes	**Cooking Time** 2 hours 25 minutes	**Per Serving** 1036 calories, 61.6g fat (of which 9.8g saturates), 64.9g carbohydrate, 1.4g salt	**4**

Get Ahead

This dish is ideal for freezing. Freeze leftover portions separately.

Complete the recipe Cool quickly immediately after adding the beans, then freeze in sealable containers.

To use Thaw overnight in the fridge. Preheat the oven to 170°C (150°C fan oven) mark 3. Put in a flameproof casserole, cover and bring to the boil on the hob. Transfer to the oven and cook for 45 minutes.

Braised Lamb Shanks with Cannellini Beans

3 tbsp olive oil

6 lamb shanks

1 large onion, chopped

3 carrots, sliced

3 celery sticks, sliced

2 garlic cloves, crushed

2 x 400g cans chopped tomatoes

150ml (¼ pint) balsamic vinegar

2 bay leaves

2 x 400g cans cannellini beans, drained and rinsed

salt and ground black pepper

crusty bread to serve

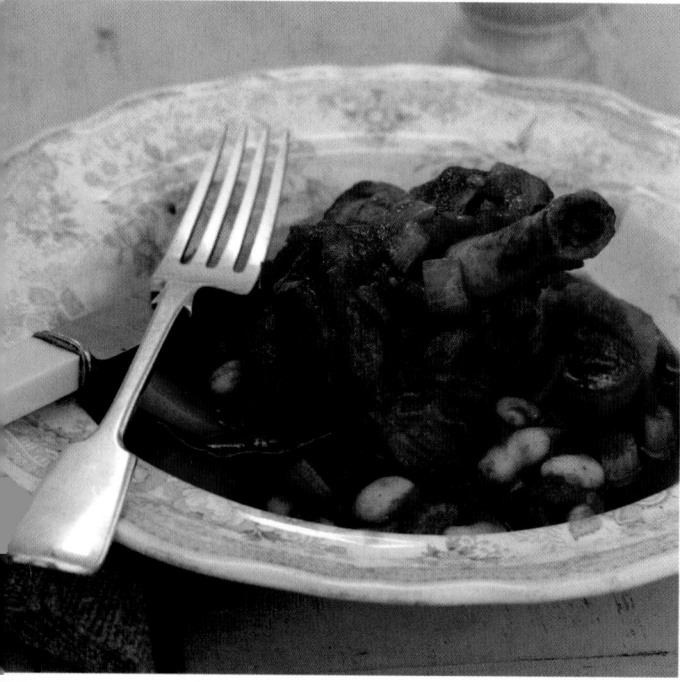

1 Preheat the oven to 170°C (150°C fan oven) mark 3. Heat the olive oil in a large flameproof casserole. Add the lamb shanks in batches and brown all over. Remove from the pan and set aside.

2 Add the onion, carrots, celery and garlic to the pan and cook gently until beginning to colour. Return the lamb to the pan. Add the tomatoes and balsamic vinegar to the pan, stirring well. Season with salt and pepper and add the bay leaves. Bring to the boil, cover and cook for 5 minutes on the hob, then transfer to the oven for 1½–2 hours or until the shanks are nearly tender.

3 Remove the dish from the oven and add the beans. Cover and put back in the oven for a further 30 minutes. Serve with crusty bread.

Serves 6	EASY		NUTRITIONAL INFORMATION	
	Preparation Time 15 minutes	**Cooking Time** 3 hours	**Per Serving** 434 calories, 21.6g fat (of which 8g saturates), 26.8g carbohydrate, 1.6g salt	Gluten free • Dairy free

Cook's Tip

Use leftover roast chicken in salads and stir-fries, soups and curries. Use the stripped carcass to make chicken stock.

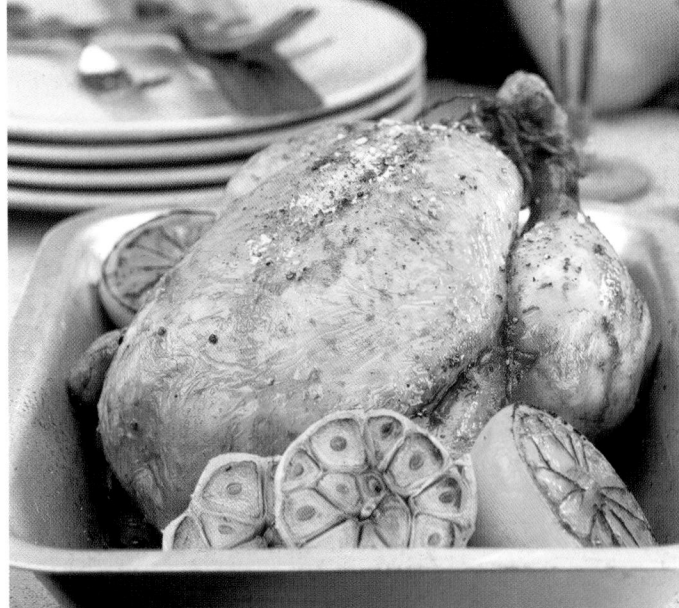

Perfect Roast Chicken

1.8kg (4lb) chicken
25g (1oz) butter, softened
2 tbsp olive oil
1 lemon, cut in half
1 small head of garlic, cut in half horizontally
salt and ground black pepper
roast potatoes and vegetables to serve

1 Preheat the oven to 220°C (200°C fan oven) mark 7. Put the chicken in a roasting tin just large enough to hold it comfortably. Spread the butter all over the chicken, then drizzle with the olive oil and season with salt and pepper.

2 Squeeze the lemon juice over it, then put one lemon half inside the chicken. Put the other half and the garlic into the roasting tin.

3 Put the chicken into the oven for 15 minutes, then turn the heat down to 190°C (170°C fan oven) mark 5 and cook for a further 45 minutes–1 hour until the leg juices run clear when pierced with a skewer. Baste from time to time with the pan juices. Add a splash of water to the tin if the juices dry out.

4 Put the chicken on a warm plate, cover with foil and 'rest' for 10 minutes, so the juices settle back into the meat, making it moist and easier to slice. Mash some of the garlic into the pan juices and serve the gravy with the chicken, with potatoes and vegetables.

EASY		NUTRITIONAL INFORMATION		Serves
Preparation Time 5 minutes	**Cooking Time** 1 hour–1¼ hours, plus resting	**Per Serving** 639 calories, 46g fat (of which 13g saturates), 0g carbohydrate, 0.6g salt	Gluten free	**4**

Italian Lamb

2 half-leg knuckles of lamb

2 tbsp olive oil

75g (3oz) butter

275g (10oz) onions, finely chopped

175g (6oz) carrots, finely chopped

175g (6oz) celery, finely chopped

2 tbsp dried porcini pieces or 125g (4oz) finely chopped brown-cap mushrooms

9 pieces sun-dried tomato, finely chopped

150g (5oz) Italian spicy sausage or salami, thickly sliced

600ml (1 pint) red wine

400g (14oz) passata

600ml (1 pint) vegetable stock

125g (4oz) dried pasta shapes

15g (1/2oz) freshly grated Parmesan

fresh flat-leafed parsley sprigs to garnish

Get Ahead

This dish is ideal for freezing. Freeze leftover portions separately.

Complete the recipe to the end of step 4. Cool quickly, then freeze for up to three months.

To use Thaw overnight at cool room temperature. Put in a flameproof casserole, cover and bring to the boil on the hob. Complete the recipe from step 6.

1 Preheat the oven to 240°C (220°C fan oven) mark 9. Put the lamb in a large roasting tin and drizzle 1 tbsp olive oi over it. Roast for 35 minutes.

2 Meanwhile, melt the butter with the remaining oil in a large flameproof casserole. Stir in the onions, carrots and celery and cook, stirring, for 10–15 minutes until golden and soft. Stir in the porcini pieces or mushrooms and cook for a further 2–3 minutes.

3 Add the sun-dried tomatoes, sausage, wine, passata and stock to the pan, then bring to the boil and simmer for 10 minutes.

4 Lift the lamb from the roasting tin, add to the tomato sauce and cover with a tight-fitting lid. Reduce the temperature to 170°C (150°C fan oven) mark 3 and cook for a further 3 hours or until the lamb is falling off the bone.

5 Lift the lamb from the casserole on to a deep, heatproof serving dish. Cover loosely with foil and keep warm in a low oven.

6 Put the casserole on the hob, stir in the pasta and bring back to the boil. Simmer for 10 minutes or until the pasta is tender. Stir in the Parmesan just before serving.

7 Carve the lamb into large pieces and serve with the pasta sauce, garnished with parsley.

Serves 4	A LITTLE EFFORT		NUTRITIONAL INFORMATION
	Preparation Time 35 minutes	**Cooking Time** 3³/₄ hours	**Per Serving** 785 calories, 52.3g fat (of which 17.6g saturates), 20.1g carbohydrate, 3.2g salt

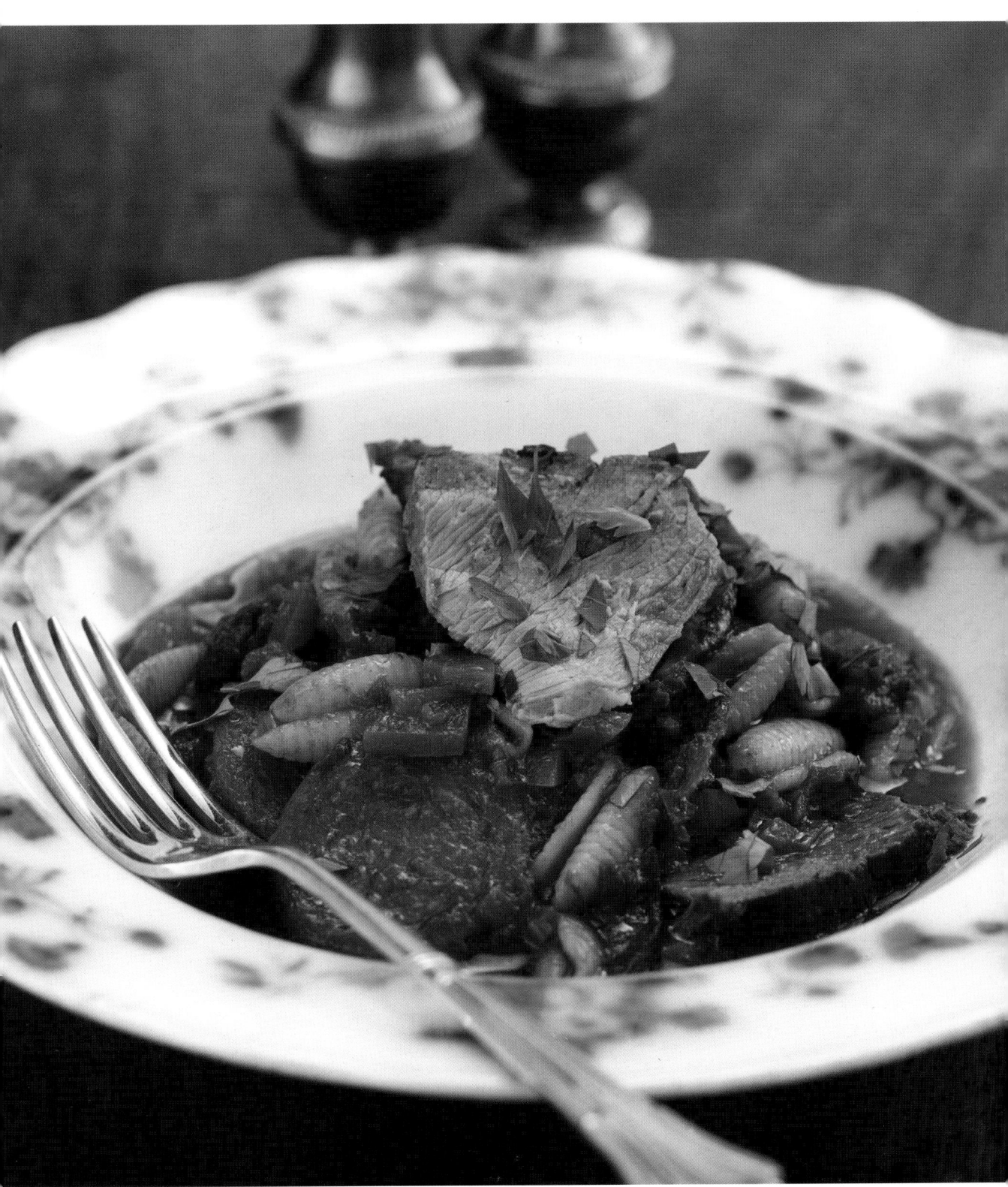

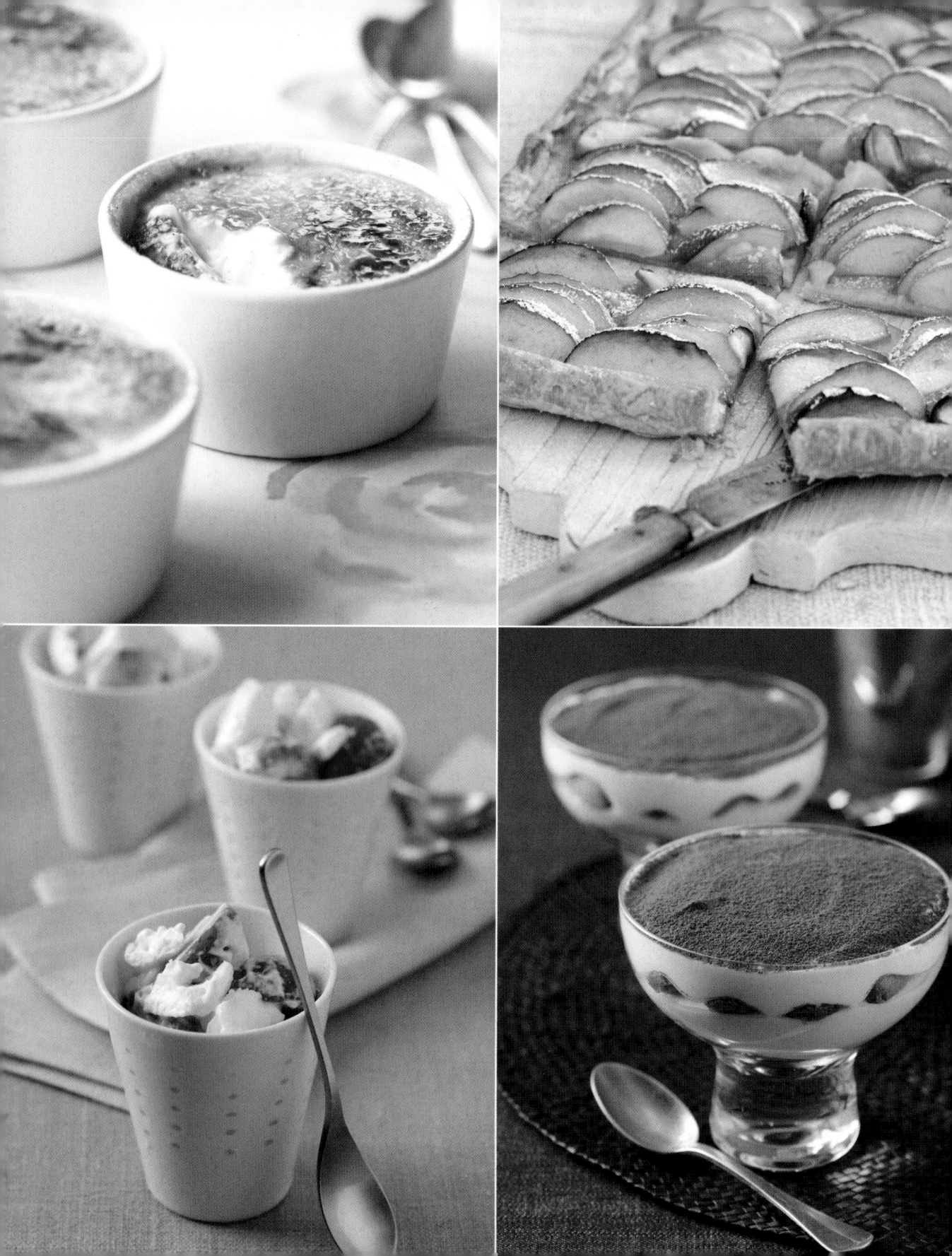

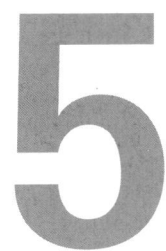

Speedy Puddings

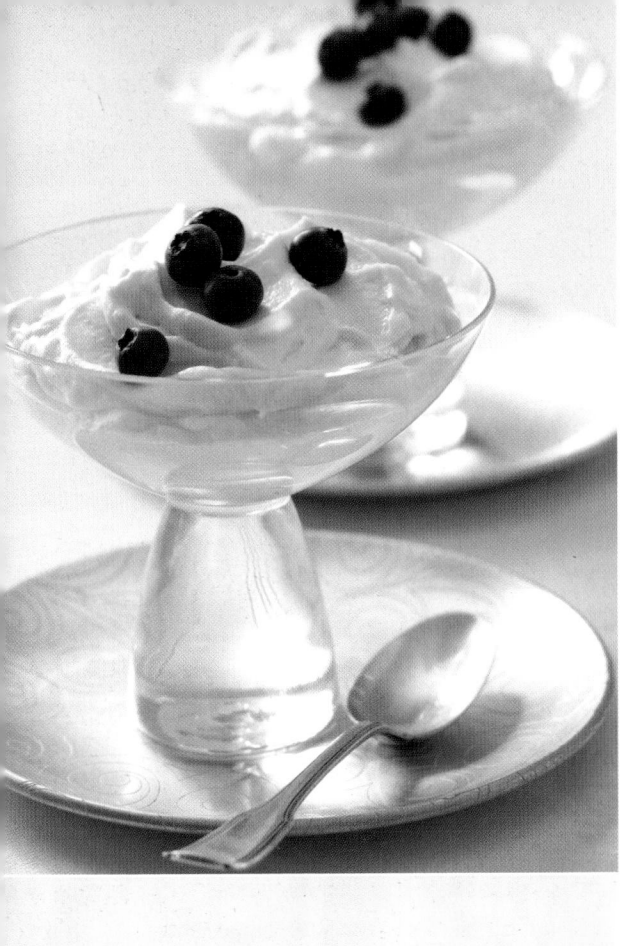

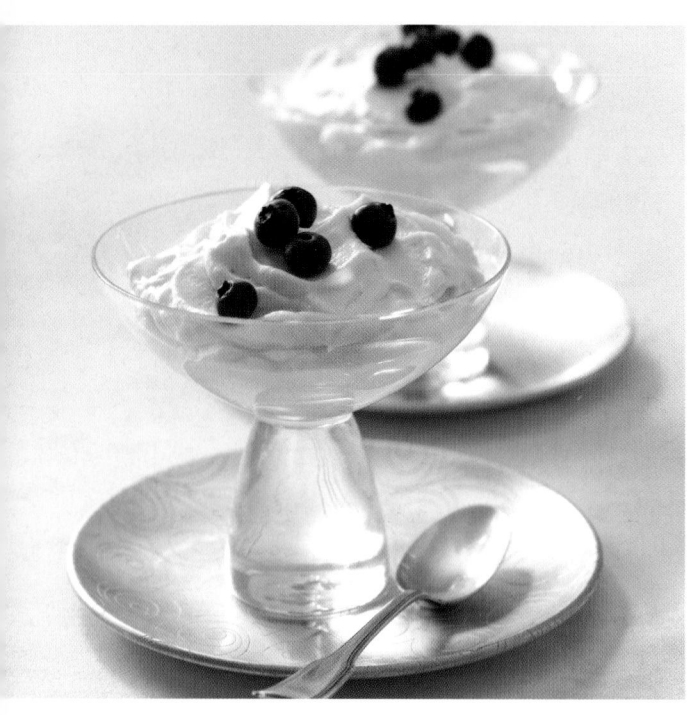

Quick Lemon Mousse

6 tbsp lemon curd

300ml (½ pint) double cream, whipped

fresh blueberries to decorate

1 Gently stir the lemon curd through the double cream until combined, and decorate with blueberries.

Serves	EASY		NUTRITIONAL INFORMATION	
4	**Preparation Time** 1–2 minutes		**Per Serving** 334 calories, 30g fat (of which 18g saturates), 16g carbohydrate, 0.1g salt	Vegetarian Gluten free

Try Something Different

Replace the brandy with Grand Marnier and use orange-flavoured plain chocolate.

Chocolate Crêpes with a Boozy Sauce

100g (3½oz) plain flour, sifted

a pinch of salt

1 medium egg

300ml (½ pint) milk

sunflower oil for frying

50g (2oz) plain chocolate (at least 70 per cent cocoa solids), roughly chopped

100g (3½oz) unsalted butter

100g (3½oz) light muscovado sugar, plus extra to sprinkle

4 tbsp brandy

1 Put the flour and salt in a bowl, make a well in the centre and add the egg. Use a balloon whisk to mix the egg with a little of the flour, then gradually add the milk to make a smooth batter. Cover and leave to stand for about 20 minutes.

2 Pour the batter into a jug. Heat 1 tsp oil in a 23cm (9in) frying pan, then pour in 100ml (3½fl oz) batter, tilting the pan so that the mixture coats the bottom, and fry for 1–2 minutes until golden underneath. Turn carefully and fry the other side. Tip on to a plate, cover with greaseproof paper and repeat with the remaining batter, using more oil as needed.

3 Divide the chocolate among the crêpes. Fold each crêpe in half, and then in half again.

4 Put the butter and sugar in a heavy-based frying pan over a low heat. Add the brandy and stir. Slide the crêpes into the pan and cook for 3–4 minutes to melt the chocolate. Serve drizzled with sauce and sprinkled with sugar.

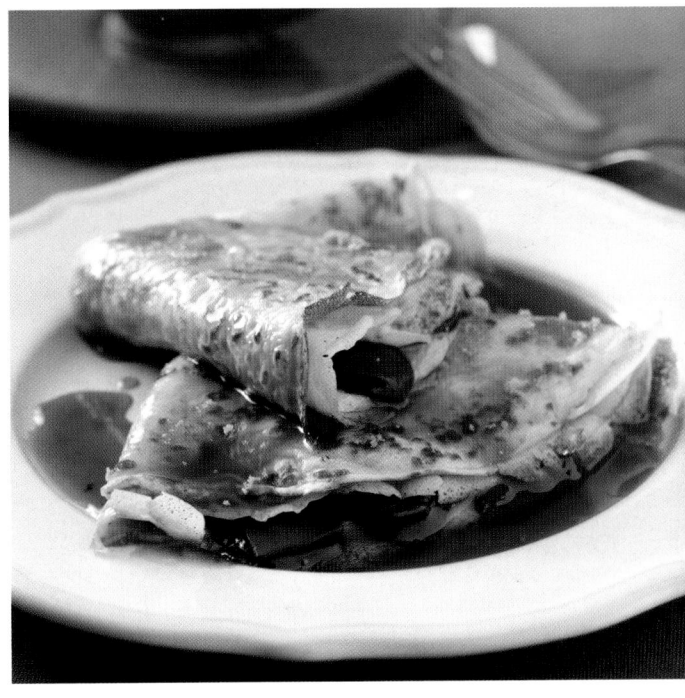

EASY		NUTRITIONAL INFORMATION		Serves
Preparation Time 5 minutes, plus 20 minutes standing	**Cooking Time** 20 minutes	**Per Serving** 594 calories, 35g fat (of which 17g saturates), 35g carbohydrate, 0.5g salt	Vegetarian	**4**

Pear and Blackberry Crumble

450g (1lb) pears, peeled, cored and chopped, tossed with the juice of 1 lemon

225g (8oz) golden caster sugar

1 tsp mixed spice

450g (1lb) blackberries

cream, custard or ice cream to serve

For the crumble topping

100g (3½oz) butter, chopped, plus extra to grease

225g (8oz) plain flour

75g (3oz) ground almonds

1 Put the pears and lemon juice in a bowl, add 100g (3½oz) sugar and the mixed spice, then add the blackberries and toss thoroughly to coat.

2 Preheat the oven to 200°C (180°C fan oven) mark 6. Lightly butter a 1.8 litre (3¼ pint) shallow ovenproof dish, then carefully tip the fruit into the dish in an even layer.

3 Put the butter, flour, ground almonds and the remaining sugar in a food processor and pulse until the mixture begins to resemble breadcrumbs. Tip into a bowl. (Alternatively, rub the butter into the flour in a large bowl by hand or using a pastry cutter. Stir in the ground almonds and the remaining sugar.) Bring parts of the mixture together with your hands to make lumps.

4 Spoon the crumble topping evenly over the fruit, then bake for 35–45 minutes until the fruit is tender and the crumble is golden and bubbling. Serve with cream, custard or ice cream.

Cook's Tip

A versatile recipe which can be popped in the oven while you whip up your main course.

Make double the amount of crumble topping and freeze half for an easy pudding another day.

Crumble is a great way to use leftover, slightly overripe fruit. Replace the pears with apples, or omit the blackberries and use 700g (1½lb) plums or rhubarb instead. You could also use gooseberries (omit the spice), or try 450g (1lb) rhubarb with 450g (1lb) strawberries.

Serves 6	EASY		NUTRITIONAL INFORMATION	
	Preparation Time 20 minutes	**Cooking Time** 35–45 minutes	**Per Serving** 525 calories, 21g fat (of which 9g saturates), 81g carbohydrate, 0.3g salt	Vegetarian

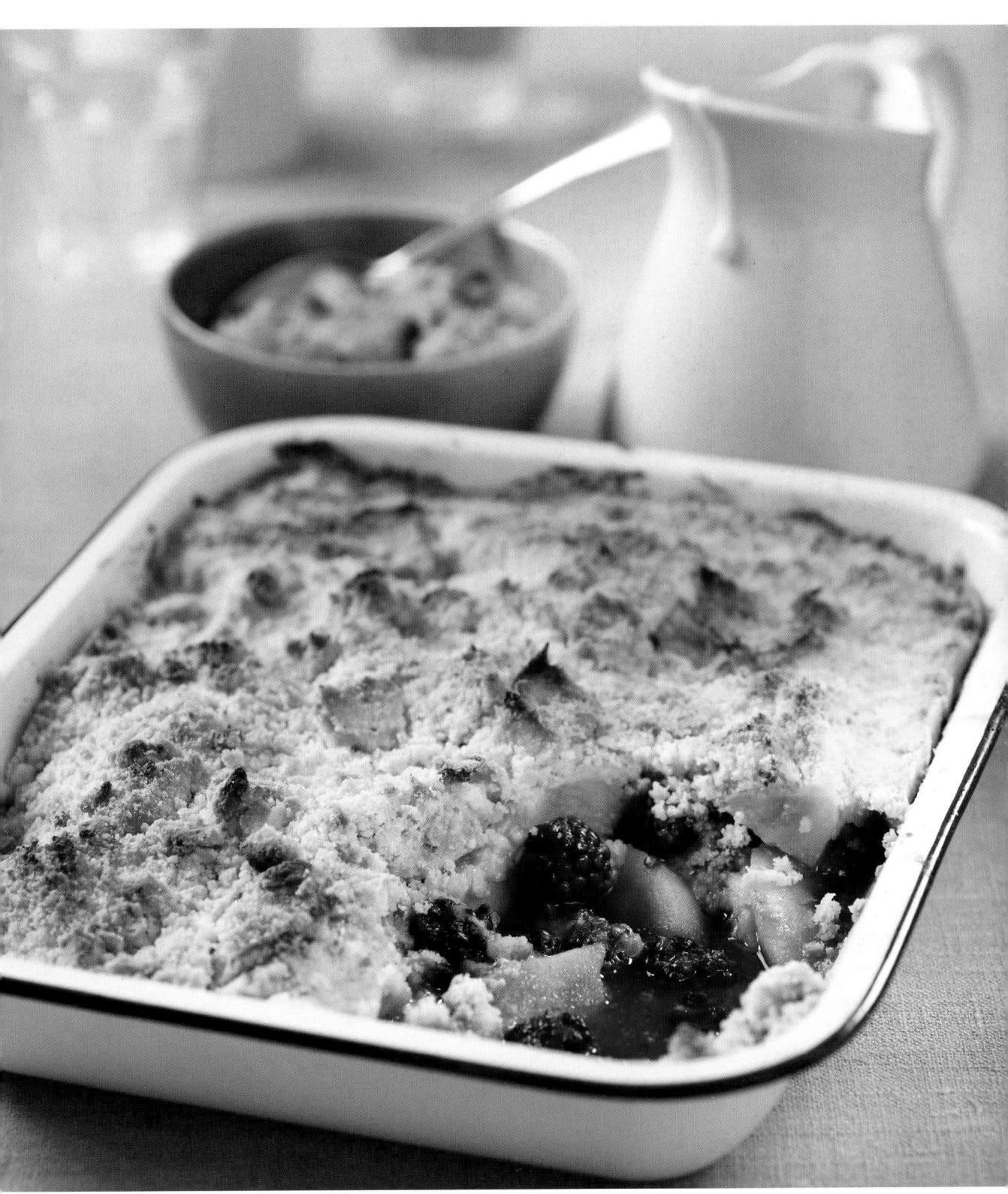

Try Something Different

Use raspberries or blueberries instead of the strawberries.

Strawberry Brûlée

250g (9oz) strawberries, hulled and sliced

2 tsp golden icing sugar

1 vanilla pod

400g (14oz) Greek yogurt

100g (3½oz) golden caster sugar

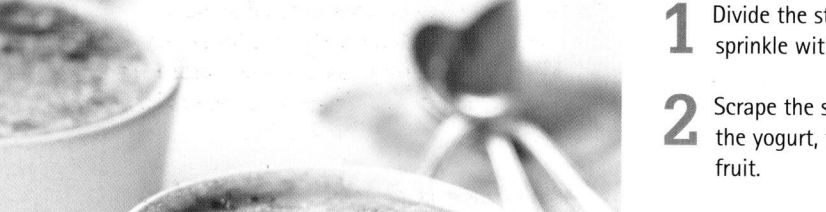

1 Divide the strawberries among four ramekins and sprinkle with icing sugar.

2 Scrape the seeds from the vanilla pod and stir into the yogurt, then spread the mixture evenly over the fruit.

3 Preheat the grill to high. Sprinkle the caster sugar evenly over the yogurt until it's well covered.

4 Put the ramekins on a baking sheet or into the grill pan and grill until the sugar turns dark brown and caramelises. Leave for 15 minutes or until the caramel is cool enough to eat, or chill for up to 2 hours before serving.

Serves 4	EASY		NUTRITIONAL INFORMATION	
	Preparation Time 15 minutes, plus chilling	**Cooking Time** 5 minutes	**Per Serving** 240 calories, 10g fat (of which 5g saturates), 35g carbohydrate, 0.2g salt	Vegetarian • Gluten free

Cook's Tip

To freeze bananas, peel and slice them thinly, then put the slices on a large non-stick baking tray and put into the freezer for 1 hour or until frozen. Transfer to a plastic bag and store in the freezer until needed.
Slightly over-ripe bananas are ideal for this recipe.

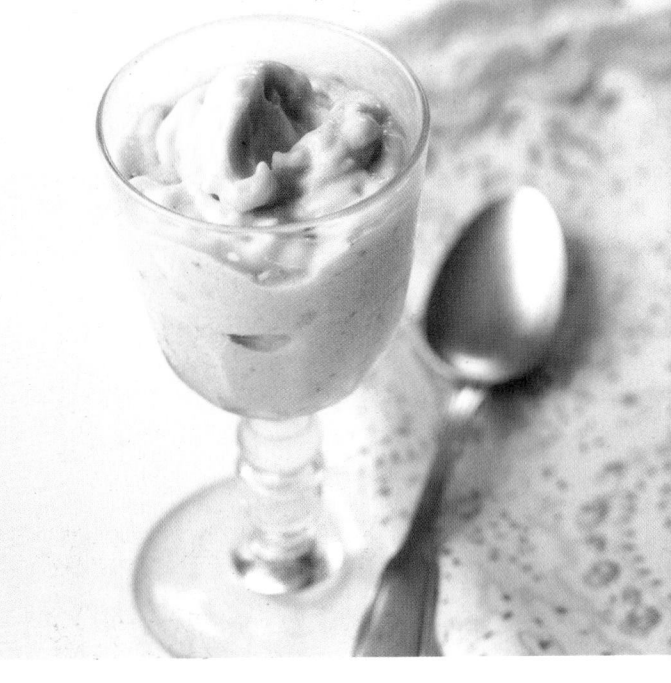

Instant Banana Ice Cream

6 ripe bananas, about 700g (1½lb), peeled, cut into thin slices and frozen (see Cook's Tip)

1–2 tbsp virtually fat-free fromage frais

1–2 tbsp orange juice

1 tsp vanilla extract

a splash of rum or Cointreau (optional)

a few drops of lime juice to taste

1　Leave the frozen bananas to stand at room temperature for 2–3 minutes. Put the still-frozen pieces in a food processor or blender with 1 tbsp fromage frais, 1 tbsp orange juice, the vanilla extract and the rum or liqueur, if you like.

2　Whiz until smooth, scraping down the sides of the bowl and adding more fromage frais and orange juice as necessary to give a creamy consistency. Add lime juice to taste and serve at once or tip into a freezer container and freeze for up to one month.

EASY	NUTRITIONAL INFORMATION		Serves
Preparation Time 5 minutes, plus about 1 hour freezing	**Per Serving** 171 calories, 0.5g fat (of which 0.2g saturates), 41.3g carbohydrate, 0g salt	Vegetarian • Gluten free	**4**

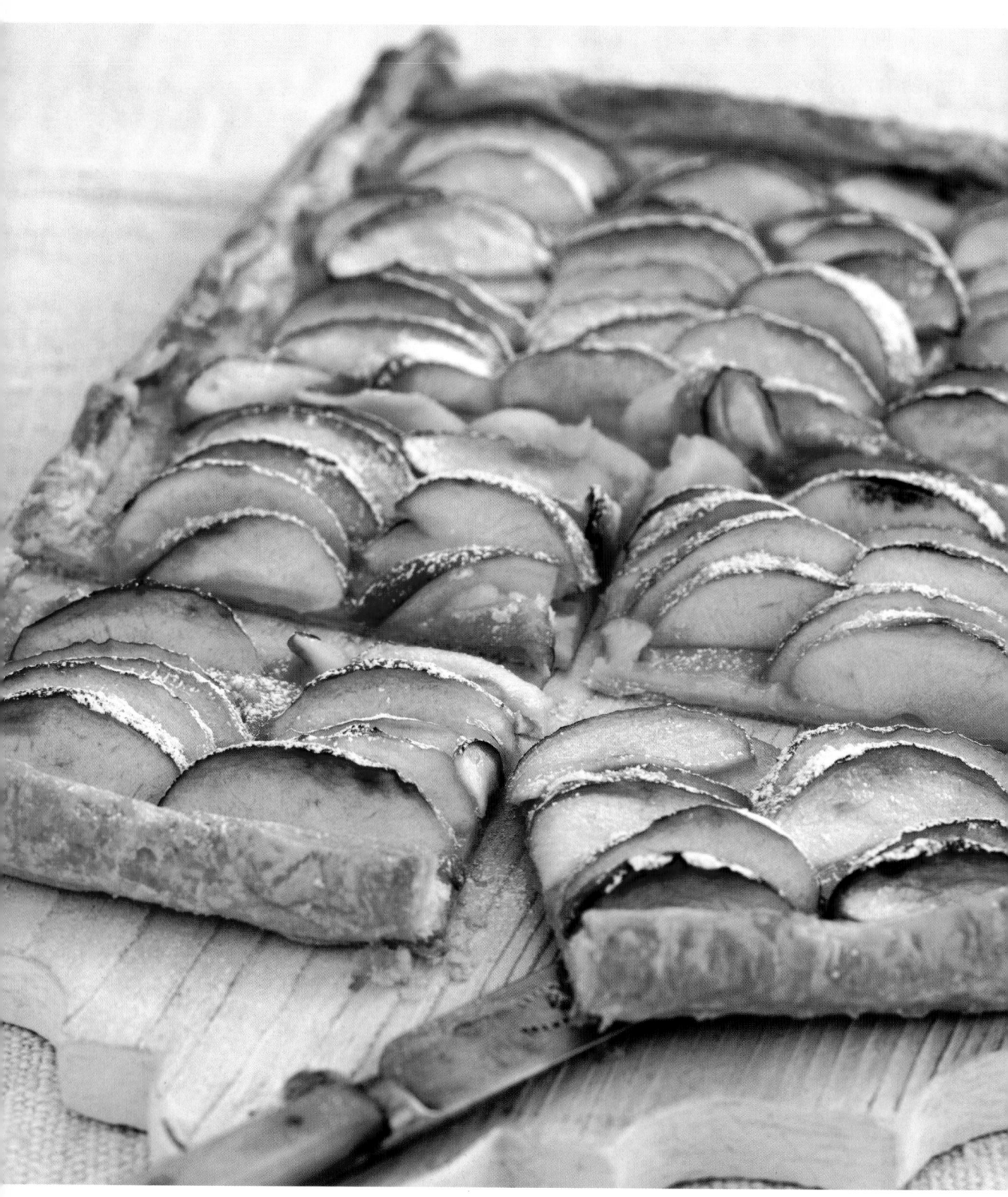

Express Apple Tart

375g pack ready-rolled puff pastry

500g (1lb 2oz) dessert apples, such as Cox's, cored and thinly sliced, then tossed in the juice of 1 lemon

golden icing sugar to dust

1 Preheat the oven to 200°C (180°C fan oven) mark 6. Put the pastry on to a 28 x 38cm (11 x 15in) baking sheet and lightly roll over it with a rolling pin to smooth down the pastry. Score lightly around the edge, leaving a 3cm (1¼in) border.

2 Put the apple slices on top of the pastry within the border. Turn the edge of the pastry halfway over to reach the edge of the apples, press down and use your fingers to crimp the edge.

3 Dust heavily with icing sugar. Bake for 20 minutes or until the pastry is cooked and the sugar has caramelised. Serve warm, dusted with more icing sugar.

EASY		NUTRITIONAL INFORMATION		Serves
Preparation Time 10 minutes	**Cooking Time** 20 minutes	**Per Serving** 197 calories, 11.6g fat (of which 0g saturates), 22.9g carbohydrate, 0.4g salt	Vegetarian	**8**

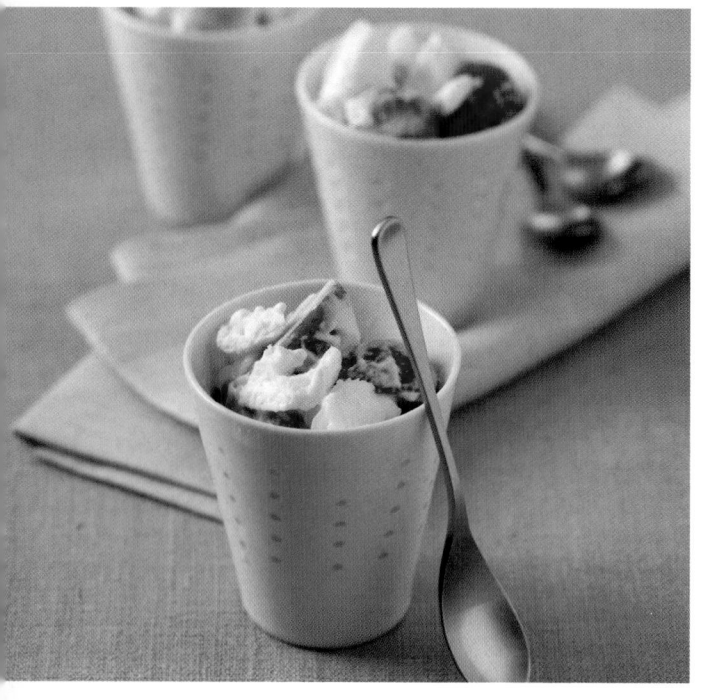

Try Something Different

Caribbean Crush: replace the sugar and liqueur with dulce de leche toffee sauce and the strawberries with sliced bananas.

Eton Mess

200g (7oz) fromage frais, chilled
200g (7oz) low-fat Greek yogurt, chilled
1 tbsp golden caster sugar
2 tbsp strawberry liqueur
6 meringues, roughly crushed
350g (12oz) strawberries, hulled and halved

1 Put the fromage frais and yogurt into a large bowl and stir to combine.

2 Add the sugar, strawberry liqueur, meringues and strawberries. Mix together gently and divide among six serving dishes.

Serves 6	EASY	NUTRITIONAL INFORMATION	
	Preparation Time 10 minutes	Per Serving 198 calories, 5g fat (of which 3g saturates), 33g carbohydrate, 0.1g salt	Vegetarian • Gluten free

Cook's Tip

Quark is a smooth soft white cheese, with a texture between yogurt and fromage frais. Fromage frais can be used instead.

250ml (9fl oz) cold coffee

2 tbsp coffee liqueur, such as Kahlúa or Tia Maria

24 sponge fingers

2 medium eggs, separated

3 tbsp icing sugar

500g (1lb 2oz) quark (see Cook's Tip)

1 tsp vanilla extract

cocoa powder to dust

Tiramisù

1 Pour the cold coffee and coffee liqueur into a bowl. Dip 12 of the sponge fingers into the liquid, and put into six serving dishes or one large dish.

2 Put the egg whites into a clean, grease-free bowl and whisk until they form soft peaks. In a separate bowl, whisk together the egg yolks, icing sugar, quark and vanilla. Fold in the whites.

3 Spoon half the quark mixture over the sponges. Dip the remaining sponge fingers in the coffee mixture, then put on top. Cover with the remaining quark mixture. Dust with cocoa powder and serve.

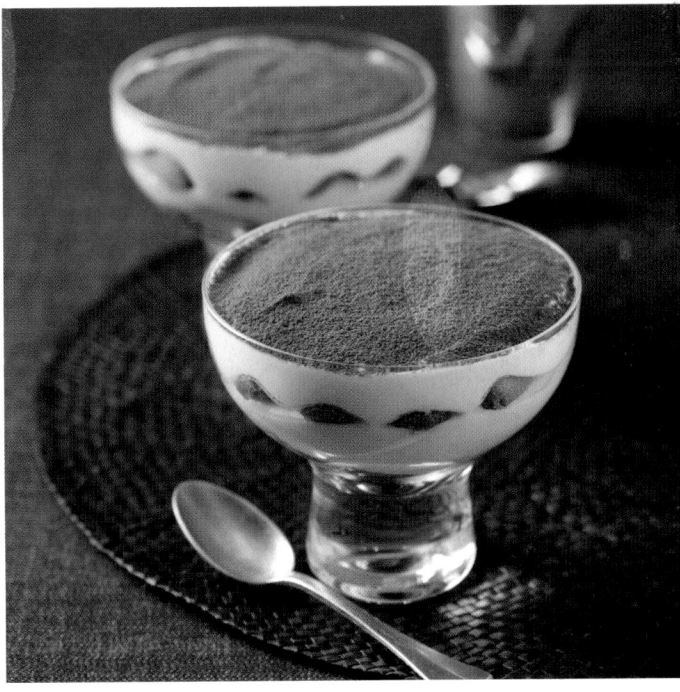

EASY	NUTRITIONAL INFORMATION		Serves
Preparation Time 20 minutes	**Per Serving** 344 calories, 16g fat (of which 4g saturates), 39g carbohydrate, 0.5g salt	Vegetarian	**6**

Fruity Fool

500g carton summer fruit compote

500g carton fresh custard

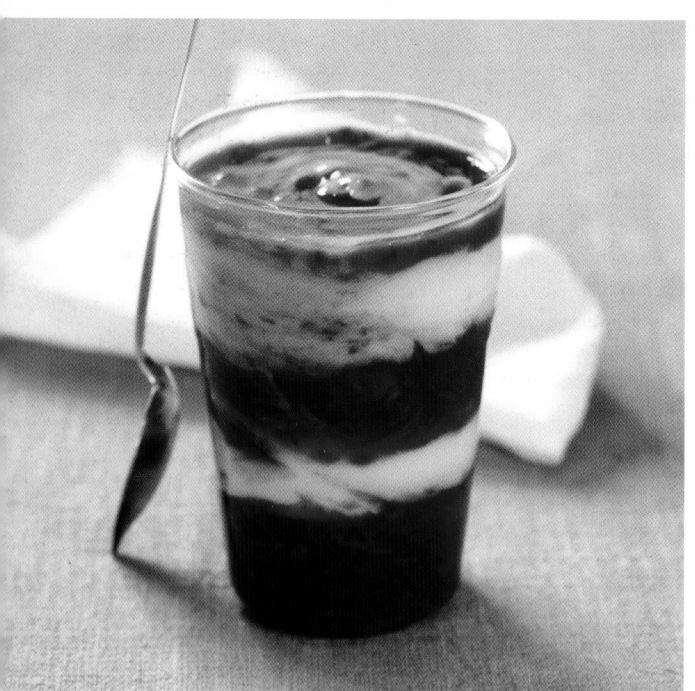

1 Divide half the compote among six serving glasses, then add a thin layer of custard. Repeat the process until all the compote and custard have been used.

2 Stir each fool once to swirl the custard and compote together, then serve.

Serves 6	EASY	NUTRITIONAL INFORMATION	
	Preparation Time 1–2 minutes	**Per Serving** 159 calories, 2g fat (of which trace saturates), 31g carbohydrate, 0.1g salt	Vegetarian • Gluten free

Cook's Tip

Slightly over-ripe bananas are ideal for this recipe.

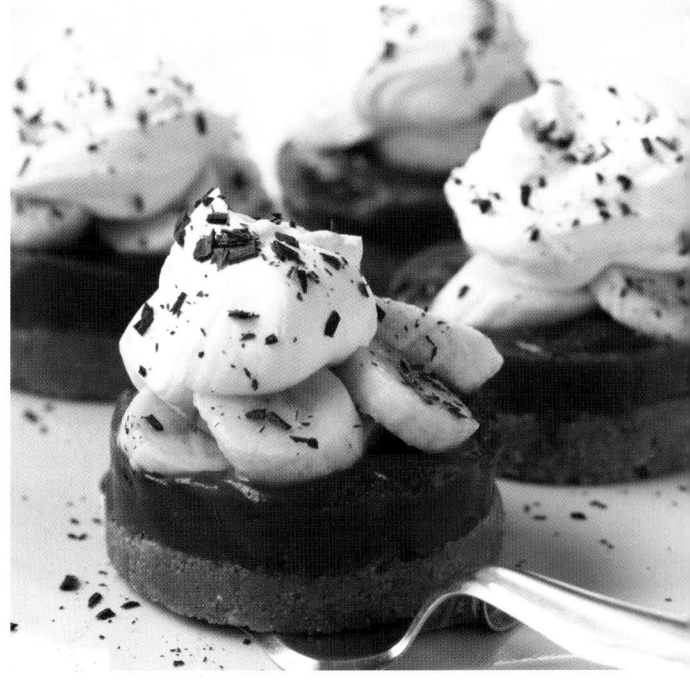

Sticky Banoffee Pies

150g (5oz) digestive biscuits

75g (3oz) unsalted butter, melted, plus extra to grease

1 tsp ground ginger (optional)

450g (1lb) dulce de leche toffee sauce

4 bananas, peeled, sliced and tossed in the juice of 1 lemon

300ml (½ pint) double cream, lightly whipped

plain chocolate shavings

1 Put the biscuits in a food processor and whiz until they resemble fine crumbs. (Alternatively, put them in a plastic bag and crush with a rolling pin. Transfer to a bowl.) Add the melted butter and ginger, if using, then process, or stir well, for 1 minute to combine.

2 Butter six 10cm (4in) rings or tartlet tins and line with greaseproof paper. Press the biscuit mixture into each ring. Divide the toffee sauce equally among the rings and top with the bananas. Pipe or spoon on the cream, sprinkle with chocolate shavings and chill. Remove from the rings or tins to serve.

EASY	NUTRITIONAL INFORMATION		Serves
Preparation Time 15 minutes, plus chilling	**Per Serving** 827 calories, 55g fat (of which 32g saturates), 84g carbohydrate, 1.2g salt	Vegetarian	**6**

Microwave Sticky Toffee Puddings

75g (3oz) mixed dried fruit

75g (3oz) pitted dates, roughly chopped

$^3/_4$ tsp bicarbonate of soda

150g (5oz) light muscovado sugar

75g (3oz) butter, softened, plus extra to grease

2 medium eggs, beaten

$^1/_2$ tsp vanilla extract

175g (6oz) self-raising flour

For the toffee sauce

125g (4oz) butter

175g (6oz) light muscovado sugar

4 tbsp double cream

25g (1oz) pecan nuts, roughly chopped

1 Grease and baseline six 250ml (9fl oz) cups. Put the dried fruit and bicarbonate of soda in a bowl and pour over 175ml (6fl oz) boiling water. Set side.

2 In a separate bowl, beat the sugar and butter for 1–2 minutes until light and fluffy. Beat in the eggs and vanilla extract, then sift over the flour and fold it into the fruit mixture.

3 Spoon into the cups. Cover very loosely with microwave film and cook three cups on Medium or 600W for 6 minutes in the microwave. Remove the microwave film from the puddings and leave to stand for 1 minute. Repeat with the remaining cups.

4 To make the sauce, put the butter, sugar and cream in a pan and heat gently, stirring well. Pour the sauce over the puddings and sprinkle on the chopped nuts.

Cook's Tip

The puddings can also be baked in a conventional oven, although this takes a little longer. Preheat the oven to 200°C (180°C fan oven) mark 6. Spoon the mixture into buttered heatproof cups, cover with foil, and put on to a baking sheet. Bake for 30 minutes or until soft and springy and a skewer comes out clean.

Serves 6	EASY		NUTRITIONAL INFORMATION	
	Preparation Time 15 minutes	**Cooking Time** 12 minutes	**Per Serving** 720 calories, 37.7g fat (of which 21.7g saturates), 96.2g carbohydrate, 1g salt	Vegetarian

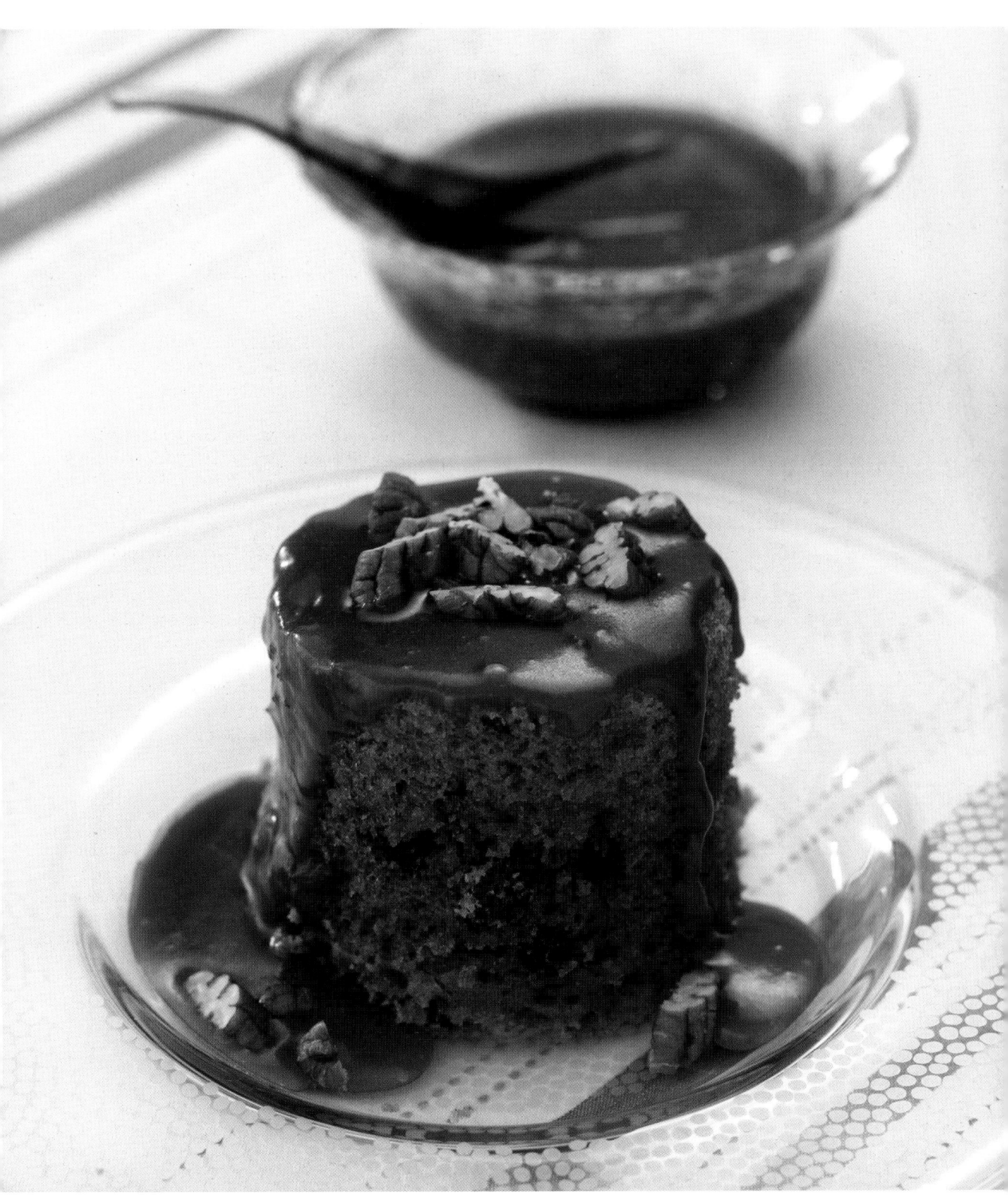

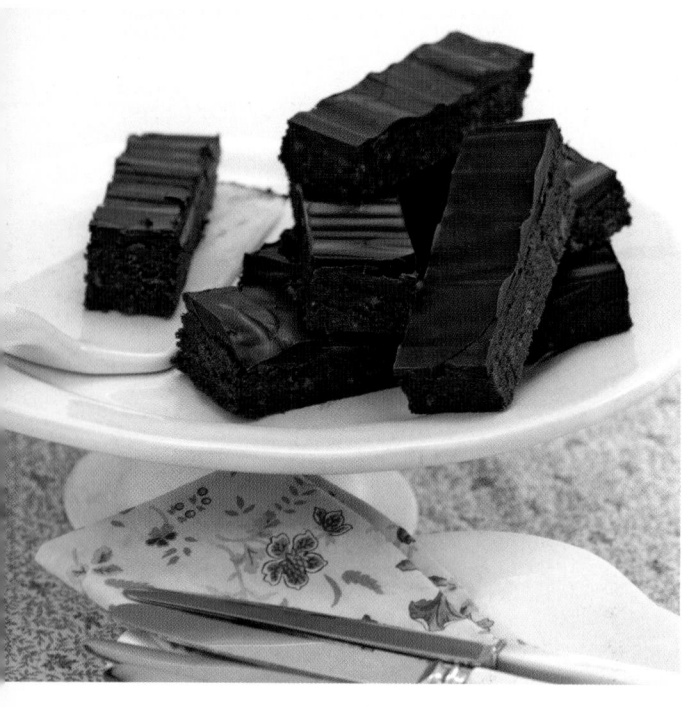

Quick Chocolate Slices

225g (8oz) butter or olive oil spread

3 tbsp golden syrup

50g (2oz) cocoa, sifted

300g pack digestive biscuits, crushed

400g (14oz) plain chocolate (at least 70 per cent cocoa solids), broken into pieces

1 Put the butter or olive oil spread in a bowl and add the golden syrup and cocoa. Melt in a 900W microwave on High for 20 seconds, or until melted. Alternatively, melt in a pan over a very low heat. Mix everything together.

2 Remove from the heat and stir in the biscuits. Mix well until thoroughly coated in chocolate, crushing down any large pieces of biscuit.

3 Turn into a greased 25.5 x 16.5cm (10 x 6½in) rectangular tin. Cool, cover and chill for 20 minutes.

4 Melt the chocolate in a heatproof bowl in a 900W microwave on High for 1 minute 40 seconds, stirring twice. Alternatively melt over a pan of gently simmering water. Stir once more and pour over the chocolate biscuit base, then chill for 20 minutes. Cut in half lengthways and cut each half into 20 rectangular fingers.

Makes 40	EASY		NUTRITIONAL INFORMATION	
	Preparation Time 10 minutes	**Cooking Time** 2 minutes	**Per Slice** 137 calories, 9.3g fat (of which 5.5g saturates), 12.7g carbohydrate, 0.3g salt	Vegetarian

Try Something Different

Serve the mixture warm as a sauce for vanilla ice cream.

Cheat's Chocolate Pots

500g carton fresh custard

200g (7oz) plain chocolate (at least 50 per cent cocoa solids), broken into pieces

1 Put the custard in a small pan with the chocolate pieces. Heat gently, stirring all the time, until the chocolate has melted.

2 Pour the mixture into four small coffee cups and chill in the fridge for 30 minutes to 1 hour before serving.

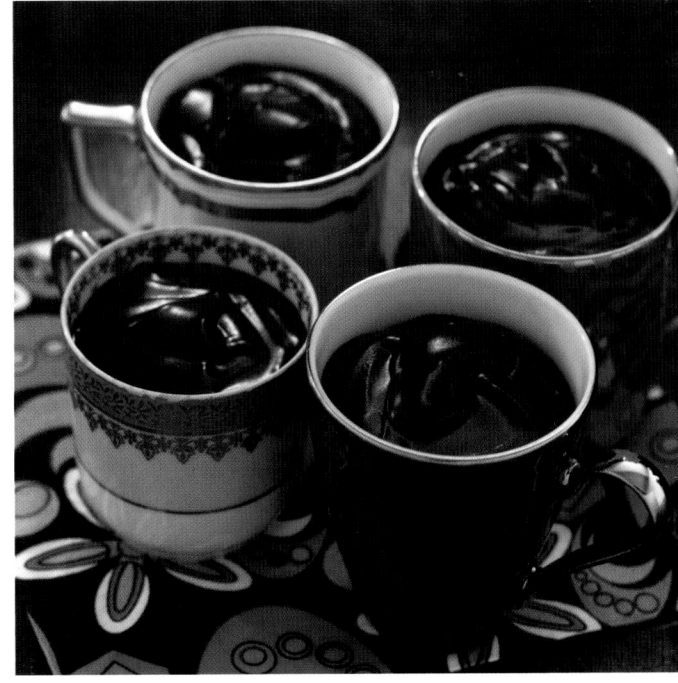

EASY		NUTRITIONAL INFORMATION		Serves
Preparation Time 5 minutes, plus chilling	**Cooking Time** 5 minutes	**Per Serving** 385 calories, 16.9g fat (of which 8.5g saturates), 52.8g carbohydrate, 0.1g salt	Vegetarian	**4**

Mango Gratin with Sabayon

3 large ripe mangoes, peeled, stoned and sliced

5 medium egg yolks

6 tbsp golden caster sugar

300ml (½ pint) champagne or sparkling wine

6 tbsp dark muscovado sugar to sprinkle

crisp sweet biscuits to serve

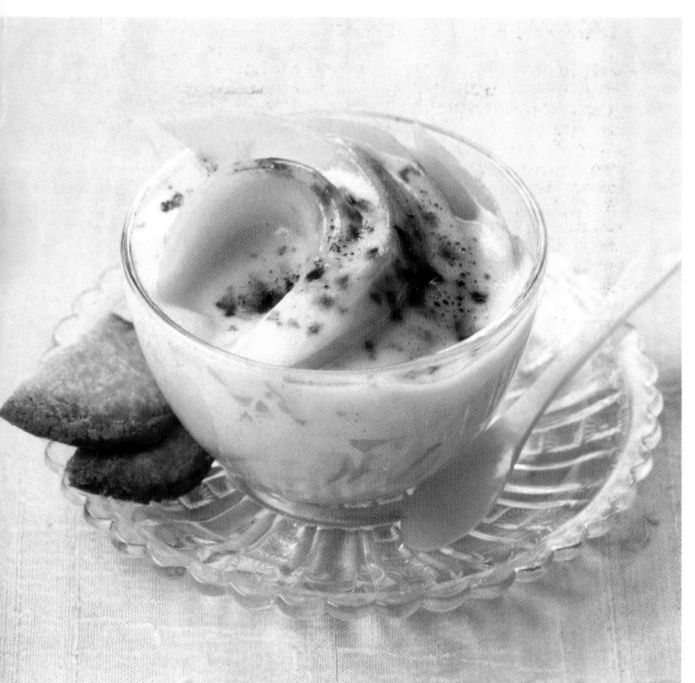

1 Arrange the mangoes in six serving glasses. Whisk the egg yolks and sugar in a large heatproof bowl over a pan of gently simmering water until the mixture is thick and falls in soft ribbon shapes. Add the champagne or sparkling wine and continue to whisk until the mixture is thick and foamy again. Remove from the heat.

2 Spoon the sabayon over the mangoes, sprinkle with the muscovado sugar, then leave for 10 minutes to go fudgey. Serve with biscuits.

Serves 6	A LITTLE EFFORT		NUTRITIONAL INFORMATION	
	Preparation Time 5 minutes, plus optional 10 minutes resting	**Cooking Time** 10 minutes	**Per Serving** 249 calories, 5g fat (of which 1g saturates), 45g carbohydrate, 0g salt	Vegetarian • Dairy free

Index